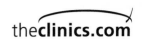
the**clinics.com**

PEDIATRIC CLINICS
OF NORTH AMERICA

Pediatric Critical Care

GUEST EDITOR
James P. Orlowski, MD, FAAP, FCCP, FCCM

June 2008 • Volume 55 • Number 3

An Imprint of Elsevier, Inc.
PHILADELPHIA   LONDON   TORONTO   MONTREAL   SYDNEY   TOKYO

W.B. SAUNDERS COMPANY
A Division of Elsevier Inc.

1600 John F. Kennedy Boulevard • Suite 1800 • Philadelphia, Pennsylvania 19103

http://www.theclinics.com

THE PEDIATRIC CLINICS OF NORTH AMERICA   Volume 55, Number
June 2008   ISSN 0031-395
Editor: Carla Holloway   ISBN-13: 978-1-4160-5792-
      ISBN-10: 1-4160-5792-

The Pediatric Clinics of North America (ISSN 0031-3955) is published bi monthly by Elsevier Inc., 360 Par
Avenue South, New York, NY 10010-1710. Months of publication are February, April, June, August, Octc
ber, and December. Business and Editorial Offices: 1600 John F. Kennedy Blvd., Suite 1800, Philadelphia
PA 19103-2899. Customer Service Office: 6277 Sea Harbor Drive, Orlando, FL 32887-4800. Periodicals post
age paid at New York, NY and additional mailing offices. Subscription prices are $149.00 per year (U
individuals), $315.00 per year (US institutions), $202.00 per year (Canadian individuals), $411.00 per yea
(Canadian institutions), $226.00 per year (international individuals), $411.00 per year (international institu
tions), $72.00 per year (US students), $119.00 per year (Canadian students), and $119.00 per year (foreig
students). To receive students/resident rare, orders must be accompanied by name of affiliated institutior
date of term, and the signature of program/residency coordinator on institution letterhead. Orders will b
billed at individual rate until proof of status is received. Foreign air speed delivery is included in all Clinic
subscription prices. All prices are subject to change without notice. POSTMASTER: Send address change
to *The Pediatric Clinics of North America*, Elsevier Journals Customer Service, 6277 Sea Harbor Drive
Orlando, FL 32887-4800. **Customer Service: 1-800-654-2452 (US). From outside of the United States, ca**
1-407-563-6020. Fax: 1-407-363-9661. E-mail: JournalsCustomerService-usa@elsevier.com.

The Pediatric Clinics of North America is also published in Spanish by McGraw-Hill Inter-americana Editore
S.A., Mexico City, Mexico; in Portuguese by Riechmann and Affonso Editores, Rua Comandante Coelh
1085, CEP 21250, Rio de Janeiro, Brazil; and in Greek by Althayia SA, Athens, Greece.

The Pediatric Clinics of North America is covered in *MEDLINE/PubMed (Index Medicus), Excerpta Medica, Cu
rent Contents, Current Contents/Clinical Medicine, Science Citation Index, ASCA, ISI/BIOMED*, and *BIOSIS*.

Printed in the United States of America.

GOAL STATEMENT

The goal of the *Pediatric Clinics of North America* is to keep practicing physicians and residents up to date with current clinical practice in pediatrics by providing timely articles reviewing the state-of-the-art in patient care.

ACCREDITATION

The *Pediatric Clinics of North America* is planned and implemented in accordance with the Essential Areas and Policies of the Accreditation Council for Continuing Medical Education (ACCME) through the joint sponsorship of the University of Virginia School of Medicine and Elsevier. The University of Virginia School of Medicine is accredited by the ACCME to provide continuing medical education for physicians.

The University of Virginia School of Medicine designates this educational activity for a maximum of 15 *AMA PRA Category 1 Credits*™. Physicians should only claim credit commensurate with the extent of their participation in the activity.

The American Medical Association has determined that physicians not licensed in the US who participate in this CME activity are eligible for 15 *AMA PRA Category 1 Credits*™.

Credit can be earned by reading the text material, taking the CME examination online at http://www.theclinics.com/home/cme, and completing the evaluation. After taking the test, you will be required to review any and all incorrect answers. Following completion of the test and evaluation, your credit will be awarded and you may print your certificate.

FACULTY DISCLOSURE/CONFLICT OF INTEREST

The University of Virginia School of Medicine, as an ACCME accredited provider, endorses and strives to comply with the Accreditation Council for Continuing Medical Education (ACCME) Standards of Commercial Support, Commonwealth of Virginia statutes, University of Virginia policies and procedures, and associated federal and private regulations and guidelines on the need for disclosure and monitoring of proprietary and financial interests that may affect the scientific integrity and balance of content delivered in continuing medical education activities under our auspices.

The University of Virginia School of Medicine requires that all CME activities accredited through this institution be developed independently and be scientifically rigorous, balanced and objective in the presentation/discussion of its content, theories and practices.

All authors/editors participating in an accredited CME activity are expected to disclose to the readers relevant financial relationships with commercial entities occurring within the past 12 months (such as grants or research support, employee, consultant, stock holder, member of speakers bureau, etc.). The University of Virginia School of Medicine will employ appropriate mechanisms to resolve potential conflicts of interest to maintain the standards of fair and balanced education to the reader. Questions about specific strategies can be directed to the Office of Continuing Medical Education, University of Virginia School of Medicine, Charlottesville, Virginia.

The authors/editors listed below have identified no financial or professional relationships for themselves or their spouse/partner:
Jeffrey S. Barrett, PhD, FCP; Marc D. Berg, MD; Desmond Bohn, MD; Frank Bowyer, MD; Joseph A. Carcillo, MD; Patricia R. Chess, MD; Lowell Clark, MD; Gillian Colville, MPhil; Cheryl L. Cramer, RN, MSN, ARNP; Lucian K. DeNicola, MD, FAAP, FCCM; Denis Devictor, MD, PhD; Dermot R. Doherty, MD; Mariano R. Fiallos, MD; W. Joshua Frazier, MD; Mark W. Hall, MD; Usama A. Hanhan, MD; Jan A. Hazelzet, MD, PhD, FCCM; Carla Holloway (Acquisitions Editor); James S. Hutchison, MD; Niranjan Kissoon, MD; Jos M. Latour, RN, MSN; Vinay M. Nadkarni, MD; Mark A. Nichter, MD; Robert H. Notter, MD, PhD; James P. Orlowski, MD, FAAP, FCCP, FCCM (Guest Editor); Catherine Preissig, MD; Karen S. Rheuban, MD (Test Author); Mark R. Rigby, MD, PhD; Peter C. Rimensberger, MD; Pierre Tissières, MD; Johannes B. van Goudoever, MD, PhD; Mathias Zuercher, MD; and Athena F. Zuppa, MD, MSCE, FAAP, FCP.

The authors/editors listed below identified the following professional or financial affiliations for themselves or their spouse/partner:
Robert A. Berg, MD is an independent contractor for Laerdal Medical AS and Medtronic.
Douglas F. Willson, MD is an independent contractor for ONY, Inc. of Amherst, N.Y.

Disclosure of Discussion of Non-FDA Approved Uses for Pharmaceutical and/or Medical Devices:
The University of Virginia School of Medicine, as an ACCME provider, requires that all authors identify and disclose any "off label" uses for pharmaceutical and medical device products. The University of Virginia School of Medicine recommends that each physician fully review all the available data on new products or procedures prior to clinical use.

TO ENROLL

To enroll in the *Pediatric Clinics of North America* Continuing Medical Education program, call customer service at 1-800-654-2452 or visit us online at www.theclinics.com/home/cme. The CME program is available to subscribers for an additional fee of $195.00.

GUEST EDITOR

JAMES P. ORLOWSKI, MD, FAAP, FCCP, FCCM, Chief of Pediatrics and Director, Pediatric Intensive Care Unit, University Community Hospital, Tampa, Florida

CONTRIBUTORS

JEFFREY S. BARRETT, PhD, FCP, Research Associate Professor of Pediatrics and Director, Pediatric Pharmacology Research Unit, Laboratory for Applied PK/PD, Division of Clinical Pharmacology and Therapeutics; Kinetic Modeling and Simulation, University of Pennsylvania; and The Children's Hospital of Philadelphia, Philadelphia, Pennsylvania

MARC D. BERG, MD, Associate Professor of Clinical Pediatrics, Division of Pediatric Clinical Care Medicine, Department of Pediatrics, Steele Memorial Research Center and Sarver Heart Center, The University of Arizona College of Medicine; and Medical Director, Pediatric Intensive Care Unit, Tucson Medical Center, Tucson, Arizona

ROBERT A. BERG, MD, Associate Dean for Clinical Affairs and Professor of Pediatrics, Division of Pediatric Clinical Care Medicine, Department of Pediatrics, Steele Memorial Research Center and Sarver Heart Center, The University of Arizona College of Medicine, Tucson, Arizona

DESMOND BOHN, MD, Professor and Chief, Critical Care Medicine, Hospital for Sick Children, Toronto, Ontario, Canada

FRANK BOWYER, MD, Professor of Pediatrics and Thomas B. and Doris E. Black Chair, Mercer University School of Medicine; and Medical Center of Central Georgia, Macon, Georgia

JOSEPH A. CARCILLO, MD, MOSES Investigators; Pediatric Critical Care, Children's Hospital of Pittsburgh, Pittsburgh, Pennsylvania

PATRICIA R. CHESS, MD, Associate Professor of Pediatrics and Biomedical Engineering, University of Rochester School of Medicine, Rochester, New York

LOWELL CLARK, MD, Associate Professor of Pediatrics, Mercer University School of Medicine; and Medical Center of Central Georgia, Macon, Georgia

GILLIAN COLVILLE, MPhil, Honorary Research Fellow, St. George's University of London; and Consultant Clinical Psychologist, Paediatric Psychology Service, St. George's Hospital, London, United Kingdom

CHERYL L. CRAMER, RN, MSN, ARNP, Pediatric Critical Care Nurse Practitioner, Pediatric Intensive Care Unit, University Community Hospital, Tampa, Florida

LUCIAN K. DENICOLA, MD, FAAP, FCCM, Jacksonville, Florida

DENIS DEVICTOR, MD, PhD, Medical Director, Pediatric Intensive Care Unit, Hopital de Bicetre, AP–HP, Department of Research on Ethics, Bicetre, France

DERMOT R. DOHERTY, MB, Assistant Professor of Anesthesia, Department of Anesthesia, University of Ottawa; and Pediatric Intensivist, Children's Hospital of Eastern Ontario, Ottawa, Ontario, Canada

MARIANO R. FIALLOS, MD, Assistant Director, Pediatric Intensive Care Unit, University Community Hospital, Tampa, Florida

W. JOSHUA FRAZIER, MD, Assistant Professor of Pediatrics, Critical Care Medicine; and The Research Institute, Nationwide Children's Hospital; Department of Pediatrics, Section of Critical Care Medicine, The Ohio State University College of Medicine, Columbus, Ohio

MARK W. HALL, MD, Assistant Professor of Pediatrics, Critical Care Medicine; and The Research Institute, Nationwide Children's Hospital; Department of Pediatrics, Section of Critical Care Medicine, The Ohio State University College of Medicine, Columbus, Ohio

USAMA A. HANHAN, MD, Assistant Director, Pediatric Intensive Care Unit, Division of Pediatrics, Department of Critical Care Medicine, University Community Hospital, Tampa; and Clinical Assistant Professor, Department of Pediatrics, Nova Southeastern University, Fort Lauderdale, Florida

JAN A. HAZELZET, MD, PhD, FCCM, Consultant, Pediatric Intensive Care, Department of Pediatrics, Division of Neonatology, Erasmus Medical Center–Sophia Children's Hospital; and Chief Medical Information Officer, Erasmus Medical Center, Rotterdam, the Netherlands

JAMES S. HUTCHISON, MD, Associate Professor, Department of Critical Care Medicine, University of Toronto and Hospital for Sick Children; Director of Acute Care Research, Hospital for Sick Children Research Institute; and Scientist, Neuroscience and Mental Health Research Program, Hospital for Sick Children Research Institute, Toronto, Ontario, Canada

NIRANJAN KISSOON, MD, Senior Medical Director, Acute and Critical Care Programs, British Columbia Children's Hospital; and Professor and Associate Head, Department of Pediatrics, University of British Columbia, Vancouver, British Columbia, Canada

JOS M. LATOUR, RN, MSN, Nurse Scientist, Division of Pediatric Intensive Care, Department of Pediatrics, Erasmus Medical Center–Sophia Children's Hospital, Rotterdam, the Netherlands

VINAY M. NADKARNI, MD, Associate Professor of Pediatrics, Department of Anesthesiology and Critical Care Medicine; and Medical Director, Center for Simulation, Advanced Education, and Innovation, The Children's Hospital of Philadelphia; Associate Director, Center for Resuscitation Science, University of Pennsylvania School of Medicine, Philadelphia, Pennsylvania

MARK A. NICHTER, MD, Associate Affiliate Professor of Pediatrics, University of South Florida School of Medicine; and Florida Pediatric Associates, St. Petersburg, Florida

ROBERT H. NOTTER, MD, PhD, Professor of Pediatrics and Environmental Medicine, University of Rochester School of Medicine, Rochester, New York

JAMES P. ORLOWSKI, MD, FAAP, FCCP, FCCM, Chief of Pediatrics and Director, Pediatric Intensive Care Unit, University Community Hospital, Tampa, Florida

CATHERINE PREISSIG, MD, Pediatric Critical Care Medicine, Emory University School of Medicine, Children's Healthcare of Atlanta at Egleston, Atlanta, Georgia

MARK R. RIGBY, MD, PhD, Assistant Professor of Pediatrics and Surgery, Departments of Pediatrics and Surgery; and Director of Research, Critical Care Medicine, Emory University School of Medicine, Children's Healthcare of Atlanta at Egleston, Atlanta, Georgia

PETER C. RIMENSBERGER, MD, Pediatric and Neonatal Intensive Care Unite, Department of Pediatrics, University Children's Hospital of Geneva, Geneva, Switzerland

PIERRE TISSIÈRES, MD, Associate Medical Director, Pediatric Intensive Care Unit, Hopital de Bicetre, AP–HP, Department of Research on Ethics, Bicetre, France

JOHANNES B. van GOUDOEVER, MD, PhD, Medical Director of Neonatology and Vice-Chairman of Pediatrics, Department of Pediatrics, Division of Neonatology, Erasmus Medical Center–Sophia Children's Hospital, Rotterdam, the Netherlands

DOUGLAS F. WILLSON, MD, Professor of Pediatrics and Medical Director, Pediatric Intensive Care Unit and Division of Pediatric Critical Care, University of Virginia Children's Medical Center, University of Virginia Health Sciences System, Charlottesville, Virginia

MATHIAS ZUERCHER, MD, Department of Anesthesia and Intensive Care, University Hospital, Basel, Switzerland; Sarver Heart Center, The University of Arizona School of Medicine, Tucson, Arizona

ATHENA F. ZUPPA, MD, MSCE, FAAP, FCP, Assistant Professor of Pediatrics, Division of Clinical Pharmacology, Department of Pediatrics; and Assistant Professor of Anesthesia and Critical Care, Division of Pediatric Critical Care Medicine, Department of Anesthesia and Critical Care Medicine, The Children's Hospital of Philadelphia, Philadelphia, Pennsylvania

CONTENTS

multiple organ system failure. These therapies have optimum benefit if: (1) the underlying disease is reversible; (2) the therapies are performed expertly and are monitored to prevent and minimize systemic hemolysis; and (3) the therapies are provided in a goal-directed manner. These therapies represent a significant advance in pediatric critical care medicine. This article provides a framework for this multidisciplinary team approach for implementing these therapies.

Proper immunologic balance between pro- and anti-inflammatory forces is necessary for recovery from critical illness. Persistence of a marked compensatory anti-inflammatory innate immune response after an insult is termed immunoparalysis. Critically ill patients demonstrating prolonged, severe reductions in monocyte HLA-DR expression or ex vivo tumor necrosis factor α production are at high risk for nosocomial infection and death. Reversal of immunoparalysis can be accomplished through the administration of immunostimulatory agents or tapering of exogenous immuno-suppression. Evidence suggests that this may be associated with improved clinical outcomes. Immune-monitoring protocols are needed to identify patients who may benefit from immunomodu-latory trials.

Acutely poisoned children remain a common problem facing pediatricians working in acute care medicine in the United States and worldwide. The management of such children continues to be challenging, and their care has evolved throughout the years. The concept of gastric decontamination in acute poisoning has significantly changed over the past 10 years, and many of the previously used techniques have been abandoned or fallen out of favor for lack of evidence to their benefit or unacceptable serious risks and side effects. Supportive care continues to be the cornerstone in managing most poisoned children. Only a few patients benefit from antidotes or specific interventions.

This article explores the use of physician extenders in the pediatric ICU setting. The Libby Zion case is highlighted because of its impact on the use of manpower in the hospital setting. The history of physician extenders, including the hospitalist, physician assistant (PA), and nurse practitioner (NP), is discussed. Findings indicate a positive impact within the pediatric intensive care setting with the use of NPs and PAs. The American Academy of Pediatrics has supported the use of physician extenders in the care of hospitalized children.

intensive care by parental empowerment through parent satisfaction with care. Incorporating the concepts of family-centered care and parental needs and experiences into a parent satisfaction instrument may provide quality improvement projects based on the empowerment of parents and eventually may facilitate the implementation and evaluation of quality initiatives.

Most deaths in the pediatric intensive care unit occur after a decision to withhold or withdraw life-sustaining treatments. The management of children at the end of life can be divided into three steps. The first concerns the decision-making process. The second concerns the actions taken once a decision has been made to forego life-sustaining treatments. The third regards the evaluation of the decision and its implementation. The mission of pediatric intensive care has expanded to provide the best possible care to dying children and their families. Improving the quality of care received by dying children remains an ongoing challenge for every pediatric intensive care unit team member.

This article reviews selected issues of endocrine concerns in the pediatric intensive care unit, exclusive of diabetic ketoacidosis. The sympathoadrenergic arm of the neuroendocrine stress response is described, followed by discussions of two topics of particular current concern: critical illness hyperglycemia and relative adrenal insufficiency. A selected set of common scenarios encountered in the daily practice of intensive care follows.

FORTHCOMING ISSUES

RECENT ISSUES

THE CLINICS ARE NOW AVAILABLE ONLINE!

Access your subscription at
www.theclinics.com

ELSEVIER
SAUNDERS

PEDIATRIC CLINICS
OF NORTH AMERICA

Pediatr Clin N Am 55 (2008) xv–xvi

Preface

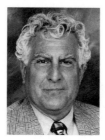

James P. Orlowski, MD, FAAP, FCCP, FCCM
Guest Editor

Just when one thinks that everything that could be known in pediatric critical care has been discovered and published, exciting new developments appear. It has been seven years since we last published an issue of the *Pediatric Clinics of North America* on pediatric critical care. In that time period, a number of exciting new or rejuvenated therapies have entered the armamentarium of pediatric critical care. Hypothermia for the cerebral resuscitation of cardiac arrest victims has become established therapy in adults and is gaining momentum in pediatrics. Surfactant therapy, which is the standard of care in neonatology, has been shown to benefit some children with acute lung injury and the acute respiratory distress syndrome. We are now capable of supporting multiple organ system failures extracorporeally in critically ill children, buying time for recovery of these organ systems. A new concept of immunoparalysis in critical illness is being recognized and the use of immuno-stimulation to reverse this state is gaining ground. There have even been dramatic changes in how we ventilate and support failed lungs in the pediatric intensive care unit (PICU). New developments in pharmacokinetics and pharmacodynamics are changing the way we prescribe and utilize medications in the PICU, and are impacting the treatment of diabetic ketoacidosis, poisonings, endocrine disorders, and even pediatric cardiopulmonary resuscitation. Along with new developments in the medical areas of diagnosis and treatment are new developments in the psychosocial areas of pediatric critical care. We are now beginning to understand the psychologic impact on children and their parents of admission to the PICU, the importance of parental satisfaction with the care received, and the psychologic

doi:10.1016/j.pcl.2008.03.003

impact of having to decide to forgo life-sustaining or death-prolonging therapies in a child. We even have to change the way we provide pediatric intensive care services, with the increased use of physician-extenders in the PICU
and a new concerted effort to prevent medical errors in critical care. Life in
the PICU is always changing and will never be the same.

James P. Orlowski, MD, FAAP, FCCP, FCCM
University Community Hospital
3100 E. Fletcher Avenue
Tampa, FL 33613, USA

E-mail address: JOrlowski@mail.uch.org

PEDIATRIC CLINICS

OF NORTH AMERICA

ELSEVIER
SAUNDERS

Pediatr Clin N Am 55 (2008) 529–544

Hypothermia Therapy for Cardiac Arrest in Pediatric Patients

James S. Hutchison, MD[a,b,c,*],
Dermot R. Doherty, MB[d,e],
James P. Orlowski, MD, FAAP, FCCP, FCCM[f],
Niranjan Kissoon, MD[g]

[a]*Department of Critical Care Medicine, University of Toronto and Hospital
for Sick Children, 555 University Avenue, Toronto, ON M5G 1X8, Canada*
[b]*Hospital for Sick Children Research Institute, 555 University Avenue, Toronto,
ON M5G 1X8, Canada*
[c]*Neuroscience and Mental Health Research Program, Hospital for Sick Children
Research Institute, 555 University Avenue, Toronto, ON M5G 1X8, Canada*
[d]*Department of Anesthesia, University of Ottowa, 401 Smyth Road, Ottawa,
ON K1H 8L1, Canada*
[e]*Children's Hospital of Eastern Ontario, 401 Smyth Road, Ottawa, ON K1H 8L1, Canada*
[f]*University Community Hospital, 3100 East Fletcher Avenue, Tampa, FL 33613, USA*
[g]*Department of Pediatrics, Children's Hospital of British Columbia,
Vancouver, BC, Canada*

Hypothermia therapy was used in combination with barbiturate therapy in the 1970s and 1980s to treat children with hypoxic-ischemic brain injury after cardiac arrest [1]. It was later abandoned because this combination of therapies was thought to increase mortality and lead to an increased number of patients surviving in a persistent vegetative state [2,3]. In recent years, evidence from the laboratory in models of global ischemia and cardiac arrest and human studies in adults and newborns have suggested that hypothermia therapy is potentially beneficial [4–7]. Recent guidelines recommend that hypothermia therapy be used in adults who remain comatose following resuscitation from ventricular arrhythmia–induced cardiac arrest [8,9] and should be considered in children who remain comatose after cardiac arrest and resuscitation [10]. This recommendation for consideration of hypothermia therapy in children

This work was supported by grants from the Hospital for Sick Children Foundation Seed Grant Competition and the Heart and Stroke Foundation of Ontario (NA5360).
* Corresponding author. Department of Critical Care Medicine, Hospital for Sick Children, 555 University Avenue, Toronto, ON M5G 1X8, Canada.
E-mail address: jamie.hutchison@sickkids.ca (J.S. Hutchison).

doi:10.1016/j.pcl.2008.02.011   *pediatric.theclinics.com*

is extrapolated from the studies in newborns and adults. No randomized controlled trials of hypothermia therapy in children have been conducted.

The objectives of this article are to (1) summarize the laboratory and clinical studies of hypothermia therapy in global cerebral ischemia and cardiac arrest, (2) present methods of cooling in children after cardiac arrest with an example from our own experience, and (3) summarize the use of hypothermia therapy in other types of brain injury.

Cardiac arrest in children

Cause

The cause of cardiac arrest is different in pediatric patients compared to adults. In pediatric patients, cardiac arrest is caused most commonly by hypoxia or shock, whereas in adults, cardiac arrest is caused most commonly by ventricular fibrillation or ventricular tachycardia secondary to coronary artery disease [11].

Pathophysiology

Cardiac arrest caused by sudden arrhythmia in adults results in sudden global cerebral ischemia. In children, hypoxia and global ischemia most commonly contribute to the brain injury. During hypoxic-ischemia and after return of circulation (reperfusion), the developing brain responds differently compared to the developed brain. For example, hypothermic protection may be more pronounced in young gerbils compared to older gerbils [12].

Neuropathology

Brain injury from cardiac arrest results from cerebral hypoxic-ischemic and reperfusion injuries and leads to death of selectively vulnerable neurons and other brain cells. The pattern of neuronal loss described in patients who die after cardiac arrest is that of laminar necrosis, particularly in layers III and V of the cerebral cortex in the watershed zones between the anterior, middle, and posterior cerebral arteries [13]. Cerebral infarction and loss of neurons in CA1 and CA3 of the hippocampus, the basal ganglia, and Purkinje layer of the cerebellum also may occur. Programmed cell death or apoptosis occurs in the hippocampus up to 7 days after resuscitation as compared to necrotic cell death described in the cortex [14,15]. The selective vulnerability of the hippocampus in survivors is reflected by volume loss of the hippocampus (relative to the cortex); however, the persistent cognitive defects seen in long-term survivors suggest global rather than focal brain injury [16,17]. Infants (<1 year of age) have relative sparing of the cerebral cortex and cerebellum and have neuronal loss in the diencephalon, hippocampus, and olivary bodies as compared to older children and adults (Fig. 1) [18]. The reasons for this developmental change in neuronal

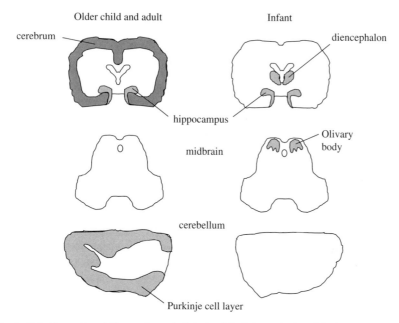

Fig. 1. Selective vulnerability to hypoxic injuries (*shaded areas*). (*Modified from* Ellison D, Love S, editors. Neuropathology: a reference text of CNS pathology. St. Louis (MO): Mosby International Ltd; 1998; with permission.)

vulnerability to hypoxic-ischemic injury are unknown. Because of this changing pattern of selective neuronal vulnerability to hypoxic-ischemic injury during development, hypothermia therapy is likely to have differing effects on the developing human brain compared to the mature brain.

Outcome

Outcome after cardiac arrest is worse in children compared to adults [19]. Survival rates vary with the location of the cardiac arrest (out-of-hospital versus in-hospital) with 12-month survival rates ranging from 7% to 53% [11,20–33]. There were large ranges in sample size, duration of follow-up, and variations in the rate of withdrawal of life support in previous studies. The outcome of out-of-hospital cardiac arrest is especially poor in children, with a survival-to-hospital-discharge rate of 7% [27]. Rate of survival from cardiac arrest in children improves when the cardiac arrest takes place in-hospital, especially when the event occurs in the critical care unit. The survival of cardiac arrest in the critical care unit at 12-month follow-up was 27% in one single-site study [33].

Survivors of cardiac arrest in the critical care unit generally have a good neurologic and functional outcome at 12-month follow-up as assessed using the 6-point pediatric cerebral performance category and pediatric overall performance category scores [33]. It is unlikely that hypothermia therapy will benefit children with the most severe hypoxic-ischemic encephalopathy after cardiac arrest. It is likely that only certain subgroups of children with mild to moderate hypoxic-ischemic encephalopathy will potentially benefit from hypothermia therapy. More research is necessary to define the features of these subgroups.

Rationale for hypothermia therapy after cardiac arrest

Animal models

Recently, research in rodent models of global cerebral ischemia demonstrated that if mild hypothermia was implemented within 1 to 6 hours after ischemia for durations of 12 to 48 hours, histologic and functional outcomes were improved [34–36]. Mild hypothermia protects against neuronal loss in the hippocampus (CA1) and improves neurobehavioral outcome after 5 minutes of global (two-vessel occlusion) cerebral ischemia in gerbils [12,34,35,37–39]. The protection against loss of CA1 neurons and memory deficits is sustained for at least 6 months after the injury [35]. Mild hypothermia is most beneficial when applied immediately after the ischemic insult and for longer durations (ie, 48 hours) [37]. Mild hypothermia of 48 hours' duration is effective even when the onset of hypothermia is delayed 6 hours after 10 minutes of severe forebrain ischemia in the rat [36].

These elegant studies of the optimal duration of hypothermia therapy provide some rationale for our choice of 48 hours' duration of hypothermia therapy in our current study of hypothermia therapy in children. Longer durations of hypothermia therapy also have been used in newborn humans [7]. Hypothermia therapy is also neuroprotective in large animal models of cardiac arrest [40]. Most of the investigations of hypothermia therapy in immature models have been in the fetal sheep model [41,42] and in the Vanucci-Rice model of cerebral hypoxic ischemia in newborn rat pups [43].

Mechanisms of neuroprotection

After cessation of cerebral blood flow in cardiac arrest, a sequence of metabolic and pathophysiologic events occurs in the minutes to days after reperfusion. A full discussion of these events is beyond the scope of this article; however, we summarize key processes in the order they occur after cardiac arrest.

Energy failure

After cessation of cerebral blood flow, glucose and glycogen are rapidly metabolized to lactate as cells switch from oxidative phosphorylation to anaerobic respiration. Lactate levels rise exponentially and proportional to plasma glucose levels and coincide with hydrolysis of ATP, causing $[H^+]$ to increase [44,45]. Hypothermia decreases cerebral metabolism approximately 6% per degree Celsius fall in temperature [44,46,47] and decreases the anoxic decline in ATP potential. This is one rationale for deep hypothermic circulatory arrest used in congenital cardiac surgery [48].

Excitotoxicity

As energy potential fails, the uncontrolled release of excitatory (predominantly glutamate) compounds acting on N-methyl-D-aspartate, alpha-amino-3-hydroxy-5-methyl-4-isoxazoleproprioniate, and Kainate receptors causes spreading depolarization and initiates release of calcium from intracellular stores. A vicious cycle of uncontrolled metabolic activity, neuronal body swelling, and further neurotransmitter release ensues [49], which further depletes cell energy stores and promote apoptosis or necrosis [50]. Calcium activates proteases, DNAses, lipases, protein kinase-C (PKC), and calpains (Ca^{2+} activated serine proteases), exacerbates excitotoxicity and neuronal excitability, and leads to excitotoxic neuronal death [51]. Hypothermia therapy attenuates several of these processes [52–54] and has been shown to decrease glutamate release in cerebral ischemia [55–58]. The neuroprotective effect of mild hypothermia cannot be explained solely by a reduction of glutamate, however [59,60].

Mitochondrial injury

Increases in cytosolic calcium can trigger the formation of membrane transport pores in the mitochondrial membrane [61]. These portals allow free passage of cytosolic compounds into the mitochondrial lumen and interfere with the inner mitochondrial membranes and elements of the respiratory chain, leading to destruction of the mitochondrion and leaking of its contents. Cytochrome-C is one of the mitochondrial compounds that leaks into the cytosol and executes the intrinsic apoptotic cascade by activating caspases [62]. Hypothermia attenuates the apoptosis cascade by decreasing cytochrome-C and activation of several of the key caspases, but it has a differential effect on the other proteins important in apoptosis, such as Bax and Bcl-2 [63,64].

Reactive oxygen species and reperfusion injury

Nitric oxide (NO) and other reactive oxygen species are generated by endothelium, neurons, and glia at the onset of ischemia. NO in particular is generated from the amino acid L-arginine and controls regional/local blood flow in the brain in proportion to neuronal activity. In the presence of reactive oxygen species generated in excess of the capacity of free radical scavengers, such as superoxide dismutase, NO combines with reactive oxygen species to generate peroxynitrite ($ONOO^-$), a volatile substance that damages DNA and other cellular components. The net amount of the reactive oxygen species generated can be inferred by the quantification of a reactive oxygen species scavenger nitrotyrosine. Hypothermia therapy reduces free radical formation in cerebral ischemia [65]. Intraischemic and postischemic hypothermia also reduces the amount of inducible nitric oxide synthase, neuronal nitric oxide synthase, and nitrotyrosine [66].

Cerebral blood flow

After global cerebral ischemia and reperfusion, there is a brief period (several minutes) of relative hyperperfusion followed by a prolonged period (several hours) of low cerebral blood flow (delayed hypoperfusion) [67]. The mechanism of delayed hypoperfusion is not clear, but there is evidence of vasoactive substances mediating vasoconstriction, adherent neutrophils, endothelial swelling, and blood hyperviscosity and platelet aggregates accumulating in microvessels. During this period of hypoperfusion there may be regional impairment of oxygen and substrate delivery, which may impair metabolic recovery. Hypothermia therapy may improve delayed hypoperfusion [68].

Cell death signaling

Mitogen-activated protein kinases, c-Jun NH2-terminal kinase (JNK), p38, and extracellular signal regulating kinases (ERKs) are key signal transducers in cellular responses to external stressors, such as oxidative stress and inflammation [69]. Their role in the activation of transcription factors of cell survival and cell death is complex, but ERK and JNK in particular are increased in the hippocampus after transient cerebral ischemia. Hypothermia therapy further increases the ERK-to-JNK ratio, which indicates a positive association with cell survival and ERK activation [70]. Inhibiting ERK does not attenuate the beneficial effect of hypothermia therapy after cardiac arrest in the rat, however, which suggests alternative mechanistic pathways of hypothermia therapy [71].

Inflammation

After cerebral ischemia there is a cellular inflammatory response, with leukocytes adhering to cerebral endothelium in the hours after reperfusion [72,73]. The role of leukocytes in neuronal cell death is not understood in transient cerebral ischemia, however. Hypothermia therapy decreases leukocyte endothelial interactions [74] and is associated with neuronal anti-inflammatory effects [56,75–77], decreased glutamate concentrations, decreased generation of free radicals and lipid peroxidation [78], and decreased heat shock protein response [39]. We have demonstrated that hypothermia therapy has selective anti-inflammatory effects, decreasing expression of nuclear factor (NF)-κB, and secretion of interleukin-8 by cerebral endothelial cells, thereby inhibiting leukocyte recruitment to the cerebral microcirculation [77].

In summary, no one single unifying mechanism explains the neuroprotective effects of hypothermia therapy. It has a large number of molecular mechanisms, which helps explain why it is potentially so effective in laboratory models and in patients with cardiac arrest and global hypoxic-ischemic encephalopathy.

Clinical experience

Children can survive with intact neurologic outcome after submersion in ice water. These outcomes were summarized by Orlowski [79] in the past, and recent reports in the literature discuss neurologically intact survivors after ice-water submersion and exposure to extremely cold environmental temperatures [80,81]. It is likely that intraischemic hypothermia is a major contributor to these good outcomes. Hypothermia therapy was used in the 1970s and 1980s to treat cerebral edema in children and adolescents after cardiac arrest caused by submersion accidents (near drowning) [1]. Bohn and Biggart and colleagues [2,3] later reported that hypothermia therapy led to increased risk of death, neutropenia, and sepsis, however, and the use of this therapy for near-drowning and cardiac arrest patients was abandoned in the late 1980s and 1990s. Potential reasons for the limitations of these studies were that historical controls were used, that the patients were cooled to temperatures that were too low (30°–33°C), that the duration of hypothermia therapy was too long (days), and that the therapy was combined with barbiturate coma, which had adverse effects that added to those of hypothermia [2]. We are using a more mild hypothermia (33°–34°C) with no addition of barbiturate-induced coma in our current trial of hypothermia therapy after cardiac arrest in children.

Recently, hypothermia therapy was shown to improve outcome after ventricular arrhythmia-induced cardiac arrest in adults [4–6]. Hypothermia therapy also has been shown to improve outcome in newborns with hypoxic-ischemic encephalopathy [7,82]. Although hypothermia therapy after cardiac arrest has not been studied using randomized controlled trials in children, the results of these controlled trials in adult and newborn humans suggest that hypothermia therapy is beneficial in children after cardiac arrest.

Potential adverse effects

Hypothermia therapy seems to be relatively safe when applied at temperatures more than 32°C for short durations (24 hours) [56]. The principal concern has been the development of arrhythmias at temperatures less than 32°C [83]. Great care must be taken when cooling because a patient's temperature can easily go below 32°C unless the core temperature is closely monitored and surface cooling techniques are stopped once the upper limit of the therapeutic temperature range (34°C) is reached. Overcooling to less than 32°C is common with surface cooling techniques and potentially deleterious after cardiac arrest in adults [84]. Mild adverse effects occur at clinically relevant temperatures and durations of hypothermia, including bradycardia and lower cardiac output, and hypotension during rewarming [85–87].

Pancreatic, metabolic, and renal abnormalities have been reported with the use of hypothermia therapy [88]. A mild coagulopathy with slight elevation of prothrombin time and partial thromboplastin time and a lower platelet count has been reported [56,85,88]. Impairment of the anterior pituitary response to exogenous administration of releasing hormones also has been reported in patients treated with hypothermia [89]. There is a risk of impairment of the immune system leading to a potentially higher incidence of pneumonia and sepsis, so patients need to be watched closely for signs of nosocomial infection [90–92]. Because of these adverse effects, lower depths ($<32°C$) or prolonged durations of hypothermia therapy are not practical or safe. The potential benefits and harms of hypothermia therapy are summarized in Table 1.

Guidelines for use of hypothermia therapy in patients

A recent advisory statement on therapeutic hypothermia after cardiac arrest was made by the Advanced Life Support Task Force of the International Liaison Committee on Resuscitation. The task force recommended that hypothermia therapy be used after ventricular fibrillation–induced cardiac arrest in adults [8,9]. The limited evidence of the use of hypothermia therapy in pediatrics is reflected in the American Heart Association guidelines, which recommend that hypothermia therapy be considered in children who remain comatose after resuscitation [10]. This recommendation is based on extrapolation from existing randomized controlled trials in adult and newborn humans, because there are no published randomized controlled trials of hypothermia therapy in children after cardiac arrest. A survey of 159 American and Canadian pediatric intensive care physicians showed that 38% sometimes use hypothermia therapy and 95% would be willing to participate in a prospective, randomized controlled trial of hypothermia therapy for cardiac arrest in children [93].

Table 1
Hypothermia therapy

Potential benefits	Potential harms
Adult and newborn human data demonstrate benefit after cardiac arrest [4,5,7,82] Adult and neonatal animal data demonstrate benefit after global cerebral ischemia [7,35,42] Stroke research (focal ischemia) shows potential benefit [103] Developmental potential: immature brain has plasticity and more recovery potential compared to adult brain	Most cardiac arrests in children are secondary to hypoxia or shock, with more profound cerebral injury and worse outcome compared to adults [19]; the gain in decreased mortality may come at the expense of increased persistent vegetative state in survivors [3] Cardiovascular: arrhythmias, bradycardia, and vasoconstriction and vasodilatation during rewarming Coagulopathy Immune suppression Pancrease, renal, metabolic, and endocrine abnormalities

Illustrative case

A 7-week-old male infant developed signs of an upper respiratory infection with coryza, cough, and poor feeding. He was previously well and was born via spontaneous vaginal delivery at term. During a coughing episode, while in his mother's arms at home, he developed cyanosis and apnea. The mother started mouth-to-mouth resuscitation and chest compressions, and the father phoned for an ambulance. When the paramedics arrived, the infant was noted to have cyanosis, apnea, and severe bradycardia, and he was pulseless. The infant was intubated, ventilated, and transported via ambulance to the local hospital. Just before arriving at the local hospital, he had return of spontaneous circulation, some irregular gasping respirations, and improved color. The duration of cardiac arrest with chest compressions was 15 minutes. An intravenous line was started, and he was transported to our institution, where he was noted to have abnormal results on his neurologic examination.

After the physicians obtained informed consent, he was entered into a randomized controlled pilot study of hypothermia therapy for cardiac arrest. He was randomized to hypothermia therapy, and cooling began within 6 hours after cardiac arrest. He was cooled rapidly using surface-cooling techniques, and lower esophageal temperature was maintained between 32.9° and 34°C for 48 hours. He was then slowly rewarmed at 0.5°C every 2 hours. His temperatures are shown in Fig. 2. Metapneumovirus and *Staphylococcus aureus* were cultured from a bronchoalveolar lavage done on admission, and the patient received a 10-day course of intravenous antibiotics. He developed acute respiratory distress syndrome, which was treated with high positive end expiratory pressure and conventional mechanical ventilation. The duration of mechanical ventilation was 8 days, and the length of stay in the pediatric intensive care unit was 9 days.

He had a normal neurologic outcome (pediatric cerebral performance category score of 1) at 6 months after cardiac arrest [94–96]. There were no adverse events, arrhythmias (aside from sinus bradycardia), nosocomial infections, or bleeding attributed to hypothermia therapy. The results of

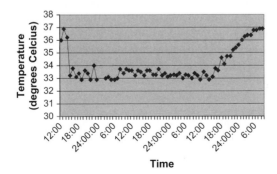

Fig. 2. Temperature of infant treated with hypothermia therapy after cardiac arrest.

randomized controlled trials will help us determine if hypothermia therapy improves mortality and neurologic outcome after cardiac arrest in children.

Methods for cooling

We use the following protocol for cooling in children after cardiac arrest. It has been modified from our protocol for cooling in children with traumatic brain injury [97]. Cooling should be started as soon as possible after the cardiac arrest because there is likely a therapeutic window:

- A cooling mattress is placed under the patient (5°C).
- Neuromuscular blocker (eg, pancuronium, 0.1 mg/kg) is administered intravenously as needed to prevent shivering.
- An esophageal temperature probe is placed, and the tip is confirmed to be in the lower third of the esophagus by chest radiograph.
- Crushed ice is placed in double plastic bags, air is removed, and the bags are sealed to prevent leakage. The bags are placed in cotton bags (pillow cases) to prevent injury to the skin. As much surface area as possible is covered with these bags of ice, and the skin is inspected frequently to prevent cold-induced injury.
- A cooling blanket (forced air) is placed over the ice and the patient.
- Once the patient's esophageal temperature reaches 34°C, the ice packs and upper cooling blanket are quickly removed, and the servo-controlled cooling mattress below the patient is on automatic at 33.5°C. Close temperature monitoring is done to prevent overcooling.
- We aim to keep the temperature between 33° and 34°C for 48 hours.
- We slowly rewarm the patient by increasing the set point on the servo-controlled cooling mattress by 0.5°C every 2 hours. Rewarming takes 14 to 18 hours.

Other methods of cooling include the cooling device used during extracorporeal membrane oxygenation, which we use after rescue extracorporeal membrane oxygenation. Ice-cold intravenous normal saline and saline ice slurry have been reported as methods of rapid cooling in adults and animal models after cardiac arrest [98,99]. To our knowledge, use of ice-cold intravenous normal saline has not yet been reported as a cooling method in children. We have used ice-cold normal saline gastric lavage in addition to surface-cooling techniques in large adolescents who are difficult to cool.

Use of hypothermia therapy in other types of brain injury in children

Hypothermia therapy has been used in severe stroke associated with cerebral edema and coma [100] and in severe traumatic brain injury in children [97,101,102]. Further study is necessary in children with stroke and traumatic brain injury to determine if hypothermia therapy improves survival and neurologic outcome.

Summary

Hypothermia therapy is neuroprotective in animal models and in new-borns and adult humans with cardiac arrest and hypoxic-ischemic encephalopathy. The American Heart Association guidelines recommend that it should be considered in children after cardiac arrest. Methods of inducing hypothermia include simple surface-cooling techniques, intravenous boluses of cold saline, gastric lavage with ice-cold normal saline, and using the temperature control device after emergency extracorporeal life support. There is a potential for overcooling and other adverse effects, including arrhythmias, coagulopathy, and immune suppression. We recommend further study before a strong recommendation can be made to use hypothermia therapy in children with cardiac arrest.

References

[1] Conn AW, Edmonds JF, Barker GA. Near-drowning in cold fresh water: current treatment regimen. Can Anaesth Soc J 1978;25:259–65.

[2] Bohn DJ, Biggar WD, Smith CR, et al. Influence of hypothermia, barbiturate therapy, and intracranial pressure monitoring on morbidity and mortality after near-drowning. Crit Care Med 1986;14:529–34.

[3] Biggart MJ, Bohn DJ. Effect of hypothermia and cardiac arrest on outcome of near-drowning accidents in children. J Pediatr 1990;117:179–83.

[4] Bernard SA, Gray TW, Buist MD, et al. Treatment of comatose survivors of out-of-hospital cardiac arrest with induced hypothermia. N Engl J Med 2002;346:557–63.

[5] The Hypothermia after Cardiac Arrest Study Group. Mild therapeutic hypothermia to improve the neurologic outcome after cardiac arrest. N Engl J Med 2002;346:549–56.

[6] Holzer M, Bernard SA, Hachimi-Idrissi S, et al. Hypothermia for neuroprotection after cardiac arrest: systematic review and individual patient data meta-analysis. Crit Care Med 2005;33:414–8.

[7] Gluckman PD, Wyatt JS, Azzopardi D, et al. Selective head cooling with mild systemic hypothermia after neonatal encephalopathy: multicentre randomised trial. Lancet 2005; 365:663–70.

[8] Nolan JP, Morley PT, Vanden Hoek TL, et al. Therapeutic hypothermia after cardiac arrest: an advisory statement by the advanced life support task force of the International Liaison Committee on Resuscitation. Circulation 2003;108:118–21.

[9] American Heart Association. 2005 guidelines for cardiopulmonary resuscitation and emergency cardiovascular care. Circulation 2005;112:IV1–203.

[10] The International Liaison Committee on Resuscitation (ILCOR). Consensus on science with treatment recommendations for pediatric and neonatal patients: pediatric basic and advanced life support. Pediatrics 2006;117:e955–77.

[11] Nadkarni VM, Larkin GL, Peberdy MA, et al. First documented rhythm and clinical outcome from in-hospital cardiac arrest among children and adults. JAMA 2006;295:50–7.

[12] Corbett D, Nurse S, Colbourne F. Hypothermic neuroprotection: a global ischemia study using 18- to 20-month-old gerbils. Stroke 1997;28:2238–42.

[13] Auer RN, Surtherland GR. Hypoxia and related conditions. In: Graham DI, Lantos PL, editors. Greenfield's neuropathology. London: Arnold, a member of the Hodder Headline Group; 2002. p. 233–80.

[14] Horn M, Schlote W. Delayed neuronal death and delayed neuronal recovery in the human brain following global ischemia. Acta Neuropathol 1992;85:79–87.

[15] Petito CK, Feldmann E, Pulsinelli WA, et al. Delayed hippocampal damage in humans following cardiorespiratory arrest. Neurology 1987;37:1281–6.
[16] Fujioka M, Nishio K, Miyamoto S, et al. Hippocampal damage in the human brain after cardiac arrest. Cerebrovasc Dis 2000;10:2–7.
[17] Drysdale EE, Grubb NR, Fox KA, et al. Chronicity of memory impairment in long-term out-of-hospital cardiac arrest survivors. Resuscitation 2000;47:27–32.
[18] Adult hypoxic and ischemic lesions. In: Ellison D, Love S, editors. Neuropathology: a reference text of CNS pathology. St. Louis (MO): Mosby International Ltd; 1998.
[19] Engdahl J, Axelsson A, Bang A, et al. The epidemiology of cardiac arrest in children and young adults. Resuscitation 2003;58(2):131–8.
[20] Slonim AD, Patel KM, Ruttimann UE, et al. Cardiopulmonary resuscitation in pediatric intensive care units. Crit Care Med 1997;25:1951–5.
[21] Parra DA, Totapally BR, Zahn E, et al. Outcome of cardiopulmonary resuscitation in a pediatric cardiac intensive care unit. Crit Care Med 2000;28:3296–300.
[22] Bos AP, Polman A, van der Voort E, et al. Cardiopulmonary resuscitation in paediatric intensive care patients. Intensive Care Med 1992;18:109–11.
[23] Von Seggern K, Egar M, Fuhrman BP. Cardiopulmonary resuscitation in a pediatric ICU. Crit Care Med 1986;14:275–7.
[24] Gillis J, Dickson D, Rieder M, et al. Results of inpatient pediatric resuscitation. Crit Care Med 1986;14(5):469–71.
[25] Suominen P, Olkkola KT, Voipio V, et al. Utstein style reporting of in-hospital paediatric cardiopulmonary resuscitation. Resuscitation 2000;45:17–25.
[26] Torres A Jr, Pickert CB, Firestone J, et al. Long-term functional outcome of inpatient pediatric cardiopulmonary resuscitation. Pediatr Emerg Care 1997;13:369–73.
[27] Schindler MB, Bohn D, Cox PN, et al. Outcome of out-of-hospital cardiac or respiratory arrest in children. N Engl J Med 1996;335:1473–9.
[28] Sirbaugh PE, Pepe PE, Shook JE, et al. A prospective, population-based study of the demographics, epidemiology, management, and outcome of out-of-hospital pediatric cardiopulmonary arrest. Ann Emerg Med 1999;33:174–84.
[29] Fiser DH, Wrape V. Outcome of cardiopulmonary resuscitation in children. Pediatr Emerg Care 1987;3:235–8.
[30] Zaritsky A, Nadkarni V, Getson P, et al. CPR in children. Ann Emerg Med 1987;16:1107–11.
[31] Samson RA, Nadkarni VM, Meaney PA, et al. Outcomes of in-hospital ventricular fibrillation in children. N Engl J Med 2006;354:2328–39.
[32] Perondi MB, Reis AG, Paiva EF, et al. A comparison of high-dose and standard-dose epinephrine in children with cardiac arrest. N Engl J Med 2004;350:1722–30.
[33] de Mos N, van Litsenburg RR, McCrindle B, et al. Pediatric in-intensive-care-unit cardiac arrest: incidence, survival, and predictive factors. Crit Care Med 2006;34:1209–15.
[34] Colbourne F, Corbett D. Delayed and prolonged post-ischemic hypothermia is neuroprotective in the gerbil. Brain Res 1994;654:265–72.
[35] Colbourne F, Corbett D. Delayed postischemic hypothermia: a six month survival study using behavioral and histological assessments of neuroprotection. J Neurosci 1995;15:7250–60.
[36] Colbourne F, Li H, Buchan AM. Indefatigable CA1 sector neuroprotection with mild hypothermia induced 6 hours after severe forebrain ischemia in rats. J Cereb Blood Flow Metab 1999;19:742–9.
[37] Colbourne F, Sutherland GR, Auer RN. Electron microscopic evidence against apoptosis as the mechanism of neuronal death in global ischemia. J Neurosci 1999;19:4200–10.
[38] Colbourne F, Auer RN, Sutherland GR. Characterization of postischemic behavioral deficits in gerbils with and without hypothermic neuroprotection. Brain Res 1998;803:69–78.
[39] Hicks SD, DeFranco DB, Callaway CW. Hypothermia during reperfusion after asphyxial cardiac arrest improves functional recovery and selectively alters stress-induced protein expression. J Cereb Blood Flow Metab 2000;20:520–30.

[40] Leonov Y, Sterz F, Safar P, et al. Moderate hypothermia after cardiac arrest of 17 minutes in dogs: effect on cerebral and cardiac outcome. Stroke 1990;21:1600–6.

[41] Gunn AJ, Gunn TR, de Haan HH, et al. Dramatic neuronal rescue with prolonged selective head cooling after ischemia in fetal lambs. J Clin Invest 1997;99:248–56.

[42] Gunn AJ, Gunn TR, Gunning MI, et al. Neuroprotection with prolonged head cooling started before postischemic seizures in fetal sheep. Pediatrics 1998;102:1098–106.

[43] Yager JY, Asselin J. Effect of mild hypothermia on cerebral energy metabolism during the evolution of hypoxic-ischemic brain damage in the immature rat. Stroke 1996;27: 919–25.

[44] Katsura K, Asplund B, Ekholm A, et al. Extra- and intracellular pH in the brain during ischaemia, related to tissue lactate content in normo- and hypercapnic rats. Eur J Neurosci 1992;4:166–76.

[45] Park WS, Chang YS, Lee M. Effects of hyperglycemia or hypoglycemia on brain cell membrane function and energy metabolism during the immediate reoxygenation-reperfusion period after acute transient global hypoxia-ischemia in the newborn piglet. Brain Res 2001;901:102–8.

[46] Steen PA, Newberg L, Milde JH, et al. Hypothermia and barbiturates: individual and combined effects on canine cerebral oxygen consumption. Anesthesiology 1983;58: 527–32.

[47] Young L. A 22-month-old victim of near drowning. J Emerg Nurs 1992;18:197–8.

[48] Amir G, Ramamoorthy C, Riemer RK, et al. Neonatal brain protection and deep hypothermic circulatory arrest: pathophysiology of ischemic neuronal injury and protective strategies. Ann Thorac Surg 2005;80:1955–64.

[49] Lee JM, Grabb MC, Zipfel GJ, et al. Brain tissue responses to ischemia. J Clin Invest 2000; 106:723–31.

[50] Ankarcrona M, Dypbukt JM, Bonfoco E, et al. Glutamate-induced neuronal death: a succession of necrosis or apoptosis depending on mitochondrial function. Neuron 1995;15:961–73.

[51] Siman R, Noszek JC. Excitatory amino acids activate calpain I and induce structural protein breakdown in vivo. Neuron 1988;1:279–87.

[52] Ji X, Luo Y, Ling F, et al. Mild hypothermia diminishes oxidative DNA damage and prodeath signaling events after cerebral ischemia: a mechanism for neuroprotection. Front Biosci 2007;12:1737–47.

[53] Harada K, Maekawa T, Tsuruta R, et al. Hypothermia inhibits translocation of CaM kinase II and PKC-alpha, beta, gamma isoforms and fodrin proteolysis in rat brain synaptosome during ischemia-reperfusion. J Neurosci Res 2002;67:664–9.

[54] Liebetrau M, Burggraf D, Martens HK, et al. Delayed moderate hypothermia reduces calpain activity and breakdown of its substrate in experimental focal cerebral ischemia in rats. Neurosci Lett 2004;357:17–20.

[55] Suehiro E, Fujisawa H, Ito H, et al. Brain temperature modifies glutamate neurotoxicity in vivo. J Neurotrauma 1999;16:285–97.

[56] Marion DW, Penrod LE, Kelsey SF, et al. Treatment of traumatic brain injury with moderate hypothermia. N Engl J Med 1997;336:540–6.

[57] Busto R, Dietrich WD, Globus MY, et al. The importance of brain temperature in cerebral ischemic injury. Stroke 1989;20:1113–4.

[58] Zhao H, Asai S, Kanematsu K, et al. Real-time monitoring of the effects of normothermia and hypothermia on extracellular glutamate re-uptake in the rat following global brain ischemia. Neuroreport 1997;8:2389–93.

[59] Yamamoto H, Mitani A, Cui Y, et al. Neuroprotective effect of mild hypothermia cannot be explained in terms of a reduction of glutamate release during ischemia. Neuroscience 1999;91:501–9.

[60] Takadera T, Ohyashiki T. Temperature-dependent N-methyl-D-aspartate receptor-mediated cytotoxicity in cultured rat cortical neurons. Neurosci Lett 2007;423:24–8.

[61] Smaili SS, Russell JT. Permeability transition pore regulates both mitochondrial membrane potential and agonist-evoked Ca2+ signals in oligodendrocyte progenitors. Cell Calcium 1999;26:121–30.

[62] MacManus JP, Linnik MD. Gene expression induced by cerebral ischemia: an apoptotic perspective. J Cereb Blood Flow Metab 1997;17:815–32.

[63] Yenari MA, Iwayama S, Cheng D, et al. Mild hypothermia attenuates cytochrome c release but does not alter Bcl-2 expression or caspase activation after experimental stroke. J Cereb Blood Flow Metab 2002;22:29–38.

[64] Xu L, Yenari MA, Steinberg GK, et al. Mild hypothermia reduces apoptosis of mouse neurons in vitro early in the cascade. J Cereb Blood Flow Metab 2002;22:21–8.

[65] Kil HY, Zhang J, Piantadosi CA. Brain temperature alters hydroxyl radical production during cerebral ischemia/reperfusion in rats. J Cereb Blood Flow Metab 1996; 16:100–6.

[66] Karabiyikoglu M, Han HS, Yenari MA, et al. Attenuation of nitric oxide synthase isoform expression by mild hypothermia after focal cerebral ischemia: variations depending on timing of cooling. J Neurosurg 2003;98:1271–6.

[67] Tsuchidate R, He QP, Smith ML, et al. Regional cerebral blood flow during and after 2 hours of middle cerebral artery occlusion in the rat. J Cereb Blood Flow Metab 1997; 17:1066–73.

[68] Karibe H, Zarow GJ, Graham SH, et al. Mild intraischemic hypothermia reduces postischemic hyperperfusion, delayed postischemic hypoperfusion, blood-brain barrier disruption, brain edema, and neuronal damage volume after temporary focal cerebral ischemia in rats. J Cereb Blood Flow Metab 1994;14:620–7.

[69] Cohen P. The search for physiological substrates of MAP and SAP kinases in mammalian cells. Trends Cell Biol 1997;7:353–61.

[70] Hicks SD, Parmele KT, DeFranco DB, et al. Hypothermia differentially increases extracellular signal-regulated kinase and stress-activated protein kinase/c-Jun terminal kinase activation in the hippocampus during reperfusion after asphyxial cardiac arrest. Neuroscience 2000;98:677–85.

[71] D'Cruz BJ, Logue ES, Falke E, et al. Hypothermia and ERK activation after cardiac arrest. Brain Res 2005;1064:108–18.

[72] Hallenbeck JM, Dutka AJ, Tanishima T, et al. Polymorphonuclear leukocyte accumulation in brain regions with low blood flow during the early postischemic period. Stroke 1986;17:246–53.

[73] Ishikawa M, Cooper D, Russell J, et al. Molecular determinants of the prothrombogenic and inflammatory phenotype assumed by the postischemic cerebral microcirculation. Stroke 2003;34:1777–82.

[74] Toyoda T, Suzuki S, Kassell NF, et al. Intraischemic hypothermia attenuates neutrophil infiltration in the rat neocortex after focal ischemia-reperfusion injury. Neurosurgery 1996;39:1200–5.

[75] Smith SL, Hall ED. Mild pre- and posttraumatic hypothermia attenuates blood-brain barrier damage following controlled cortical impact injury in the rat. J Neurotrauma 1996;13:1–9.

[76] Whalen MJ, Carlos TM, Clark RS, et al. The relationship between brain temperature and neutrophil accumulation after traumatic brain injury in rats. Acta Neurochir Suppl (Wien) 1997;70:260–1.

[77] Sutcliffe IT, Smith HA, Stanimirovic D, et al. Effects of moderate hypothermia on IL-1 beta-induced leukocyte rolling and adhesion in pial microcirculation of mice and on proinflammatory gene expression in human cerebral endothelial cells. J Cereb Blood Flow Metab 2001;21:1310–9.

[78] Lei B, Tan X, Cai H, et al. Effect of moderate hypothermia on lipid peroxidation in canine brain tissue after cardiac arrest and resuscitation. Stroke 1994;25:147–52.

[79] Orlowski JP. Drowning, near-drowning, and ice-water submersions. Pediatr Clin North Am 1987;34:75–92.

[80] de Caen A. Management of profound hypothermia in children without the use of extracorporeal life support therapy. Lancet 2002;360:1394–5.

[81] Eich C, Brauer A, Kettler D. Recovery of a hypothermic drowned child after resuscitation with cardiopulmonary bypass followed by prolonged extracorporeal membrane oxygenation. Resuscitation 2005;67:145–8.

[82] Shankaran S, Laptook AR, Ehrenkranz RA, et al. Whole-body hypothermia for neonates with hypoxic-ischemic encephalopathy. N Engl J Med 2005;353:1574–84.

[83] Clifton GL, Allen S, Berry J, et al. Systemic hypothermia in treatment of brain injury. J Neurotrauma 1992;9:S487–95.

[84] Merchant RM, Abella BS, Peberdy MA, et al. Therapeutic hypothermia after cardiac arrest: unintentional overcooling is common using ice packs and conventional cooling blankets. Crit Care Med 2006;34:S490–4.

[85] Clifton GL, Miller ER, Choi SC, et al. Lack of effect of induction of hypothermia after acute brain injury. N Engl J Med 2001;344:556–63.

[86] Kuwagata Y, Ogura H, Tasaki O, et al. Left ventricular wall velocity assessment by Doppler imaging in patients with severe head injury undgergoing therapeutic hypothermia. International Journal of Intensive Care 1997;82–7.

[87] Kuwagata Y, Oda J, Ninomiya N, et al. Changes in left ventricular performance in patients with severe head injury during and after mild hypothermia. J Trauma 1999;47:666–72.

[88] Metz C, Holzschuh M, Bein T, et al. Moderate hypothermia in patients with severe head injury: cerebral and extracerebral effects. J Neurosurg 1996;85:533–41.

[89] Hayshi S, Isayama K, Teramoto A. Anterior pituitary functions in patients with severe head injuries treated with moderate hypothermia. Brain Nerve 1997;49:145–50.

[90] Yokota H, Fuse A, Ninomiya N, et al. Complications of the hemodynamic and respiratory systems during hypothermal treatment for severe head injury. Japanese Journal of Neurosurgery 1998;7:9–13.

[91] Bernard SA, MacJanes B, Buist M. Experience with prolonged induced hypothermia in severe head injury. Crit Care 1999;3:167–72.

[92] Ishikawa K, Tanaka H, Shiozaki T, et al. Characteristics of infection and leukocyte count in severely head-injured patients treated with mild hypothermia. J Trauma 2000;49:912–22.

[93] Haque IU, Latour MC, Zaritsky AL. Pediatric critical care community survey of knowledge and attitudes toward therapeutic hypothermia in comatose children after cardiac arrest. Pediatr Crit Care Med 2006;7:7–14.

[94] Fiser DH. Assessing the outcome of pediatric intensive care. J Pediatr 1992;121:68–74.

[95] Fiser DH, Long N, Roberson PK, et al. Relationship of pediatric overall performance category and pediatric cerebral performance category scores at pediatric intensive care unit discharge with outcome measures collected at hospital discharge and 1- and 6-month follow-up assessments. Crit Care Med 2000;28:2616–20.

[96] Fiser DH, Tilford JM, Roberson PK. Relationship of illness severity and length of stay to functional outcomes in the pediatric intensive care unit: a multi-institutional study. Crit Care Med 2000;28:1173–9.

[97] Hutchison J, Ward R, Lacroix J, et al. Hypothermia pediatric head injury trial: the value of a pretrial clinical evaluation phase. Dev Neurosci 2006;28:291–301.

[98] Bernard S, Buist M, Monteiro O, et al. Induced hypothermia using large volume, ice-cold intravenous fluid in comatose survivors of out-of-hospital cardiac arrest: a preliminary report. Resuscitation 2003;56:9–13.

[99] Vanden Hoek TL, Kasza KE, Beiser DG, et al. Induced hypothermia by central venous infusion: saline ice slurry versus chilled saline. Crit Care Med 2004;32:S425–31.

[100] Hutchison JS, Ichord R, Guerguerian AM, et al. Cerebrovascular disorders. Semin Pediatr Neurol 2004;11:139–46.

[101] Biswas AK, Bruce DA, Sklar FH, et al. Treatment of acute traumatic brain injury in children with moderate hypothermia improves intracranial hypertension. Crit Care Med 2002;30:2742–51.

[102] Adelson PD, Ragheb J, Kanev P, et al. Phase II clinical trial of moderate hypothermia after severe traumatic brain injury in children. Neurosurgery 2005;56:740–54.

[103] Feigin VL, Anderson CS, Rodgers A, et al. The emerging role of induced hypothermia in the management of acute stroke. J Clin Neurosci 2002;9:502–7.

ELSEVIER
SAUNDERS

PEDIATRIC CLINICS
OF NORTH AMERICA

Pediatr Clin N Am 55 (2008) 545–575

Surfactant for Pediatric Acute Lung Injury

Douglas F. Willson, MD[a],*, Patricia R. Chess, MD[b],
Robert H. Notter, MD, PhD[b]

[a]Pediatric ICU and Division of Pediatric Critical Care, University of Virginia Children's
Medical Center, UVA Health Sciences System, Box 800386,
Charlottesville, VA 22908-0386, USA
[b]University of Rochester School of Medicine, 601 Elmwood Avenue,
Rochester, NY 14642, USA

Because of their extensive alveolar network and capillary vasculature, the lungs have significant exposure and susceptibility to injury from toxins and pathogens present either in the circulation or in the external environment. The medical consequences of acute pulmonary injury in pediatric and adult patients frequently are defined as the syndromes of acute lung injury (ALI) and acute respiratory distress syndrome (ARDS). The American-European Consensus Conference in 1994 defined ALI as respiratory failure of acute onset with a ratio of partial pressure of arterial oxygen to fraction of inspired oxygen (PaO_2/FIO_2) of 300 mm Hg or lower (regardless of the level of positive end expiratory pressure), bilateral infiltrates on frontal chest radiograph, and a pulmonary capillary wedge pressure lower than 18 mm Hg (if measured) or no evidence of left atrial hypertension [1]. ARDS is defined identically except for a lower PaO_2/FIO_2 limit of less than 200 mm Hg [1]. The Consensus Committee definitions of ALI/ARDS are widely used clinically, supplemented by lung injury or critical care scores such as the Murray [2] or APACHE II [3] scores in adults, or the Pediatric Risk of Mortality [4,5], Pediatric Index of Mortality [6], or Oxygenation Index [7] scores in children.

The incidence of ALI/ARDS has been reported variably to be 50,000 to 190,000 cases per year in the United States [1,8–14]. The incidence of ALI in two recent studies has been estimated at 22 to 86 cases per 100,000 persons per year [13,14], with 40% to 43% of these patients having ARDS [13].

This work was supported in part by grant HL-56176 from the National Institutes of Health.
    * Corresponding author.
    E-mail address: dfw4m@virginia.edu (D.F. Willson).

These studies primarily considered adults; the incidence of ALI/ARDS has been reported to be significantly lower, at 2 to 8 cases per 100,000 persons per year, in the pediatric age group [15–19]. Survival statistics for patients who have ALI/ARDS vary depending on specific lung injury etiology and age, but overall mortality rates in both adult and pediatric patients remain very substantial despite sophisticated intensive care [1,8–14,16–19]. Mortality rates reported in a series of studies in pediatric patients who had ALI/ARDS are given in Table 1 [15,19–25]. The practical significance of distinguishing between the two clinical syndromes is uncertain, because a meta-analysis of 102 studies before 1996 suggested little or no difference in mortality rates between patients meeting criteria for ALI and those meeting the criteria for ARDS [9]. Rubenfeld and colleagues [13] reached the same conclusion in a recent article in *The New England Journal of Medicine*, which reported mortality rates of 38.5% for ALI and 41% for ARDS, with an estimated 74,500 deaths per year and an aggregate 3.6 million hospital days of care in the United States.

There clearly is a significant need for improved treatments for ALI/ARDS in all age groups. This article focuses on the potential utility of exogenous surfactant replacement therapy. Although the clinical syndromes of ALI and ARDS encompass a broad spectrum of etiologies, it is important to consider specific etiologies in targeting surfactant therapy. In particular, it is important to distinguish between ALI/ARDS from direct pulmonary causes as opposed to systemic (indirect, nonpulmonary) causes. Direct pulmonary causes of ALI/ARDS include lung viral or bacterial infections, gastric aspiration, blunt thoracic trauma with lung contusion, meconium aspiration (in infants), near-drowning, thoracic radiation, hyperoxia, and the inhalation of smoke or other toxicants. Indirect (systemic) causes of ALI/ARDS include sepsis, closed space burn injury, hypovolemic shock, nonthoracic trauma, multiple transfusions, and pancreatitis. The pathology of ALI/ARDS is particularly complex in indirect insults like sepsis, where multiorgan involvement is common, and extrapulmonary inflammation is severe and pervasive. The multifaceted systemic pathology of ALI/ARDS from

Table 1
Mortality rates reported in a series of studies in pediatric acute lung injury/acute respiratory distress syndrome

Study	Year	# Patients	Mortality (%)
Pfenninger et al [15]	1982	20	40
DeBruin et al [21][a]	1992	100	72
Timmons et al [22]	1995	470	43
Dahlem et al [23]	2003	44	27.3
Curley et al [24]	2005	102	8
Willson et al [25]	2005	152	28
Flori et al [19]	2005	328	22
Pediatric Study Group (ANZICS) [20]	2007	117	35

[a] Patients consisted of mostly immunocompromised children.

nonpulmonary causes of lung injury probably renders therapy with exogenous surfactant less effective than in direct pulmonary ALI/ARDS. As detailed later, post hoc analyses in two recent clinical trials of surfactant therapy in ALI/ARDS suggest greater efficacy in direct than in indirect pulmonary injury [25,26]. In all forms of ALI/ARDS, the major rationale for surfactant therapy is the presence of surfactant dysfunction in the injured lungs (Fig. 1). Although ALI/ARDS can include chronic lung injury in its later fibroproliferative phase, surfactant dysfunction is most prominent in the acute phase of ALI/ARDS, as described later.

Surfactant dysfunction in acute pulmonary injury

Total lavaged phospholipid is either unchanged or increased in most animal models of ALI/ARDS, including models of direct pulmonary injury such as gastric aspiration or respiratory infection [27–32]. Although surfactant deficiency potentially can occur during the course of ALI/ARDS (eg, from type II cell injury), surfactant dysfunction in association with inflammation and permeability injury generally is much more prominent. Impairments in lung surfactant activity and reductions in the content or composition of active large surfactant aggregates have been reported in bronchoalveolar lavage, edema fluid, or tracheal aspirates from patients who have ALI/ARDS or other diseases involving lung injury [33–45]. Research during the last 2 decades has identified a number of pathways and mechanisms contributing to surfactant dysfunction in acute pulmonary injury (for review, see [27,46,47]).

One prevalent pathway of surfactant dysfunction in lung injury is through biophysical or chemical interactions with substances present in the alveoli as a result of permeability edema or inflammation. Biophysical studies in vitro have shown that the surface activity of lung surfactant can be impaired by multiple injury-related inhibitors including plasma and blood proteins [48–55], meconium [56], cell membrane lipids [50,55,57], fluid free fatty acids [55,58–60], reactive oxidants [58,61–63], and lytic enzymes including proteases [64] and phospholipases [65,66]. Surfactant dysfunction associated with inhibitory substances in the lungs also has been demonstrated widely in animal models of acute inflammatory lung injury [27–32,46,67–69]. In terms of physicochemical mechanisms of action, albumin and other blood proteins impair the surface activity of lung surfactant primarily by competitive adsorption that reduces the entry of active surfactant components into the air–water interface [52,70]. In contrast, cell membrane lipids, lysophospholipids, or fatty acids act at least in part by mixing into the surface film and compromising its ability to reach low surface tension during dynamic compression [50,55,59,70]. Also, phospholipases, proteases, and reactive oxygen-nitrogen species can act to degrade essential surfactant lipids or proteins chemically or alter them functionally [64,66,71]. It is well documented that surfactant activity deficits from these various

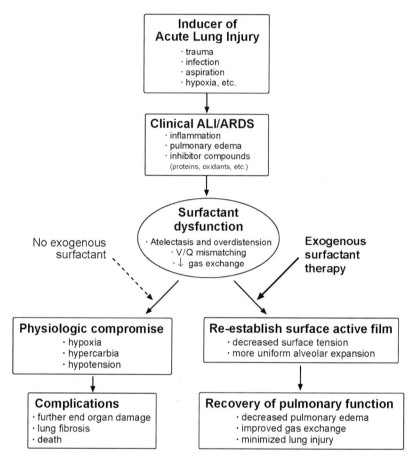

Fig. 1. Schematic of the rationale for exogenous surfactant therapy to mitigate surfactant dysfunction in acute lung injury (ALI)/acute respiratory distress syndrome (ARDS). The pathophysiology of acute inflammatory lung injury includes surfactant dysfunction, which contributes to respiratory failure in term infants, children, and adults who have clinical ALI and ARDS. Surfactant dysfunction reduces lung volumes and compliance, causes atelectasis and overdistension, increases ventilation/perfusion (V/Q) mismatching, and reduces gas exchange. In addition, surfactant dysfunction and lung injury can be present in the clinical course of premature infants being treated with mechanical ventilation and supplemental oxygen for surfactant-deficient lung disease in association with the neonatal respiratory distress syndrome. Scientific understanding indicates that surfactant dysfunction in lung injury can, at least in principle, be ameliorated by exogenous surfactant therapy, as discussed in this article. (*Data from* Seeger W, Grube C, Günther A, et al. Surfactant inhibition by plasma proteins: differential sensitivity of various surfactant preparations. Eur Respir J 1993;6:9719–77.)

mechanisms can be overcome or at least mitigated in vitro by increasing the concentration of active surfactant, even if inhibitor substances are still present [27,46,47].

Another pathway by which surfactant activity can be reduced during lung injury is by depletion or alteration of active large aggregates. Surfactant exists in the alveolar hypophase in a size-distributed microstructure of aggregates, the largest of which typically have the greatest surface activity and the highest apoprotein content [60,72–78]. The percentage of large aggregates and their content of surfactant protein A (SP-A) and surfactant protein B (SP-B) are reduced in bronchoalveolar lavage from patients who have ARDS [38–40]. Animal studies of ALI/ARDS indicate that large surfactant aggregates can be depleted or reduced in activity by molecular interactions with inhibitor substances as well as by changes in surfactant aggregate metabolism in the alveoli or involving altered reuptake or recycling in type II cells [30,60,79–81]. Although large aggregates are depleted or compromised in many forms of ALI/ARDS, information on total surfactant pools is inconsistent, with both decreased [35,37] and unchanged amounts [34,36] reported.

The ability of exogenous surfactant therapy to reverse or mitigate acute respiratory pathology in animal models of ALI/ARDS also has been documented extensively (Box 1). Examples of animal studies showing benefits in acute lung function or mechanics following surfactant therapy include acid aspiration [82–84], meconium aspiration [85–88], anti-lung serum [89], bacterial or endotoxin injury [90–95], bilateral vagotomy [96], hyperoxia [97–101], in vivo lavage [102–107], N-nitroso-N-methylurethane (NNNMU) injury [108–110], and viral pneumonia [111,112]. These acute animal model studies typically did not address long-term outcomes. Significant improvements in respiratory function would be expected to lead to improved long-term outcomes in patients who have ALI/ARDS, provided that untreated elements of pathology do not blunt this effect. As noted earlier, these improvements are most likely to be seen in direct pulmonary forms of ALI/ARDS.

Clinical exogenous surfactant drugs

Although endogenous surfactant contains similar chemical constituents across mammalian species, exogenous surfactant drugs do not. The degree

---

Box 1. Animal models of acute lung injury/acute respiratory distress syndrome lung injury that have been shown to respond acutely to exogenous surfactant therapy

Aspiration of acid [82–84] or meconium [85–88]
Anti-lung serum infusion [89]
Bacterial or endotoxin-induced injury [90–95]
Bilateral vagotomy [96]
Hyperoxic lung injury [97–101]
In vivo lung lavage with mechanical ventilation [102–107]
N-nitroso-N-methylurethane–induced lung injury [108–110]
Viral pneumonia [111,112]

to which pharmaceutical surfactants resemble native surfactant is highly variable and has direct consequences for surface and physiologic activity. Pharmaceutical surfactants comprise three functionally relevant classifications (Box 2): (1) organic solvent extracts of lavaged lung surfactant from animals; (2) organic solvent extracts of processed animal lung tissue with or without additional synthetic additives; and (3) synthetic preparations formulated in vitro without material from animal lungs. Organic solvent extracts of lavaged alveolar surfactant (category 1) contain all the hydrophobic lipid and protein components of endogenous surfactant, although specific compositional details can vary depending on the method of preparation. Extracts of minced or homogenized lung tissue (category 2) necessarily contain some nonsurfactant components and require more extensive processing that can alter composition further compared with native surfactant. The synthetic surfactants

---

Box 2. Clinical exogenous surfactant drugs for treating diseases that involve lung surfactant deficiency or dysfunction

1. Organic solvent extracts of lavaged animal lung surfactant
   Calf-lung surfactant extract (Infasurf; ONY, Inc. and Forest Laboratories)
   Bovine lung extract surfactant (bLES)
   Alveofact
2. Supplemented or unsupplemented organic solvent extracts of processed animal lung tissue
   Survanta (Abbott/Ross Laboratories)
   Surfactant-TA
   Curosurf (Chesi Farmaceutici and Dey Laboratories)
3. Synthetic exogenous lung surfactants
   Exosurf (Glaxo-Wellcome)
   Artificial lung-expanding compound (ALEC)
   KL4 (Surfaxin)
   Recombinant surfactant protein C (Venticute)

Curosurf (Chesi Farmaceutici and Dey Laboratories), Infasurf (ONY, Inc and Forest Laboratories), and Survanta (Abbott/Ross Laboratories) currently are approved by the Food and Drug Administration (FDA) in the United States, and KL4 (Surfaxin, Discovery Laboratories) is under clinical evaluation. Exosurf (Glaxo-Wellcome) also is FDA approved but is no longer used clinically. Details on the composition, activity, and efficacy of these surfactants in treating or preventing RDS in premature infants are detailed elsewhere [46]. This article focuses on their use in ALI/ARDS. See text for details.

Data from Notter RH. Lung surfactants: basic science and clinical applications. New York: Marcel Dekker, Inc; 2000; and Chess P, Finkelstein JN, Holm BA, et al. Surfactant replacement therapy in lung injury. In: Notter RH, Finkelstein JN, Holm BA, editors. Lung injury: mechanisms, pathophysiology, and therapy. Boca Raton (FL): Taylor Francis Group, Inc; 2005. p. 617–63.

in category 3 that have been studied most widely are Exosurf (Glaxo-Wellcome) and artificial lung-expanding compound (ALEC), although neither of these two preparations is in active clinical use because they have been shown to have inferior activity compared with animal-derived surfactants [46,51,113–117]. Two additional synthetic surfactants, KL4 (Surfaxin, Discovery Laboratories) and a recombinant surfactant protein C (SP-C), (Venticute), presently are undergoing clinical evaluation, and new synthetic lipid:peptide exogenous surfactants currently are under development.

Four exogenous surfactant preparations currently are licensed for clinical use in respiratory distress syndrome (RDS) in the United States: Infasurf (ONY, Inc. and Forest Laboratories), Survanta (Abbott/Ross Laboratories), Curosurf (Chesi Farmaceutici and Dey Laboratories), and Exosurf (no longer in use). As reviewed elsewhere [46,118,119], Infasurf is a direct chloroform:methanol extract of large-aggregate surfactant obtained by bronchoalveolar lavage from calf lungs. Survanta is an extract of minced bovine lung tissue to which synthetic dipalmitoyl phosphatidylcholine (DPPC), tripalmitin, and palmitic acid are added. Curosurf is prepared from minced porcine lung tissue by a combination of washing, chloroform-methanol extraction, and liquid-gel chromatography. In addition, KL4 surfactant (Surfaxin), which is under consideration for approval by the Food and Drug Administration, is made up of a 21–amino acid peptide that has repeating units of one leucine (K) and four lysine (L) residues and is combined at 3% by weight with a 3:1 mixture of DPPC and palmitoyl-oleoyl phosphatidylglycerol plus 15% palmitic acid. The synthetic surfactant Venticute, which also has been studied in ARDS, contains synthetic lipids and palmitic acid plus a 34–amino acid modified human recombinant SP-C that has substitutions of phenylalanine for cysteine at two positions and isoleucine for methionine at another [46].

Current studies on surfactant replacement therapy in patients who have acute lung injury/acute respiratory distress syndrome

A significant number of clinical studies have reported benefits following the instillation of exogenous surfactants in term infants, children, or adults who have ALI/ARDS or related acute respiratory failure [25,120–135] (Table 2). Many of these studies, however, are small case series or pilot studies and found improvements only in acute lung function (oxygenation). Controlled trials of surfactant therapy in patients who have ALI/ARDS have met with mixed success, particularly in adults who have sepsis-associated ARDS [136,137]. The clinical experience with exogenous surfactant therapy in term infants, children, and adults is summarized here.

The best-studied application of surfactant therapy in term infants who had acute pulmonary injury is in meconium aspiration syndrome [129–133]. Meconium obstructs and injures the lungs when aspirated and is known to cause surfactant dysfunction [56,138]. Auten and colleagues [129], Khammash and

Table 2
Clinical studies reporting benefits of exogenous surfactant therapy in acute respiratory failure

Study	Patients (N)	Disease or Syndrome	Surfactant	Outcomes
Günther et al [120]	Adults (27)	ARDS	Alveofact	Improved surfactant function
Walmrath et al [155]	Adults (10)	ARDS from sepsis	Alveofact	Improved oxygenation
Spragg et al [122]	Adults (6)	ARDS from multiple causes	Curosurf	Improved oxygenation and biophysical function
Wiswell et al [123]	Adults (12)	ARDS from multiple causes	Surfaxin	Improved oxygenation
Willson et al [124,125]	Children (29 and 42)	ARDS from multiple causes	Infasurf	Improved oxygenation
Willson et al [25]	Children (152)	ARDS from multiple causes	Infasurf	Improved survival, and improved oxygenation
Lopez-Herce et al [126]	Children (20)	ARDS + post-op-cardiac	Curosurf	Improved oxygenation
Hermon et al [127]	Children (19)	ARDS + post-op-cardiac	Curosurf or Alveofact	Improved oxygenation
Herting et al [128]	Children (8)	Pneumonia	Curosurf	Improved oxygenation
Auten et al [129]	Infants (14)	Meconium aspiration or pneumonia	CLSE (Infasurf)	Improved oxygenation
Lotze et al [130,131]	Infants (28 and 328)	ECMO, multiple indications	Survanta	Improved oxygenation, decreased ECMO
Khammash et al [132]	Infants (20)	Meconium aspiration	bLES	Improved oxygenation in 75% of patients
Findlay et al [133]	Infants (40)	Meconium aspiration	Survanta	Improved oxygenation, decreased pneumothorax and mechanical ventilation
Luchetti et al [134,135]	Infants (20 and 40)	RSV bronchiolitis	Curosurf	Improved oxygenation

Tabulated clinical studies include both controlled and noncontrolled trials.
Abbreviations: ALI, acute lung injury; ARDS, acute respiratory distress syndrome; bLES, bovine lavage extract surfactant; CLSE, calf-lung surfactant extract; ECMO, extracorporeal membrane oxygenation; RSV, respiratory syncytial virus.

colleagues [132], and Findlay and colleagues [133] have reported significant improvement from surfactant administration in infants who had meconium aspiration. The randomized, controlled study of Findlay and colleagues [133] found reductions in the incidence of pneumothorax, duration of mechanical ventilation and oxygen therapy, time of hospitalization, and requirements for extracorporeal membrane oxygenation (ECMO) in 20 term infants treated with Survanta compared with controls. Lotze and colleagues [130,131] also reported favorable results using Survanta in a controlled trial in term infants referred for ECMO because of severe respiratory failure (meconium aspiration was a prevalent diagnosis in both studies). Twenty-eight infants treated with four doses of Survanta (150 mg/kg) had improved pulmonary mechanics, decreased duration of ECMO treatment, and a lower incidence of complications after ECMO than control infants [130]. A subsequent multicenter controlled trial in 328 term infants also reported significant improvements in respiratory status and the need for ECMO following surfactant treatment [131]. Surfactant therapy also has been found to be beneficial to lung function or respiratory outcome in several studies in infants who had respiratory syncytial virus (RSV) infection [134,135,139]. Luchetti and colleagues [134] reported that 10 infants who had RSV bronchiolitis treated with tracheally instilled porcine-derived surfactant (Curosurf, 50 mg/kg body weight) had improved gas exchange and a reduced time on mechanical ventilation and in the pediatric ICU compared with an equal number of control infants not treated with exogenous surfactant. A subsequent multicenter controlled trial in 40 patients also found that surfactant therapy with Curosurf improved gas exchange and respiratory mechanics and shortened the duration of mechanical ventilation and hospitalization in infants who had acute respiratory failure from RSV bronchiolitis [135]. Also, Tibby and colleagues [139] have reported that nine infants who had severe RSV bronchiolitis who received two doses of Survanta (100 mg/kg) had a more rapid improvement in oxygenation and ventilation indices in the first 60 hours than 10 control infants receiving air-placebo. Exogenous surfactant therapy now is used in neonatal ICUs at many institutions to treat respiratory failure in term infants who have meconium aspiration or pulmonary viral/bacterial infection. Surfactant therapy also has been studied in infants who have congenital diaphragmatic hernia, but its use remains controversial in this context [140,141].

Studies of surfactant therapy in children and adults who have ALI/ARDS show positive results in a number of case reports or relatively small pilot trials [120,121,124–128]. Controlled clinical trials have been less successful, however, particularly in adults. By far the largest prospective, controlled study of surfactant therapy in adults who had ARDS was definitively negative [136]. Anzueto and colleagues [136] administered nebulized Exosurf or placebo to 725 adults who had ARDS secondary to sepsis and found no improvement in any measure of oxygenation and no effect on morbidity or mortality. The interpretation of these negative results is confounded, however, because both laboratory and clinical studies have documented that Exosurf has low activity compared with animal-derived surfactants [51,113–117,142–145], and aerosolization has not been shown to be as effective as airway instillation in delivering surfactant. Gregory and colleagues [137] reported small benefits in oxygenation in a controlled trial in adults who had ARDS who received four 100-mg/kg doses of Survanta but found no overall advantage in survival in the 43 surfactant-treated patients studied. A more recent study by Spragg and colleagues [26] using recombinant SP-C surfactant (Venticute) in adults who had ARDS showed immediate improvements in oxygenation but no longer-term improvement in duration of mechanical ventilation, lengths of stay, or mortality. Post hoc analysis did suggest, however, that the response in the subgroup of patients who had ARDS caused by "direct lung injury" was positive, and a follow-up prospective study in this group of patients is underway.

Controlled studies of surfactant therapy in children up to age 21 years who have ALI/ARDS have been more encouraging. A randomized but unblinded controlled trial at eight centers by Willson and colleagues [125] in 42 children who had ALI/ARDS showed that those receiving Infasurf (70 mg/kg) had immediate improvement in oxygenation and fewer ventilator days and days in intensive care (Fig. 2). This unblinded trial followed an initial open-label study by the same group demonstrating improved oxygenation in 29 children (0.1–16 years) treated with instilled Infasurf [124]. In addition, a clinical trial by Moller and colleagues [146] reported that children who had ARDS showed an immediate improvement in oxygenation and less need for rescue therapy following treatment with Survanta, although this

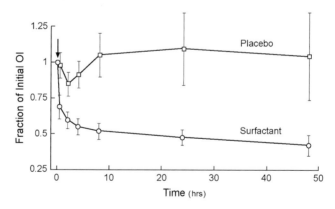

Fig. 2. Improvements in oxygenation index (OI) after instillation of exogenous surfactant in children who have acute lung injury/acute respiratory distress syndrome. Patients ranging in age from 1 day through 18 years in eight pediatric ICUs were assigned randomly to surfactant or control groups. Surfactant-treated patients received a dose of Infasurf of 80 mL/m^2 body surface (70 mg/kg body weight) by tracheal instillation during hand ventilation with 100% oxygen (*arrow*). Control patients received hand ventilation and 100% oxygen alone. Ten of 21 surfactant-treated patients received a second dose 12 or more hours after the first. Significant improvements were found in lung function in patients receiving exogenous surfactant therapy. OI is defined as $100 \times MAP \times FIO_2/PaO_2$, where MAP is the mean airway pressure; FIO_2 is the fraction of inspired oxygen; PaO_2 is the arterial partial pressure of oxygen. (*From* Willson DF, Bauman LA, Zaritsky A, et al. Instillation of calf lung surfactant extract (calfactant) is beneficial in pediatric acute hypoxemic respiratory failure. Crit Care Med 1999;27:188–95.)

latter study was underpowered for more definitive outcomes. Most recently, a large blinded, randomized, controlled study by Willson and colleagues [25] in 152 pediatric patients who had ALI/ARDS (77 surfactant treated and 75 placebo) yielded very positive results, showing both immediate improvements in oxygenation and a significant survival advantage for patients receiving calfactant (Infasurf) relative to placebo (Table 3). Patients aged 1 week through 21 years in this 21-center study were enrolled within 48 hours of endotracheal intubation with radiographic evidence of bilateral lung disease and an oxygenation index greater than 7. Patients who had pre-existing lung, cardiac, or central nervous system disease were excluded. Ventilator-free days and mortality were primary outcomes. Surfactant treatment resulted in decreased oxygenation index, decreased mortality, and a higher percentage of response to conventional mechanical ventilation compared with air-placebo (See Table 3). A post hoc analysis indicated that the great majority of these beneficial effects were confined to patients who had direct injury forms of ALI/ARDS (Table 4).

None of these studies in infants, children, or adults showed any significant adverse long-term effects from surfactant administration, although transient hypoxia and some hemodynamic instability surrounding

Table 3
Clinical outcomes from a recent controlled study using exogenous surfactant (Infasurf; calfactant) in pediatric patients who had acute lung injury/acute respiratory distress syndrome

Outcome	Calfactant (n = 77)	Placebo (n =75)	P value
Mortality (primary outcome)			
Died in hospital	15 (19%)	27 (36%)	0.03
Died w/o extubation	12 (16%)	24 (32%)	0.02
Failed CMV[a]	13 (21%)	26 (42%)	0.02
ECMO	3	3	–
Use of nitric oxide	9	10	0.80
HFOV after entry	7	15	0.07
Secondary outcomes			
Pediatric ICU LOS	15.2 ± 13.3	13.6 ± 11.6	0.85
Hospital LOS	26.8 ± 26	25.3 ± 32.2	0.91
Days O_2 therapy	17.3 ± 16	18.5 ± 31	0.93
Hospital charges[b]	$205 ± 220	$213 ± 226	0.83
Hospital charges/day[b]	$7.5 ± 7.6	$7.9 ± 7.5	0.74

In addition to improving mortality and reducing the percentage of patients that failed CMV as reported in the table, instilled calfactant also significantly improved oxygenation index compared with placebo (P = .01; data not shown).

Abbreviations: CMV, conventional mechanical ventilation; ECMO, extracorporeal membrane oxygenation; HFOV, high-frequency oscillatory ventilation; iNO, inhaled nitric oxide; LOS, length of stay.

[a] Some patients that failed CMV had more than one nonconventional therapy (ECMO, iNO, or HFOV).

[b] Costs are given in thousands of dollars.

Data from Willson DF, Thomas NJ, Markovitz BP, et al. Effect of exogenous surfactant (calfactant) in pediatric acute lung injury: a randomized controlled trial. JAMA 2005;293:470–6.

Table 4
Efficacy of exogenous surfactant (Infasurf, calfactant) in direct and indirect forms of lung injury
in children up to age 21 years who had acute lung injury/acute respiratory distress syndrome

	Placebo	Calfactant	P value
Direct lung injury (n)	48	50	–
Oxygenation index ↓ 25% or more	31%	66%	0.0006
Ventilator days	17 ± 10	13 ± 9	0.05
Died	38%	8%	0.0005
Indirect lung injury (n)	27	27	–
Oxygenation index ↓ 25% or more	41%	37%	0.79
Ventilator days	17 ± 10	18 ± 10	0.75
Died	33%	41%	0.65

Percentages of patients who had a decrease in oxygenation index greater than 25%, days on
mechanical ventilation, and percentage mortality were calculated in a post hoc analysis. The efficacy of exogenous surfactant was confined to patients who had direct pulmonary forms of
ALI/ARDS.

Data from Willson DF, Thomas NJ, Markovitz BP, et al. Effect of exogenous surfactant (calfactant) in pediatric acute lung injury: a randomized controlled trial. JAMA 2005;293:470–6.

intratracheal or bronchoscopic instillation are common. Transmission of infectious agents or allergic reactions also has not been reported with any of
the exogenous surfactants currently licensed in the United States.

Considerations affecting the efficacy of exogenous surfactant therapy in acute lung injury/acute respiratory distress syndrome

Several factors increase the difficulty of developing effective surfactant
therapy for ALI/ARDS. As emphasized earlier, patients who have ALI/
ARDS share aspects of lung injury pathophysiology, but these diagnoses
are clinical syndromes that comprise a diverse set of etiologies. The occurrence of ALI/ARDS in a heterogeneous population of patients who have
varying degrees of lung injury and systemic disease significantly reduces
the resolving power of clinical trials of surfactant therapy. In addition,
edema and inflammation in patients who have acute pulmonary injury
make it more difficult to deliver and distribute exogenous surfactant to
the alveoli. Finally, meaningful evaluations of surfactant therapy in ALI/
ARDS must account for differences in surfactant drug activity that can
impact therapeutic efficacy significantly. Specific considerations for surfactant therapy in ALI/ARDS are discussed here.

Delivery methods and dosages for exogenous surfactant therapy in patients with lung injury

The primary method used to deliver exogenous surfactants to children
and adults who have ALI/ARDS is based on that shown to be most effective
in premature infants who have RDS, that is, direct intratracheal instillation

through an endotracheal tube or airway instillation through a bronchoscope. Surface-active material instilled into the airways has the capacity to spread rapidly and distribute to the periphery of the lung [147–149]. Spreading from the central airways toward the alveoli is promoted by surface tension gradients that drive transport from regions of high surfactant concentration to regions of lower surfactant concentration. A typical dose of intratracheal surfactant in premature infants is 100 mg/kg body weight. This dose represents a significant excess over the amount of surfactant phospholipid needed to cover the surface of the alveolar network with a tightly packed surfactant film (only about 3 mg/kg of surfactant phospholipid at a molecular weight of 750 d are needed to form a monomolecular film at a limiting area of 40 $\mathring{A}^2$ molecules over an alveolar surface of 1 m^2/kg body weight [46,150]). Excess instilled exogenous surfactant that reaches the alveoli provides a reservoir of material for the hypophase and interface and is available for incorporation into endogenous surfactant pools via recycling pathways.

Although instillation is an effective method of delivering exogenous surfactants, total dosages required in older children and adults who have ALI/ARDS are not trivial. To achieve a dose comparable to that used in premature infants based on body weight or body surface area, much larger total drug amounts and volumes are required. The prototypical 70-kg adult requires 7 g of exogenous surfactant at a dosage level of 100 mg/kg body weight. This dosage necessitates an instilled volume of 87.5 to 280 mL at the phospholipid concentrations of current clinical surfactant drugs in saline (25–80 mg/mL). It obviously is important to minimize instilled surfactant volumes in patients who have severe respiratory failure. At the same time, the instilled surfactant volume impacts the intrapulmonary drug distribution, which already is compromised by edema and inflammation. Studies in animal models of ALI/ARDS have indicated that the distribution of exogenous surfactant can be improved by instilling larger fluid volumes or by using associated bronchoalveolar lavage [151–154], but the feasibility and/or utility of these approaches in clinical practice is uncertain. Clinical studies on intratracheal or bronchoscopic instillation of exogenous surfactants in patients who have ALI/ARDS have used a range of instilled volumes, with doses as high as 300 mg/kg [155] and as low as 25 mg/kg [26].

An alternative to administering exogenous surfactant drugs by instillation is to deliver them in aerosol form. In theory, aerosolization could reduce the required surfactant doses significantly, because delivery can be targeted to the alveoli by controlling particle size. Phospholipid aerosols with stable particle sizes appropriate for alveolar deposition in normal lungs can be formed by ultrasonic or jet nebulization [150,156,157], and exogenous surfactants have been aerosolized to animals and patients who have surfactant deficiency or dysfunction [91,105,110,136,158–160]. The theoretic potential of aerosols to improve alveolar deposition and to reduce required surfactant doses has not been replicated in practice, however. Aerosol methodology to date has not been shown to deliver exogenous surfactants to the alveoli as effectively as instillation, although this performance may improve in the future as technology advances.

Another approach to facilitate the delivery and distribution of exogenous surfactants in injured lungs involves the use of specific modes and strategies of mechanical ventilation. For example, studies indicate that the distribution and/or efficacy of instilled exogenous surfactant can be improved by jet ventilation [161,162] and partial liquid ventilation [163–165]. Additional mechanism-based research on the impact of specific ventilation methods and strategies on the delivery, distribution, and efficacy of exogenous surfactants may be important for optimizing this therapy in ALI/ARDS. The delivery and distribution of surfactant drugs in injured lungs also potentially could be improved by the use of low-viscosity formulations to reduce transport resistance after tracheal or bronchoscopic instillation. Whole surfactant and animal-derived exogenous surfactants have complex non-Newtonian, concentration-dependent viscosities that vary significantly among preparations [166,167]. For a given surfactant preparation at fixed shear rate, viscosity can be reduced significantly by altering the physical formulation through changes in dispersion methodology, ionic environment, or temperature [166,167].

Activity and inhibition resistance of exogenous surfactant drugs

One of the most important considerations in the clinical efficacy of surfactant therapy is the relative activity of different exogenous surfactant drugs. Differences in efficacy between clinical exogenous surfactants have been demonstrated in a number of comparison trials in premature infants [114–117,142–145,168,169]. Results of these clinical comparisons indicate that surfactants derived from animal lungs (categories 1 and 2 in Box 2) have significantly greater efficacy than the protein-free synthetic surfactants Exosurf and ALEC. Retrospective meta-analyses combining clinical data from multiple surfactant trials have reached the same conclusion [170–174]. As noted earlier, the largest study of surfactant therapy in adults who had ALI/ARDS used the protein-free synthetic surfactant Exosurf and found no therapeutic benefit [136]. The hydrophobic surfactant proteins are highly active in endogenous surfactant, and finding effective substitutes for them in protein-free synthetic surfactants is extremely difficult. The addition of mixed bovine SP-B/SP-C to Exosurf greatly improves its surface activity and its efficacy in reversing surfactant-deficient pressure–volume mechanics in excised rat lungs [113], documenting that the biochemical components of this surfactant are not adequate substitutes for the hydrophobic apoproteins in activity.

Animal-derived clinical exogenous surfactants themselves also differ substantially in their surface activity and ability to resist inhibitor-induced dysfunction. The consensus of available biophysical and animal research indicates that exogenous surfactants based on extracts of lavaged large-aggregate endogenous surfactant in category 1 of Box 2 have the great-est overall surface and physiologic activity. These drugs have close composi-tional analogy to the mix of phospholipids and hydrophobic proteins in active alveolar surfactant. The surface tension–lowering ability of several clinical surfactants during dynamic cycling on a pulsating bubble apparatus (37°C, 20 cycles/minute, 50% area compression) is illustrated in Fig. 3 [51]. Suspensions of calf-lung surfactant extract (CLSE) (Infasurf) and Alveofact were found to reach the lowest minimum surface tensions at the lowest surfactant concentrations among the preparations studied. Category 1 exog-enous surfactants such as CLSE and Alveofact also resist inhibition by blood proteins more effectively than exogenous surfactants like Survanta and Cur-osurf that are processed from lung tissue (Fig. 4) [51,113].

The differences in biophysical activity found between surfactants in gen-eral reflect differences in their functional biochemical compositions. For example, the differences in activity between CLSE and Survanta seen in Figs. 3 and 4 relate primarily to differences in the content of SP-B in the two preparations [106,118,175]. Survanta has an SP-B content by ELISA of only 0.044% by weight relative to phospholipid, whereas CLSE (Infa-surf) has an SP-B content of 0.9% by weight, approaching that of lavaged whole surfactant [118]. SP-B is known to be the most active of the hydro-phobic surfactant proteins in enhancing the adsorption, dynamic surface ac-tivity, and inhibition resistance of phospholipids [118,176–184]. The addition of bovine SP-B or synthetic SP-B peptides to Survanta significantly

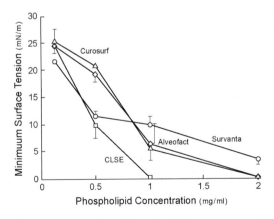

Fig. 3. Overall surface tension–lowering ability of clinical exogenous surfactants. Minimum surface tension after 5 minutes of pulsation in a bubble surfactometer (37°C, 20 cycles/minute, 50% area compression) is plotted as a function of surfactant phospholipid concentration for several clinical surfactants. The surfactants shown vary widely in overall surface tension–lowering ability, with the most active being category 1 surfactants from Box 2 (eg, Infasurf and Alveofact). (*Data from* Mizuno K, Ikegami M, Chen C-M, et al. Surfactant protein-B supplementation improves in vivo function of a modified natural surfactatnt. Pediatr Res 1995;37;271–6.)

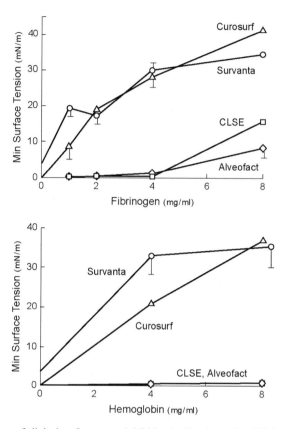

Fig. 4. Resistance of clinical surfactants to inhibition by blood proteins. Minimum surface tension after 5 minutes of pulsation in a bubble surfactometer (37°C, 20 cycles/minute, and 50% area compression) is plotted against the concentration of inhibitory blood proteins (fibrinogen and hemoglobin). The results indicate that animal-derived exogenous surfactants that closely mimic natural surfactant by being extracted from lung lavage (see category 1 surfactants from Box 2) have an improved ability to resist inhibition by plasma proteins compared with the other preparations shown. Surfactant phospholipid concentration was 2 mg/mL. (*Data from* Seeger W, Grube C, Gunther A, et al. Surfactant inhibition by plasma proteins: differential sensitivity of various surfactant preparations. Eur Respir J 1993;6:971–7.)

improves its surface and physiologic activity so that they approach that of Infasurf and whole surfactant (Fig. 5) [106,118,175]. Despite its lack of SP-B, other active components such as SP-C in Survanta allow it to have significant efficacy in some forms of ALI/ARDS, as noted earlier [130,131,133]. Treatment with Survanta has not been found to give substantial improvements in adult patients with ARDS [137], but category 1 exogenous surfactants with the complete mix of surfactant lipids and near-endogenous amounts of both SP-B and SP-C may prove to have increased efficacy.

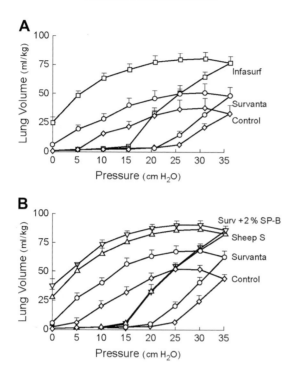

Fig. 5. Effects on physiologic activity from the addition of purified SP-B to Survanta. (*A*) Premature rabbit fetuses (27 days' gestation) treated with Survanta or Infasurf and untreated controls. (*B*) Premature rabbit fetuses treated with Survanta, Survanta plus SP-B (2% by weight by ELISA), natural surfactant from adult sheep (Sheep S), or untreated controls. Infasurf improved lung mechanics more than Survanta (*A*), and the importance of SP-B in this behavior is shown by the increased activity of Survanta plus SP-B compared with Survanta alone (*B*). Surfactants were instilled intratracheally at a dose of 100 mg/kg body weight, and quasistatic pressure–volume curves were measured following 15 minutes of mechanical ventilation. (*Data from* Mizuno K, Ikegami M, Chen C-M, et al. Surfactant protein-B supplementation improves in vivo function of a modified natural surfactant. Pediatr Res 1995;37:271–6.)

Differences in the activity of exogenous surfactants, such as shown in Figs. 3–5, generally are larger in magnitude than differences found in clinical comparison trials of surfactant drugs [114–117,142–145,168,169], because basic science studies are able to discriminate phenomena under controlled conditions and with more mechanistic detail than possible in clinical trials. Outcomes of patients (whether they are premature infants or adults who have severe acute respiratory failure) in clinical surfactant trials are influenced by multiple variables unrelated to lung surfactant activity. Patient outcomes in surfactant trials also can be affected by secondary phenomena involving drug incorporation into type II cell recycling pathways or combination with small amounts of native surfactant apoproteins in the alveoli [46]. Even placebo-controlled studies of surfactant therapy in premature infants typically required substantial numbers of patients to demonstrate improvements in survival and other long-term outcomes (as opposed to acute lung functional improvements) [46]. Mechanism-based differences in activity between exogenous surfactants in correlated biochemical, biophysical, and animal research thus are highly important in assessing and evaluating clinical findings.

Examples of research on new synthetic exogenous surfactants for acute lung injury/acute respiratory distress syndrome

In addition to investigating the activity and delivery of clinical exogenous surfactants, researchers are attempting to develop new synthetic or semisynthetic surfactants for treating lung injury ([46,47,185–188] for review). Synthetic lung surfactants manufactured under controlled conditions in the laboratory have significant potential advantages in purity, reproducibility, and quality control compared with animal-derived preparations. As biologic products, animal surfactants have significant batch-to-batch variability that increases the cost and complexity of quality control testing during manufacture. Laboratory-synthesized drugs have the potential to be significantly less expensive over time once the costs of development are recovered, and they can be produced in unlimited amounts. Synthetic surfactants also are free from concerns about animal pathogens such as prions, and they are not subject to cultural or religious issues that can affect the use of bovine- or porcine-derived preparations in some countries. Considerations relating to drug dosage described in the preceding section illustrate the practical importance of synthetic preparations in treating ALI/ARDS, where amounts 50 to 100 times larger than those used in premature infants are required in adults and older children to achieve an equivalent dose on a body weight basis. A larger total number of surfactant doses per patient also may be necessary in patients who have ALI/ARDS, further increasing the total amount of surfactant required. The cost of multiple doses of exogenous surfactant per adult patient would be prohibitive at a level even closely proportional to the expense of 100- to 200-mg vials of animal-derived surfactants currently used in infants. In theory, the production of synthetic surfactants could be scaled up to large amounts with substantially reduced expense to allow more cost-effective therapy for ALI/ARDS.

Two important conceptual approaches being followed to develop synthetic exogenous surfactants are (1) combining human-sequence recombinant proteins or synthetic amphipathic peptides with synthetic biological glycerophospholipids; and (2) combining synthetic amphipathic peptides with novel synthetic lipids designed to have favorable physicochemical properties such as high surface activity and structural resistance to inflammatory phospholipases during lung injury. KL4 (Surfaxin) [87,107,123,189–195] and recombinant SP-C surfactant (Venticute) [26,196–201] are two current examples of the first of these approaches (see Box 2). The 21-amino acid

KL4 peptide is only a very rough structural analogue to native SP-B, however, and advances in peptide molecular modeling and synthesis technology support the feasibility of preparing new SP-B peptides with significantly greater sequence and molecular-folding specificity and correspondingly higher activity ([202–204] for review). The development of new synthetic SP-B peptides is particularly important for optimal synthetic exogenous surfactants, given the greater activity of SP-B compared with SP-C in native surfactant [118,176–184]. In addition to the peptide/protein components in new synthetic surfactants, it is important to consider their lipid constituents. On a weight or molar basis, lipids are the major components of both endogenous and exogenous lung surfactants. Ester-linked glycerophospholipids of the kind found in native surfactant are the primary lipids used in current synthetic exogenous surfactants. Synthetic ether-linked lipids are now available that have direct structural analogy to lung surfactant lipids plus designed molecular behavior that enhances adsorption and spreading while maintaining very high, dynamic surface tension lowering in surface films [71,205–211]. Moreover, such lipids have structural features that make them resistant to phospholipases such as phospholipase A_2, which has been implicated in the pathology of ALI/ARDS [65,212–218]. Phospholipase-induced degradation of lung surfactant glycerophospholipids reduces the concentration of active components and also generates reaction products such as lysophosphatidylcholine and fluid free fatty acids that can decrease surface activity further by interacting biophysically with remaining surfactant at the alveolar interface [55,59,70]. Synthetic exogenous surfactants containing such phosphonolipids combined with purified surfactant proteins or synthetic peptides have very high overall surface activity plus an ability to resist phospholipases in ALI/ARDS [71,208–211,219]. Ongoing basic research is continuing to design and synthesize peptides related to SP-B and other surfactant proteins for use in highly active, fully synthetic exogenous surfactants in combination with either normal glycerophospholipids or phospholipase-resistant analogues.

Summary and future prospects for surfactant therapy in acute lung injury/acute respiratory distress syndrome

Exogenous surfactant therapy now is standard in the prevention and treatment of RDS in premature infants, and basic science and clinical evidence support its use in at least some patients who have lung injury–associated respiratory failure as described in this article. The efficacy of surfactant therapy in term infants who have meconium aspiration is sufficiently documented that this intervention is now standard in many neonatal ICUs. Surfactant therapy also is used frequently in neonatal patients who have ALI/ARDS (or related acute respiratory failure) from respiratory infections or pneumonia. Controlled trials of surfactant therapy in children who have ALI/ARDS have shown significant benefits, with significant survival advantages in direct pulmonary lung injuries as reported in the recent trial of Willson and colleagues [25]. The relative enthusiasm of pediatric intensive care specialists for surfactant therapy in respiratory failure probably reflects to some extent the fact that this intervention originally was defined for neonatal applications. The striking success of surfactant therapy in treating and preventing RDS in premature neonates and the large body of accompanying basic research on the composition and activity of exogenous surfactants thus have been particularly apparent to pediatric subspecialists.

Current clinical evidence supporting the use of surfactant in adults who have ALI/ARDS is less extensive and compelling than in infants and children. The surfactants that to date have been most widely studied in adults who have ARDS (Exosurf and Survanta) are known to have limitations in composition and activity compared with several other available preparations. Also, adult studies have not focused on direct pulmonary forms of ALI/ARDS, in which surfactant therapy is most likely to be effective as a targeted intervention. In addition, neonatal data suggest that early surfactant administration generates improved responses compared with delayed administration [220], possibly as a result of better intrapulmonary drug distribution coupled with minimized ventilator-induced lung injury. It would make sense intuitively that similar advantages might accompany early surfactant administration in patients who have ALI/ARDS. It is challenging and expensive to examine surfactant therapy in placebo-controlled clinical trials of substantial size in adults who have ALI/ARDS, but further studies of direct pulmonary forms of these conditions treated with the most active available exogenous surfactant preparations clearly are warranted, based both on pathophysiologic understanding and on extensive biophysical and animal research.

Finally, a major issue regarding surfactant therapy in ALI/ARDS involves its potential use in combination with agents or interventions that target additional aspects of the complex pathophysiology of acute pulmonary injury. Such a combination therapy approach may be particularly important in adults who have ALI/ARDS, in whom responses to exogenous surfactant so far have been disappointing. The use of multiple therapeutic agents or interventions based on specific rationales for potential synergy might enhance patient outcomes significantly in complex disease processes involving inflammatory lung injury. The potential use of exogenous surfactant therapy in the context of specific combined-modality interventions is described in detail elsewhere [119,221,222]. Examples of agents that might be synergistic with exogenous surfactant in ALI/ARDS include anti-inflammatory drugs such as steroids or receptor antagonists, antioxidants, and vasoactive drugs such as inhaled nitric oxide. In addition, it may be equally important to consider specific ventilator modalities or ventilation strategies that reduce iatrogenic lung injury in conjunction with surfactant therapy. Given the known importance of surfactant dysfunction in inflammatory lung injury, it is likely that surfactant therapy alone or in combination with other agents will be applicable for adult as well as pediatric patients who have ALI/ARDS associated with direct pulmonary injury.

References

[1] Bernard GR, Artigas A, Brigham KL, et al. The American-European Consensus Conference on ARDS: definitions, mechanisms, relevant outcomes, and clinical trial coordination. Am J Respir Crit Care Med 1994;149:818–24.

[2] Murray JF, Matthay MA, Luce JM, et al. An expanded definition of the adult respiratory distress syndrome. Am Rev Respir Dis 1988;138:720–3.

[3] American College of Chest Physicians Society of Critical Care Medicine Consensus Conference Committee. Definitions for sepsis and organ failure and guidelines for the use of innovative therapies for sepsis. Crit Care Med 1992;20:864–74.

[4] Pollack MM, Patel KM, Ruttimann UE. PRISM III: an updated pediatric risk of mortality score. Crit Care Med 1996;24:743–52.

[5] Slater A, Shann F, ANZICS Paediatric Study Group. The suitability of the Pediatric Index of Mortality (PIM), PIM2, the Pediatric Risk of Mortality (PRISM), and PRISM III for monitoring the quality of pediatric intensive care in Australia and New Zealand. Pediatr Crit Care Med 2004;5:447–54.

[6] Shann F, Pearson G, Slater A, et al. Paediatric Index of Mortality (PIM): a mortality prediction model for children in intensive care. Intensive Care Med 1997;23:201–7.

[7] Trachsel D, McCrindle BW, Nakagawa S, et al. Oxygenation index predicts outcome in children with acute hypoxemic respiratory failure. Am J Respir Crit Care Med 2005;172: 206–11.

[8] Hudson LD, Milberg JA, Anardi D, et al. Clinical risks for development of the acute respiratory distress syndrome. Am J Respir Crit Care Med 1995;151:293–301.

[9] Krafft P, Fridrich P, Pernerstorfer T, et al. The acute respiratory distress syndrome; definitions, severity, and clinical outcome. An analysis of 101 clinical investigations. Intensive Care Med 1996;22:519–29.

[10] Doyle RL, Szaflarski N, Modin GW, et al. Identification of patients with acute lung injury: predictors of mortality. Am J Respir Crit Care Med 1995;152:1818–24.

[11] Ware LB, Matthay MA. The acute respiratory distress syndrome. N Engl J Med 2000;342: 1334–48.

[12] Rubenfeld GD. Epidemiology of acute lung injury. Crit Care Med 2003;31(Suppl): S276–84.

[13] Rubenfeld GD, Caldwell E, Peabody E, et al. Incidence and outcomes of acute lung injury. N Engl J Med 2005;353:1685–93.

[14] Goss CH, Brower RG, Hudson LD, et al. Incidence of acute lung injury in the United States. Crit Care Med 2003;31:1607–11.

[15] Pfenninger J, Gerber A, Tschappeler H, et al. Adult respiratory distress syndrome in children. J Pediatr 1982;101:352–7.

[16] Bindl L, Dresbach K, Lentze M. Incidence of acute respiratory distress syndrome in German children and adolescents: a population based study. Crit Care Med 2005;33:209–12.

[17] Manzano F, Yuste E, Colmenero M, et al. Incidence of acute respiratory distress syndrome and its relation to age. J Crit Care 2005;20:274–80.

[18] Randolph AG, Wypij D, Venkataraman ST, et al. Effect of mechanical ventilator weaning protocols on respiratory outcomes in infants and children. A randomized controlled trial. JAMA 2002;288:2561–8.

[19] Flori HR, Glidden DV, Rutherford GW, et al. Pediatric acute lung injury. Prospective evaluation of risk factors associated with mortality. Am J Respir Crit Care Med 2005; 171:995–1001.

[20] The Paediatric Study Group of the Australian and New Zealand Intensive Care Society (ANZICS). Acute lung injury in pediatric intensive care in Australia and New Zealand: a prospective, multicentre, observational study. Pediatr Crit Care Med 2007;8:317–23.

[21] DeBruin W, Notterman DA, Magid M, et al. Acute hypoxemic respiratory failure in infants and children: clinical and pathologic characteristics. Crit Care Med 1992;20:1223–34.

[22] Timmons OD, Havens PL, Fackler JC. Pediatric Critical Care Study Group and the Extracorporeal Life Support Organization. Predicting death in pediatric patients with acute respiratory failure. Chest 1995;108:789–97.

[23] Dahlem P, van Aalderen WMC, Hamaker ME, et al. Incidence and short-term outcome of acute lung injury in mechanically ventilated children. Eur Respir J 2003;22:980–3.

[24] Curley MAQ, Hibberd PL, Fineman LD, et al. Effect of prone positioning on clinical outcomes in children with acute lung injury. A randomized controlled trial. JAMA 2005; 294:229–37.

[25] Willson DF, Thomas NJ, Markovitz BP, et al. Effect of exogenous surfactant (calfactant) in pediatric acute lung injury: a randomized controlled trial. JAMA 2005;293:470–6.

[26] Spragg RG, Lewis JF, Wurst W, et al. Treatment of acute respiratory distress syndrome with recombinant surfactant protein C surfactant. Am J Respir Crit Care Med 2003;167:1562–6.

[27] Wang Z, Holm BA, Matalon S, et al. Surfactant activity and dysfunction in lung injury. In: Notter RH, Finkelstein JN, Holm BA, editors. Lung injury: mechanisms, pathophysiology, and therapy. Boca Raton (FL): Taylor Francis Group, Inc; 2005. p. 297–352.

[28] Russo TA, Bartholomew LA, Davidson BA, et al. Total extracellular surfactant is increased but abnormal in a rat model of gram-negative bacterial pneumonitis. Am J Physiol 2002;283:L655–63.

[29] Russo TA, Wang Z, Davidson BA, et al. Surfactant dysfunction and lung injury due to the E. coli virulence factor hemolysin in a rat pneumonia model. Am J Physiol Lung Cell Mol Physiol 2007;292:L632–43.

[30] Davidson BA, Knight PR, Wang Z, et al. Surfactant alterations in acute inflammatory lung injury from aspiration of acid and gastric particulates. Am J Physiol Lung Cell Mol Physiol 2005;288:L699–708.

[31] Wright TW, Notter RH, Wang Z, et al. Pulmonary inflammation disrupts surfactant function during P. carinii pneumonia. Infect Immun 2001;69:758–64.

[32] Bruckner L, Gigliotti F, Wright TW, et al. Pneumocystis carinii infection sensitizes the lung to radiation-induced injury after syngeneic marrow transplantation: role of CD4+ T-cells. Am J Physiol Lung Cell Mol Physiol 2006;290:L1087–96.

[33] Petty T, Reiss O, Paul G, et al. Characteristics of pulmonary surfactant in adult respiratory distress syndrome associated with trauma and shock. Am Rev Respir Dis 1977;115:531–6.

[34] Hallman M, Spragg R, Harrell JH, et al. Evidence of lung surfactant abnormality in respiratory failure. J Clin Invest 1982;70:673–83.

[35] Seeger W, Pison U, Buchhorn R, et al. Surfactant abnormalities and adult respiratory failure. Lung 1990;168(Suppl):891–902.

[36] Pison U, Seeger W, Buchhorn R, et al. Surfactant abnormalities in patients with respiratory failure after multiple trauma. Am Rev Respir Dis 1989;140:1033–9.

[37] Gregory TJ, Longmore WJ, Moxley MA, et al. Surfactant chemical composition and biophysical activity in acute respiratory distress syndrome. J Clin Invest 1991;88:1976–81.

[38] Günther A, Siebert C, Schmidt R, et al. Surfactant alterations in severe pneumonia, acute respiratory distress syndrome, and cardiogenic lung edema. Am J Respir Crit Care Med 1996;153:176–84.

[39] Veldhuizen RAW, McCaig LA, Akino T, et al. Pulmonary surfactant subfractions in patients with the acute respiratory distress syndrome. Am J Respir Crit Care Med 1995; 152:1867–71.

[40] Griese M. Pulmonary surfactant in health and human lung diseases: state of the art. Eur Respir J 1999;13:1455–76.

[41] Mander A, Langton-Hewer S, Bernhard W, et al. Altered phospholipid composition and aggregate structure of lung surfactant is associated with impaired lung function in young children with respiratory infections. Am J Respir Cell Mol Biol 2002;27:714–21.

[42] Schmidt R, Meier U, Markart P, et al. Altered fatty acid composition of lung surfactant phospholipids in interstitial lung disease. Am J Physiol 2002;283:L1079–85.

[43] Skelton R, Holland P, Darowski M, et al. Abnormal surfactant composition and activity in severe bronchiolitis. Acta Paediatr 1999;88:942–6.

[44] LeVine AM, Lotze A, Stanley S, et al. Surfactant content in children with inflammatory lung disease. Crit Care Med 1996;24:1062–7.

[45] Dargaville PA, South M, McDougall PN. Surfactant abnormalities in infants with severe viral bronchiolitis. Arch Dis Child 1996;75:133–6.

[46] Notter RH. Lung surfactants: basic science and clinical applications. New York: Marcel Dekker, Inc; 2000.

[47] Notter RH, Wang Z. Pulmonary surfactant: physical chemistry, physiology and replacement. Rev Chem Eng 1997;13:1–118.

[48] Holm BA, Notter RH, Finkelstein JH. Surface property changes from interactions of albumin with natural lung surfactant and extracted lung lipids. Chem Phys Lipids 1985; 38:287–98.

[49] Seeger W, Stohr G, Wolf HRD, et al. Alteration of surfactant function due to protein leakage: special interaction with fibrin monomer. J Appl Physiol 1985;58:326–38.

[50] Holm BA, Notter RH. Effects of hemoglobin and cell membrane lipids on pulmonary surfactant activity. J Appl Physiol 1987;63:1434–42.

[51] Seeger W, Grube C, Günther A, et al. Surfactant inhibition by plasma proteins: differential sensitivity of various surfactant preparations. Eur Respir J 1993;6:971–7.

[52] Holm BA, Enhorning G, Notter RH. A biophysical mechanism by which plasma proteins inhibit lung surfactant activity. Chem Phys Lipids 1988;49:49–55.

[53] Fuchimukai T, Fujiwara T, Takahashi A, et al. Artificial pulmonary surfactant inhibited by proteins. J Appl Physiol 1987;62:429–37.

[54] Keough KWM, Parsons CS, Tweeddale MG. Interactions between plasma proteins and pulmonary surfactant: pulsating bubble studies. Can J Physiol Pharmacol 1989;67:663–8.

[55] Wang Z, Notter RH. Additivity of protein and non-protein inhibitors of lung surfactant activity. Am J Respir Crit Care Med 1998;158:28–35.

[56] Moses D, Holm BA, Spitale P, et al. Inhibition of pulmonary surfactant function by meconium. Am J Obstet Gynecol 1991;164:477–81.

[57] Cockshutt A, Possmayer F. Lysophosphatidylcholine sensitizes lipid extracts of pulmonary surfactant to inhibition by plasma proteins. Biochim Biophys Acta 1991;1086:63–71.

[58] Seeger W, Lepper H, Hellmut RD, et al. Alteration of alveolar surfactant function after exposure to oxidant stress and to oxygenated and native arachidonic acid in vitro. Biochim Biophys Acta 1985;835:58–67.

[59] Hall SB, Lu ZR, Venkitaraman AR, et al. Inhibition of pulmonary surfactant by oleic acid: mechanisms and characteristics. J Appl Physiol 1992;72:1708–16.

[60] Hall SB, Hyde RW, Notter RH. Changes in subphase surfactant aggregates in rabbits injured by free fatty acid. Am J Respir Crit Care Med 1994;149:1099–106.

[61] Hickman-Davis JM, Fang FC, Nathan C, et al. Lung surfactant and reactive oxygen-nitrogen species: antimicrobial activity and host-pathogen interactions. Am J Physiol 2001;281:L517–23.

[62] Haddad IY, Ischiropoulos H, Holm BA, et al. Mechanisms of peroxynitrite-induced injury to pulmonary surfactants. Am J Physiol 1993;265:L555–64.

[63] Amirkhanian JD, Merritt TA. Inhibitory effects of oxyradicals on surfactant function: utilizing in vitro Fenton reaction. Lung 1998;176:63–72.

[64] Pison U, Tam EK, Caughey GH, et al. Proteolytic inactivation of dog lung surfactant-associated proteins by neutrophil elastase. Biochim Biophys Acta 1989;992:251–7.

[65] Holm BA, Kelcher L, Liu M, et al. Inhibition of pulmonary surfactant by phospholipases. J Appl Physiol 1991;71:317–21.

[66] Enhorning G, Shumel B, Keicher L, et al. Phospholipases introduced into the hypophase affect the surfactant film outlining a bubble. J Appl Physiol 1992;73:941–5.

[67] Lewis JF, Jobe AH. Surfactant and the adult respiratory distress syndrome. Am Rev Respir Dis 1993;147:218–33.

[68] Seeger W, Günther A, Walmrath HD, et al. Alveolar surfactant and adult respiratory distress syndrome. Pathogenic role and therapeutic prospects. Clin Invest 1993;71: 177–90.

[69] Lachmann B, van Daal G-J. Adult respiratory distress syndrome: animal models. In: Robertson B, van Golde LMG, Batenburg JJ, editors. Pulmonary surfactant: from molecular biology to clinical practice. Amsterdam: Elsevier Science Publishers; 1992. p. 635–63.

[70] Holm BA, Wang Z, Notter RH. Multiple mechanisms of lung surfactant inhibition. Pediatr Res 1999;46:85–93.

[71] Wang Z, Schwan AL, Lairson LL, et al. Surface activity of a synthetic lung surfactant containing a phospholipase-resistant phosphonolipid analog of dipalmitoyl phosphatidylcholine. Am J Physiol 2003;285:L550–9.

[72] Magoon MW, Wright JR, Baritussio A, et al. Subfractionation of lung surfactant: implications for metabolism and surface activity. Biochim Biophys Acta 1983;750:18–31.

[73] Wright JR, Benson BJ, Williams MC, et al. Protein composition of rabbit alveolar surfactant subfractions. Biochim Biophys Acta 1984;791:320–32.

[74] Gross NJ, Narine KR. Surfactant subtypes in mice: characterization and quantitation. J Appl Physiol 1989;66:342–9.

[75] Putz G, Goerke J, Clements JA. Surface activity of rabbit pulmonary surfactant subfractions at different concentrations in a captive bubble. J Appl Physiol 1994;77:597–605.

[76] Putman E, Creuwels LAJM, Van Golde LMG, et al. Surface properties, morphology and protein composition of pulmonary surfactant subtypes. Biochem J 1996;320:599–605.

[77] Veldhuizen RAW, Hearn SA, Lewis JF, et al. Surface-area cycling of different surfactant preparations: SP-A and SP-B are essential for large aggregate integrity. Biochem J 1994; 300:519–24.

[78] Gross NJ. Extracellular metabolism of pulmonary surfactant: the role of a new serine protease. Annu Rev Physiol 1995;57:135–50.

[79] Lewis JF, Ikegami M, Jobe AH. Altered surfactant function and metabolism in rabbits with acute lung injury. J Appl Physiol 1990;69:2303–10.

[80] Putman E, Boere AJ, van Bree L, et al. Pulmonary surfactant subtype metabolism is altered after short-term ozone exposure. Toxicol Appl Pharmacol 1995;134:132–8.

[81] Atochina EN, Beers MF, Scanlon ST, et al. P. carinii induces selective alterations in component expression and biophysical activity of lung surfactant. Am J Physiol 2000; 278:L599–609.

[82] Kobayashi T, Ganzuka M, Taniguchi J, et al. Lung lavage and surfactant replacement for hydrochloric acid aspiration in rabbits. Acta Anaesthesiol Scand 1990;34:216–21.

[83] Zucker A, Holm BA, Wood LDH, et al. Exogenous surfactant with PEEP reduces pulmonary edema and improves lung function in canine aspiration pneumonitis. J Appl Physiol 1992;73:679–86.

[84] Schlag G, Strohmaier W. Experimental aspiration trauma: comparison of steroid treatment versus exogenous natural surfactant. Exp Lung Res 1993;19:397–405.

[85] Al-Mateen KB, Dailey K, Grimes MM, et al. Improved oxygenation with exogenous surfactant administration in experimental meconium aspiration syndrome. Pediatr Pulmonol 1994;17:75–80.

[86] Sun B, Curstedt T, Robertson B. Exogenous surfactant improves ventilation efficiency and alveolar expansion in rats with meconium aspiration. Am J Respir Crit Care Med 1996;154: 764–70.

[87] Cochrane CG, Revak SD, Merritt TA, et al. Bronchoalveolar lavage with KL4-surfactant in models of meconium aspiration syndrome. Pediatr Res 1998;44:705–15.

[88] Sun B, Curstedt T, Song GW, et al. Surfactant improves lung function and morphology in newborn rabbits with meconium aspiration. Biol Neonate 1993;63:96–104.

[89] Lachmann B, Hallman M, Bergman K-C. Respiratory failure following anti-lung serum: study on mechanisms associated with surfactant system damage. Exp Lung Res 1987;12: 163–80.

[90] Nieman G, Gatto L, Paskanik A, et al. Surfactant replacement in the treatment of sepsis-induced adult respiratory distress syndrome in pigs. Crit Care Med 1996;24: 1025–33.

[91] Lutz C, Carney D, Finck C, et al. Aerosolized surfactant improves pulmonary function in endotoxin-induced lung injury. Am J Respir Crit Care Med 1998;158:840–5.

[92] Lutz CJ, Picone A, Gatto LA, et al. Exogenous surfactant and positive end-expiratory pressure in the treatment of endotoxin-induced lung injury. Crit Care Med 1998;26: 1379–89.

[93] Tashiro K, Li W-Z, Yamada K, et al. Surfactant replacement reverses respiratory failure induced by intratracheal endotoxin in rats. Crit Care Med 1995;23:149–56.

[94] Eijking EP, van Daal GJ, Tenbrinck R, et al. Effect of surfactant replacement on Pneumocystis carinii pneumonia in rats. Intensive Care Med 1990;17:475–8.

[95] Sherman MP, Campbell LA, Merritt TA, et al. Effect of different surfactants on pulmonary group B streptococcal infection in premature rabbits. J Pediatr 1994;125:939–47.

[96] Berry D, Ikegami M, Jobe A. Respiratory distress and surfactant inhibition following vagotomy in rabbits. J Appl Physiol 1986;61:1741–8.

[97] Matalon S, Holm BA, Notter RH. Mitigation of pulmonary hyperoxic injury by administration of exogenous surfactant. J Appl Physiol 1987;62:756–61.

[98] Loewen GM, Holm BA, Milanowski L, et al. Alveolar hyperoxic injury in rabbits receiving exogenous surfactant. J Appl Physiol 1989;66:1987–92.

[99] Engstrom PC, Holm BA, Matalon S. Surfactant replacement attenuates the increase in alveolar permeability in hyperoxia. J Appl Physiol 1989;67:688–93.

[100] Matalon S, Holm BA, Loewen GM, et al. Sublethal hyperoxic injury to the alveolar epithelium and the pulmonary surfactant system. Exp Lung Res 1988;14:1021–33.

[101] Novotny WE, Hudak BB, Matalon S, et al. Hyperoxic lung injury reduces exogenous surfactant clearance in vitro. Am J Respir Crit Care Med 1995;151:1843–7.

[102] Lachmann B, Fujiwara T, Chida S, et al. Surfactant replacement therapy in experimental adult respiratory distress syndrome (ARDS). In: Cosmi EV, Scarpelli EM, editors. Pulmonary surfactant system. Amsterdam: Elsevier; 1983. p. 221–35.

[103] Kobayashi T, Kataoka H, Ueda T, et al. Effect of surfactant supplementation and end expiratory pressure in lung-lavaged rabbits. J Appl Physiol 1984;57:995–1001.

[104] Berggren P, Lachmann B, Curstedt T, et al. Gas exchange and lung morphology after surfactant replacement in experimental adult respiratory distress induced by repeated lung lavage. Acta Anaesthesiol Scand 1986;30:321–8.

[105] Lewis JF, Goffin J, Yue P, et al. Evaluation of exogenous surfactant treatment strategies in an adult model of acute lung injury. J Appl Physiol 1996;80:1156–64.

[106] Walther FJ, Hernandez-Juviel J, Bruni R, et al. Spiking Survanta with synthetic surfactant peptides improves oxygenation in surfactant-deficient rats. Am J Respir Crit Care Med 1997;156:855–61.

[107] Walther F, Hernandez-Juviel J, Bruni R, et al. Protein composition of synthetic surfactant affects gas exchange in surfactant-deficient rats. Pediatr Res 1998;43:666–73.

[108] Harris JD, Jackson F, Moxley MA, et al. Effect of exogenous surfactant instillation on experimental acute lung injury. J Appl Physiol 1989;66:1846–51.

[109] Lewis JF, Ikegami M, Jobe AH. Metabolism of exogenously administered surfactant in the acutely injured lungs of adult rabbits. Am Rev Respir Dis 1992;145:19–23.

[110] Lewis J, Ikegami M, Higuchi R, et al. Nebulized vs. instilled exogenous surfactant in an adult lung injury model. J Appl Physiol 1991;71:1270–6.

[111] van Daal GJ, So KL, Gommers D, et al. Intratracheal surfactant administration restores gas exchange in experimental adult respiratory distress syndrome associated with viral pneumonia. Anesth Analg 1991;72:589–95.

[112] van Daal GJ, Bos JAH, Eijking EP, et al. Surfactant replacement therapy improves pulmonary mechanics in end-stage influenza A pneumonia in mice. Am Rev Respir Dis 1992;145:859–63.

[113] Hall SB, Venkitaraman AR, Whitsett JA, et al. Importance of hydrophobic apoproteins as constituents of clinical exogenous surfactants. Am Rev Respir Dis 1992;145:24–30.

[114] Hudak ML, Farrell EE, Rosenberg AA, et al. A multicenter randomized masked compar-ison of natural vs synthetic surfactant for the treatment of respiratory distress syndrome. J Pediatr 1996;128:396–406.

[115] Hudak ML, Martin DJ, Egan EA, et al. A multicenter randomized masked comparison trial of synthetic surfactant versus calf lung surfactant extract in the prevention of neonatal respiratory distress syndrome. Pediatrics 1997;100:39–50.

[116] Vermont-Oxford Neonatal Network. A multicenter randomized trial comparing synthetic surfactant with modified bovine surfactant extract in the treatment of neonatal respiratory distress syndrome. Pediatrics 1996;97:1–6.

[117] Horbar JD, Wright LL, Soll RF, et al. A multicenter randomized trial comparing two surfactants for the treatment of neonatal respiratory distress syndrome. J Pediatr 1993; 123:757–66.

[118] Notter RH, Wang Z, Egan EA, et al. Component-specific surface and physiological activity in bovine-derived lung surfactants. Chem Phys Lipids 2002;114:21–34.

[119] Chess P, Finkelstein JN, Holm BA, et al. Surfactant replacement therapy in lung injury. In: Notter RH, Finkelstein JN, Holm BA, editors. Lung injury: mechanisms, pathophysiology, and therapy. Boca Raton (FL): Taylor Francis Group, Inc; 2005. p. 617–63.

[120] Gunther A, Schmidt R, Harodt J, et al. Bronchoscopic administration of bovine natural surfactant in ARDS and septic shock: impact on biophysical and biochemical surfactant properties. Eur Respir J 2002;10:797–804.

[121] Walmrath D, Gunther A, Ghofrani HA, et al. Bronchoscopic surfactant administration in patients with severe adult respiratory distress syndrome and sepsis. Am J Respir Crit Care Med 1996;154:57–62.

[122] Spragg R, Gilliard N, Richman P, et al. Acute effects of a single dose of porcine surfactant on patients with the adult respiratory distress syndrome. Chest 1994;105:195–202.

[123] Wiswell TE, Smith RM, Katz LB, et al. Bronchopulmonary segmental lavage with Surfaxin (KL(4) - surfactant) for acute respiratory distress syndrome. Am J Respir Crit Care Med 1999;160:1188–95.

[124] Willson DF, Jiao JH, Bauman LA, et al. Calf lung surfactant extract in acute hypoxemic respiratory failure in children. Crit Care Med 1996;24:1316–22.

[125] Willson DF, Bauman LA, Zaritsky A, et al. Instillation of calf lung surfactant extract (calfactant) is beneficial in pediatric acute hypoxemic respiratory failure. Crit Care Med 1999;27:188–95.

[126] Lopez-Herce J, de Lucas N, Carrillo A, et al. Surfactant treatment for acute respiratory distress syndrome. Arch Dis Child 1999;80:248–52.

[127] Hermon MM, Golej J, Burda H, et al. Surfactant therapy in infants and children: three years experience in a pediatric intensive care unit. Shock 2002;17:247–51.

[128] Herting E, Moller O, Schiffman JH, et al. Surfactant improves oxygenation in infants and chil-dren with pneumonia and acute respiratory distress syndrome. Acta Paediatr 2002;91:1174–8.

[129] Auten RL, Notter RH, Kendig JW, et al. Surfactant treatment of full-term newborns with respiratory failure. Pediatrics 1991;87:101–7.

[130] Lotze A, Knight GR, Martin GR, et al. Improved pulmonary outcome after exogenous surfactant therapy for respiratory failure in term infants requiring extracorporeal mem-brane oxygenation. J Pediatr 1993;122:261–8.

[131] Lotze A, Mitchell BR, Bulas DI, et al. Multicenter study of surfactant (beractant) use in the treatment of term infants with severe respiratory failure. J Pediatr 1998;132:40–7.

[132] Khammash H, Perlman M, Wojtulewicz J, et al. Surfactant therapy in full-term neonates with severe respiratory failure. Pediatrics 1993;92:135–9.

[133] Findlay RD, Taeusch HW, Walther FJ. Surfactant replacement therapy for meconium aspiration syndrome. Pediatrics 1996;97:48–52.

[134] Luchetti M, Casiraghi G, Valsecchi R, et al. Porcine-derived surfactant treatment of severe bronchiolitis. Acta Anaesthesiol Scand 1998;42:805–10.

[135] Luchetti M, Ferrero F, Gallini C, et al. Multicenter, randomized, controlled study of porcine surfactant in severe respiratory syncytial virus-induced respiratory failure. Pediatr Crit Care Med 2002;3:261–8.

[136] Anzueto A, Baughman RP, Guntupalli KK, et al. Aerosolized surfactant in adults with sepsis-induced acute respiratory distress syndrome. N Engl J Med 1996;334:1417–21.

[137] Gregory TJ, Steinberg KP, Spragg R, et al. Bovine surfactant therapy for patients with acute respiratory distress syndrome. Am J Respir Crit Care Med 1997;155:109–31.

[138] Clark DA, Nieman GF, Thompson JE, et al. Surfactant displacement by meconium free fatty acids: an alternative explanation for atelectasis in meconium aspiration syndrome. J Pediatr 1987;110:765–70.

[139] Tibby SM, Hatherill M, Wright SM, et al. Exogenous surfactant supplementation in infants with respiratory syncytial virus bronchiolitis. Am J Respir Crit Care Med 2000;162:1251–6.

[140] Ivascu FA, Hirschl RB. New approaches to managing congenital diaphragmatic hernia. Semin Perinat 2004;28:185–98.

[141] Van Meurs K, the Congenital Diaphragmatic Hernia Study Group. Is surfactant therapy beneficial in the treatment of the term newborn infants with congenital diaphragmatic hernia? J Pediatr 2004;145:312–6.

[142] Bloom BT, Kattwinkel J, Hall RT, et al. Comparison of Infasurf (calf lung surfactant extract) to Survanta (beractant) in the treatment and prevention of RDS. Pediatrics 1997;100:31–8.

[143] Rollins M, Jenkins J, Tubman R, et al. Comparison of clinical responses to natural and synthetic surfactants. J Perinat Med 1993;21:341–7.

[144] Sehgal SS, Ewing CK, Richards T, et al. Modified bovine surfactant (Survanta) vs a protein-free surfactant (Exosurf) in the treatment of respiratory distress syndrome in preterm infants: a pilot study. J Natl Med Assoc 1994;86:46–52.

[145] Choukroun ML, Llanas B, Apere H, et al. Pulmonary mechanics in ventilated preterm infants with respiratory distress syndrome after exogenous surfactant administration: a comparison between two surfactant preparations. Pediatr Pulmonol 1994;18: 273–98.

[146] Moller JC, Schaible T, Roll C, et al. with the Surfactant ARDS Study Group. Treatment with bovine surfactant in severe acute respiratory distress syndrome in children: a randomized multicenter study. Inten Care Med 2003;29:437–46.

[147] Davis JM, Russ GA, Metlay L, et al. Short-term distribution kinetics in intratracheally administered exogenous lung surfactant. Pediatr Res 1992;31:445–50.

[148] Espinosa FF, Shapiro AH, Fredberg JJ, et al. Spreading of exogenous surfactant in an airway. J Appl Physiol 1993;75:2028–39.

[149] Grotberg JB, Halpern D, Jensen OE. Interaction of exogenous and endogenous surfactant: spreading-rate effects. J Appl Physiol 1995;78:750–6.

[150] Marks LB, Notter RH, Oberdoerster G, et al. Ultrasonic and jet aerosolization of phospholipids and the effects on surface activity. Pediatr Res 1984;17:742–7.

[151] Balaraman V, Meister J, Ku TL, et al. Lavage administration of dilute surfactants after acute lung injury in neonatal piglets. Am J Respir Crit Care Med 1998;158:12–7.

[152] Balaraman V, Sood SL, Finn KC, et al. Physiologic response and lung distribution of lavage vs bolus Exosurf in piglets with acute lung injury. Am J Respir Crit Care Med 1996;153:1838–43.

[153] Gommers D, Eijking EP, van't Veen A, et al. Bronchoalveolar lavage with a diluted surfactant suspension prior to surfactant instillation improves the effectiveness of surfactant therapy in experimental acute respiratory distress syndrome (ARDS). Intensive Care Med 1998;24:494–500.

[154] van Der Beek J, Plotz F, van Overbeek F, et al. Distribution of exogenous surfactant in rabbits with severe respiratory failure: the effect of volume. Pediatr Res 1993;34:154–8.

[155] Walmrath D, Grimminger F, Pappert D, et al. Bronchoscopic administration of bovine natural surfactant in ARDS and septic shock: impact on gas exchange and haemodynamics. Eur Respir J 2002;19:805–10.

[156] Marks LB, Oberdoerster G, Notter RH. Generation and characterization of aerosols of dispersed surface active phospholipids by ultrasonic and jet nebulization. J Aerosol Sci 1983;14:683–94.

[157] Wojciak JF, Notter RH, Oberdoerster G. Size stability of phosphatidylcholine-phosphatidylglycerol aerosols and a dynamic film compression state from their interfacial impaction. J Colloid Interface Sci 1985;106:547–57.

[158] Dijk PH, Heikamp A, Bambang-Oetomo S. Surfactant nebulization versus instillation during high frequency ventilation in surfactant-deficient rabbits. Pediatr Res 1998;44: 699–704.

[159] Ellyett KM, Broadbent RS, Fawcett ER, et al. Surfactant aerosol treatment of respiratory distress syndrome in the spontaneously breathing rabbit. Pediatr Res 1996;39:953–7.

[160] Zelter M, Escudier BJ, Hoeffel JM, et al. Effects of aerosolized artificial surfactant on repeated oleic acid injury in sheep. Am Rev Respir Dis 1990;141:1014–9.

[161] Davis JM, Richter SE, Kendig JW, et al. High frequency jet ventilation and surfactant treatment of newborns in severe respiratory failure. Pediatr Pulmonol 1992;13:108–12.

[162] Davis JM, Notter RH. Lung surfactant replacement for neonatal pathology other than primary repiratory distress syndrome. In: Boynton B, Carlo W, Jobe A, editors. New therapies for neonatal respiratory failure: a physiologic approach. Cambridge: Cambridge University Press; 1994. p. 81–92.

[163] Leach CL, Greenspan JS, Rubenstein SD, et al. Partial liquid ventilation with perflubron in premature infants with severe respiratory distress syndrome. N Engl J Med 1996;335:761–7.

[164] Leach CL, Holm BA, Morin FC, et al. Partial liquid ventilation in premature lambs with respiratory distress syndrome: efficacy and compatibility with exogenous surfactant. J Pediatr 1995;126:412–20.

[165] Chappell SE, Wolfson MR, Shaffer TH. A comparison of surfactant delivery with conventional mechanical ventilation and partial liquid ventilation in meconium aspiration injury. Respir Med 2001;95:612–7.

[166] King DM, Wang Z, Kendig JW, et al. Concentration-dependent, temperature-dependent non-newtonian viscosity of lung surfactant dispersions. Chem Phys Lipids 2001;112:11–9.

[167] King DM, Wang Z, Palmer HJ, et al. Bulk shear viscosities of endogenous and exogenous lung surfactants. Am J Physiol 2002;282:L277–84.

[168] Bloom BT, Delmore P, Rose T, et al. Human and calf lung surfactant: a comparison. Neonatal Intensive Care 1993;31–5.

[169] Speer CP, Gefeller O, Groneck P, et al. Randomised clinical trial of two treatment regimens of natural surfactant preparations in neonatal respiratory distress syndrome. Arch Dis Child 1995;72:F8–13.

[170] Soll RF, Merritt TA, Hallman M. Surfactant in the prevention and treatment of respiratory distress syndrome. In: Boynton BR, Carlo WA, Jobe AH, editors. New therapies for neonatal respiratory failure. New York: Cambridge University Press; 1994. p. 49–80.

[171] Kattwinkel J. Surfactant: evolving issues. Clin Perinatol 1998;25:17–32.

[172] Halliday HL. Overview of clinical trials comparing natural and synthetic surfactants. Biol Neonate 1995;67(Suppl):32–47.

[173] Halliday HL. Controversies—synthetic or natural surfactant—the case for natural surfactant. J Perinat Med 1996;24(5):417–26.

[174] Soll RF. Surfactant therapy in the USA: trials and current routines. Biol Neonate 1997;71: 1–7.

[175] Mizuno K, Ikegami M, Chen C-M, et al. Surfactant protein-B supplementation improves *in vivo* function of a modified natural surfactant. Pediatr Res 1995;37:271–6.

[176] Curstedt T, Jornvall H, Robertson B, et al. Two hydrophobic low-molecular-mass protein fractions of pulmonary surfactant: characterization and biophysical activity. Eur J Biochem 1987;168:255–62.

[177] Oosterlaken-Dijksterhuis MA, Haagsman HP, van Golde LM, et al. Characterization of lipid insertion into monomolecular layers mediated by lung surfactant proteins SP-B and SP-C. Biochemistry 1991;30:10965–71.

[178] Oosterlaken-Dijksterhuis MA, Haagsman HP, van Golde LM, et al. Interaction of lipid vesicles with monomolecular layers containing lung surfactant proteins SP-B or SP-C. Biochemistry 1991;30:8276–81.

[179] Oosterlaken-Dijksterhuis MA, van Eijk M, van Golde LMG, et al. Lipid mixing is mediated by the hydrophobic surfactant protein SP-B but not by SP-C. Biochim Biophys Acta 1992;1110:45–50.

[180] Revak SD, Merritt TA, Degryse E, et al. The use of human low molecular weight (LMW) apoproteins in the reconstitution of surfactant biological activity. J Clin Invest 1988;81:826–33.

[181] Seeger W, Günther A, Thede C. Differential sensitivity to fibrinogen inhibition of SP-C- vs. SP-B-based surfactants. Am J Physiol 1992;261:L286–91.

[182] Wang Z, Gurel O, Baatz JE, et al. Differential activity and lack of synergy of lung surfactant proteins SP-B and SP-C in surface-active interactions with phospholipids. J Lipid Res 1996; 37:1749–60.

[183] Yu SH, Possmayer F. Comparative studies on the biophysical activities of the low-molecular-weight hydrophobic proteins purified from bovine pulmonary surfactant. Biochim Biophys Acta 1988;961:337–50.

[184] Wang Z, Baatz JE, Holm BA, et al. Content-dependent activity of lung surfactant protein B (SP-B) in mixtures with lipids. Am J Physiol 2002;283:L897–906.

[185] Johansson J, Curstedt T, Robertson B. Synthetic protein analogues in artificial surfactants. Acta Paediatr 1996;85:642–6.

[186] Johansson J, Gustafsson M, Zaltash S, et al. Synthetic surfactant protein analogs. Biol Neonate 1998;74(Suppl):9–14.

[187] Walther FJ, Gordon LM, Zasadzinski JM, et al. Surfactant protein B and C analogues. Mol Genet Metab 2000;71:342–51.

[188] Robertson B, Johansson J, Curstedt T. Synthetic surfactants to treat neonatal lung disease. Mol Med Today 2000;6:119–24.

[189] Cochrane CG, Revak SD, Merritt TA, et al. The efficacy and safety of KL4-surfactant in preterm infants with respiratory distress syndrome. Am J Respir Crit Care Med 1996; 153:404–10.

[190] Cochrane CG, Revak SD. Surfactant lavage treatment in a model of respiratory distress syndrome. Chest 1999;116(Suppl):85S–86S.

[191] Cochrane CG, Revak SD. Pulmonary surfactant protein B (SP-B): structure-function relationships. Science 1991;254:566–8.

[192] Cochrane CG, Revak SD. Protein-phospholipid interactions in pulmonary surfactant. Chest 1994;105:57S–62S.

[193] Merritt TA, Kheiter A, Cochrane CG. Positive end-expiratory pressure during KL4 surfactant instillation enhances intrapulmonary distribution in a simian model of respiratory distress syndrome. Pediatr Res 1995;38:211–7.

[194] Revak S, Merritt T, Cochrane C, et al. Efficacy of synthetic peptide-containing surfactant in the treatment of respiratory distress syndrome in preterm infant rhesus monkeys. Pediatr Res 1996;39:715–24.

[195] Revak SD, Merritt TA, Hallman M, et al. The use of synthetic peptides in the formation of biophysically and biologically active surfactants. Pediatr Res 1991;29:460–5.

[196] Ikegami M, Jobe AH. Surfactant protein-C in ventilated premature lamb lung. Pediatr Res 1998;44:860–4.

[197] Davis AJ, Jobe AH, Hafner D, et al. Lung function in premature lambs and rabbits treated with a recombinant SP-C surfactant. Am J Respir Crit Care Med 1998;157:553–9.

[198] Lewis J, McCaig L, Hafner D, et al. Dosing and delivery of a recombinant surfactant in lung-injured sheep. Am J Respir Crit Care Med 1999;159:741–7.

[199] Hafner D, Germann P-G, Hauschke D. Effects of rSP-C surfactant on oxygenation and histology in a rat-lung-lavage model of acute lung injury. Am J Respir Crit Care Med 1998;158:270–8.

[200] Spragg RG, Smith RM, Harris K, et al. Effect of recombinant SP-C surfactant in a porcine lavage model of acute lung injury. J Appl Physiol 1999;88:674–81.

[201] Spragg RG, Lewis JF, Rathgeb F, et al. Intratracheal instillation of rSP-C surfactant improves oxygenation in patients with ARDS [abstract]. Am J Respir Crit Care Med 2002;165:A22.

[202] Notter RH, Schwan AL, Wang Z, et al. Novel phospholipase-resistant lipid/peptide synthetic lung surfactants. Mini Rev Med Chem 2007;7:932–4.

[203] Waring AJ, Walther FJ, Gordon LM, et al. The role of charged amphipathic helices in the structure and function of surfactant protein B (SP-B). J Pept Res 2005;66:364–74.

[204] Walther FJ, Waring AJ, Sherman MA, et al. Hydrophobic surfactant proteins and their analogues. Neonatology 2007;91:303–10.

[205] Turcotte JG, Lin WH, Pivarnik PE, et al. Chemical synthesis and surface activity of lung surfactant phospholipid analogs. II. Racemic N-substituted diether phosphonolipids. Biochim Biophys Acta 1991;1084:1–12.

[206] Turcotte JG, Sacco AM, Steim JM, et al. Chemical synthesis and surface properties of an analog of the pulmonary surfactant dipalmitoyl phosphatidylcholine analog. Biochim Biophys Acta 1977;488:235–48.

[207] Chang Y, Wang Z, Notter RH, et al. Synthesis and interfacial behavior of sulfur-containing analogs of lung surfactant dipalmitoyl phosphatidylcholine. Bioorg Med Chem Lett 2004; 14:5983–6.

[208] Chang Y, Wang Z, Schwan AL, et al. Surface properties of sulfur- and ether-linked phosphonolipids with and without purified hydrophobic lung surfactant proteins. Chem Phys Lipids 2005;137:77–93.

[209] Notter RH, Wang Z, Wang Z, et al. Synthesis and surface activity of diether-linked phosphoglycerols: potential applications for exogenous lung surfactants. Bioorg Med Chem Lett 2007;17:113–7.

[210] Davy JA, Wang Z, Notter RH, et al. Synthesis of sulfur-containing glycerophospholipids. J Sulfur Chem 2007;28:45–72.

[211] Wang Z, Chang Y, Schwan AL, et al. Activity and inhibition resistance of a phospholipase-resistant synthetic exogenous surfactant in excised rat lungs. Am J Respir Cell Mol Biol 2007;37:387–94.

[212] Kim DK, Fukuda T, Thompson BT, et al. Bronchoalveolar lavage fluid phospholipase A_2 activities are increased in human adult respiratory distress syndrome. Am J Physiol 1995; 269:L109–18.

[213] Touqui L, Arbibe L. A role for phospholipase A_2 in ARDS pathogenesis. Molec Med Today 1999;5:244–9.

[214] Vadas P. Elevated plasma phospholipase A_2 levels: correlation with the hemodynamic and pulmonary changes in gram-negative septic shock. J Lab Clin Med 1984;104:873–81.

[215] Kostopanagiotou G, Routs C, Smyrniotis V, et al. Alterations in bronchoalveolar lavage fluid during ischemia-induced acute hepatic failure in the pig. Hepatology 2003;37:1130–8.

[216] Attalah HL, Wu Y, Alaoui-El-Azher M, et al. Induction of type-IIA secretory phospholipase A2 in animal models of acute lung injury. Eur Respir J 2003;21:1040–5.

[217] Nakos G, Kitsiouli E, Hatzidaki E, et al. Phospholipases A_2 and platelet-activating–factor acetylhydrolase in patients with acute respiratory distress syndrome. Crit Care Med 2003; 33:772–9.

[218] Ackerman SJ, Kwatia MA, Doyle CB, et al. Hydrolysis of surfactant phospholipids catalyzed by phospholipase A_2 and eosinophil lysophospholipases causes surfactant dysfunction: a mechanism for small airway closure in asthma. Chest 2003;123:255S.

[219] Walther FJ, Waring AJ, Hernandez-Juviel JM, et al. Dynamic surface activity of a fully-synthetic phospholipase-resistant lipid/peptide lung surfactant. PLoS ONE 2007;2(10): e1039.

[220] Kendig JW, Notter RH, Cox C, et al. A comparison of surfactant as immediate prophylaxis and as rescue therapy in newborns of less than 30 weeks gestation. N Engl J Med 1991;324: 865–71.

[221] Notter RH, Apostolakos M, Holm BA, et al. Surfactant therapy and its potential use with other agents in term infants, children and adults with acute lung injury. Perspectives in Neonatology 2000;1(4):4–20.

[222] Pryhuber GS, D'Angio CT, Finkelstein JN, et al. Combined-modality therapies for lung injury. In: Notter RH, Finkelstein JN, Holm BA, editors. Lung injury: mechanisms, pathophysiology, and therapy. Boca Raton (FL): Taylor Francis Group, Inc; 2005. p. 779–838.

ELSEVIER
SAUNDERS

PEDIATRIC CLINICS
OF NORTH AMERICA

Pediatr Clin N Am 55 (2008) 577–587

Diabetic Ketoacidosis in the Pediatric ICU

James P. Orlowski, MD, FAAP, FCCP, FCCM*,
Cheryl L. Cramer, RN, MSN, ARNP,
Mariano R. Fiallos, MD

*Pediatric Intensive Care Unit, University Community Hospital, 3100 East Fletcher Avenue,
Tampa, FL 33613, USA*

Diabetic ketoacidosis (DKA) in children is defined as a serum glucose concentration greater than 300 mg/dL, the presence of ketones in the blood, a blood pH below 7.3, and a serum bicarbonate level below 15 mEq/L [1]. The child who has DKA typically presents with a history of polyuria, polydipsia, polyphagia, and weight loss. The classic clinical presentation is an acutely ill child with lethargy, dehydration, hyperpnea (Kussmaul respirations), and a fruity smell (acetone) on the breath. The severity of DKA is defined by the degree of acidosis: mild is a venous pH between 7.2 and 7.3; moderate is a pH between 7.1 and 7.2; and severe is a pH less than 7.1 [2].

The younger the child, the more difficult it is to diagnose DKA, especially with new-onset or previously undiagnosed diabetes mellitus (DM). Fifteen percent to 70% of all newly diagnosed infants and children who have DM present with DKA [2]. Infants and toddlers often are misdiagnosed as having pneumonia, asthma, or bronchiolitis, and treatment may have been commenced with steroids and/or sympathomimetic agents, which only exacerbate, and compound, the metabolic derangements. Because the diagnosis of DM with DKA is not suspected in the young child, the duration of symptoms may be longer, leading to more severe dehydration and acidosis and the possibility of obtundation progressing to coma. In a carefully analyzed cohort of pediatric patients who had new-onset DM with DKA, 23.3% of the children presented with DKA. Thirty-six percent of children under 5 years of age presented with DKA as the initial diagnosis, compared with 16% of adolescents older than 14 years of age [3].

---

* Corresponding author.
  E-mail address: jorlowski@mail.uch.org (J.P. Orlowski).

0031-3955/08/$ - see front matter © 2008 Elsevier Inc. All rights reserved.
doi:10.1016/j.pcl.2008.02.015
pediatric.theclinics.com

Whereas delay in diagnosis is the major contributor to DKA in previously undiagnosed DM in younger children, omission of insulin in established DM is the leading cause of recurrent DKA and is most prevalent in adolescents. The omission of insulin may be intentional or inadvertent. There usually is an important psychosocial reason for omitting insulin in the adolescent. In adolescents, some 5% of patients account for more than 25% of all admissions for DKA [4]. DKA is more common in families who do not have ready access to medical care for social or economic reasons. Lower income and lower parental educational achievement are associated with a higher risk of DKA in the child [5]. Lack of health insurance also is associated with higher rates and greater severity of DKA at diagnosis, presumably because uninsured patients delay seeking timely medical care. The risk of DKA is increased in children who have poor control of their DM or have had previous episodes of DKA, in peripubertal and adolescent girls, in children or adolescents who have clinical depression or other psychiatric disorders, in children who have unstable home situations or family dynamics, and in children receiving insulin pump therapy [2]. The last is a significant risk factor for DKA: any malfunction in the delivery of insulin by the pump leads rapidly to complete insulin deficiency, because only short-acting insulin is used in pumps. Psychologic or physical stress or intercurrent infection also can contribute to the development of DKA in established DM, although these causes are not as common in children and adolescents who are followed closely by a diabetes care team.

Pathophysiology of diabetic ketoacidosis

A relative or absolute deficiency of insulin is the cause of DKA. The deficiency of insulin can be the result of beta-cell failure in the pancreas, omission of insulin in the established DM patient, or antagonism of its action by physiologic stress such as sepsis. With the obesity epidemic in civilized countries, cases of DKA are being seen increasingly in children who have type 2 DM with the metabolic syndrome, in which there is peripheral resistance to insulin rather than a true deficiency of insulin. A clue to the presence of type 2 DM is acanthosis nigricans [2].

Insulin is required for the active movement of glucose into cells as a source of energy. In the absence of insulin, the body goes into a catabolic state with breakdown of glycogen, protein, and fat in muscle, liver, and adipose tissue. Counterregulatory hormones such as glucagon, cortisol, growth hormone, and catecholamines stimulate glycogenolysis, gluconeogenesis, proteolysis, lipolysis, and ketogenesis in an attempt to provide more fuel to cells. Despite an excess of extracellular glucose, the cells sense a deficiency of fuel for metabolic needs. The brain, with at least 20% of the body's total metabolic demands, cannot use fatty acids as fuel and presents a large and inescapable need for either glucose or ketones as fuel. Ketones produced by the hepatic oxidation of fatty acids in a state of insulin lack and excess glucagon stimulation provide an important energy source for the brain during DKA [6–8].

The most important perturbations seen in DKA are metabolic acidosis, hyperosmolality, dehydration, and electrolyte disturbances. An important hallmark of DKA is the metabolic acidosis caused by elevated plasma concentrations of the ketoacids acetoacetate and beta-hydroxybutyrate. Lack of insulin permits lipolysis to accelerate in adipose tissue, releasing long-chain fatty acids. In the liver, these fatty acids are shunted toward beta-oxidation and ketone production because of increased glucagon levels. Ketones normally stimulate insulin release and thereby inhibit lipolysis, but in the absence of this feedback loop extreme lipemia and ketonemia occur. Nonenzymatic decarboxylation of acetoacetate produces elevated acetone concentrations in plasma. Typically in DKA the ratio of beta-hydroxybutyrate to acetoacetate is about 3:1, but it may range up to 15:1 in severe DKA [9,10]. Acetone may represent 1.5 to 4 times the molar concentration of acetoacetate [11]. Acetone fills an important role as a buffer by continuous nonenzymatic conversion of acetoacetate to acetone and carbon dioxide. Acetone then is excreted in breath and urine in a ratio of 5:1, and the carbon dioxide is excreted in breathing. This mechanism removes about one fourth of the hydrogen ions generated by hepatic ketogenesis. Lactic acidosis secondary to hypoxia and/or poor tissue perfusion, shifts acetoacetate toward beta-hydroxybutyrate, reducing the body's ability to eliminate ketoacids by the acetone route. Lactic acidosis occurs in large part from anaerobic glycolysis in hypoperfused tissues secondary to hypovolemia from osmotic diuresis. Measuring lactate and acetoacetate gives a crude indication of the relative proportions of these metabolic acids. Hyperchloremic metabolic acidosis also can be seen in DKA, most commonly as a result of aggressive intravenous fluid resuscitation with solutions containing large amounts of chloride [12]. The metabolic acidosis of DKA should not be treated with bicarbonate administration, because the hyperosmolar solution and the resultant paradoxical cerebral acidosis may contribute to the development of cerebral edema [13].

The hyperosmolar state induced by insulin deficiency is responsible for at least as much of the physiologic derangements seen in DKA as the ketoacidosis. The osmolality is estimated from the formula:

$$Osmolality = 2[Na] + [K] + [Glucose]/18 + [BUN]/2.8$$

where sodium and potassium concentrations are expressed in mEq/L and glucose and serum urea nitrogen (BUN) concentrations are expressed in mg/dL.

In the typical child who has DKA, glucose is elevated about 400 mg/dL above normal, and the BUN is elevated by about 15 mg/dL. These elevations result in an additional osmolar load of about 22 and 5 mOsm/L, respectively.

The primary fluid loss is secondary to the osmotic diuresis induced by hyperglycemia and glycosuria. The typical child who has DKA is about 10% dehydrated. Estimation of the degree of dehydration is best made by known body weights. Unfortunately, this determination is not always possible, and so estimates are made based on physical findings, which are based on extracellular fluid volume. The extracellular fluid volume in DKA is maintained by plasma hyperosmolality, however, so the deficit in total body water is easily underestimated. Loss of water through osmotic diuresis is perhaps the most dangerous process brought about by DKA. When fluid loss is severe enough to begin to impair renal function (glomerular filtration rate), the excretion of excess glucose is impaired, and hyperglycemia accelerates. The combination of rapidly rising glucose and BUN levels results in extreme hyperosmolality. Hyperosmolality has been shown to correlate better than other laboratory measurements in DKA with levels of obtundation and with electroencephalographic slowing [14]; hyperosmolality and its too rapid correction may set the stage for the rare occurrence of cerebral edema during recovery from DKA. Cardiorespiratory function can remain adequate to sustain life even at the extremes of pH and osmolality seen in DKA, but shock invariably occurs when dehydration is severe enough, and hypovolemic shock can be fatal if not reversed appropriately by volume replacement.

Hyponatremia usually is reported by the laboratory when sera from DKA patients are analyzed, and quite commonly the reported low value is an artifact. Extreme lipemia can decrease the measured sodium value simply by decreasing the aqueous phase of blood in which sodium predominantly resides. The true serum sodium can be calculated from the formula:

$$True[Na] = [measured\ Na](0.021[T] + 0.994)$$

where T equals the triglyceride level in g/dL and sodium is expressed in mEq/L [15].

Another important cause of artifactually low sodium in DKA is hyperglycemia. As the amount of glucose in the extracellular fluid increases, water shifts there from intracellular fluid, lowering the concentration of solutes, including sodium. The classic correction is to add 2.8 mEq/L to the measured sodium for every 100-mg/dL elevation of blood glucose.

Disturbed potassium homeostasis is another potentially dangerous electrolyte imbalance in DKA. Hyperkalemia commonly is found at presentation in DKA [16]. Metabolic acidosis and hyperosmolality both cause potassium to redistribute from intracellular fluid to extracellular fluid, and continued osmotic diuresis results in progressive depletion of body potassium stores. The best way to assess for intracellular potassium deficit is by looking for U-waves and flattened T-waves on the EKG [17]. Insulin and glucose are well-known treatments for hyperkalemia, facilitating the entry of potassium into muscle cells. In the absence of insulin, hyperglycemia produces hyperkalemia, which is reversed when insulin is resupplied. When insulin is supplied, hypokalemia is likely to result and at times can be profound, with the resultant risk of arrhythmias. It therefore is important to provide potassium during the early stages of treatment for DKA.

Profound hypophosphatemia caused by renal losses from osmotic diuresis is common in the presentation and early treatment of DKA. Depressed levels of red blood cell 2,3-diphosphoglycerate have been described in DKA [18,19]. The low levels of red blood cell 2,3-diphosphoglycerate will decrease the partial pressure of oxygen at which hemoglobin is 50% saturated with oxygen, an effect that initially is counterbalanced by the acidosis. As the acidosis corrects, the effects of hypophosphatemia may become more pronounced. Theoretically, hypophosphatemia can cause rhabdomyolysis, hemolysis, muscle weakness, respiratory failure, and insulin resistance. Treatment of hypophosphatemia should be part of the initial and ongoing treatment of DKA [20,21].

Overly aggressive treatment of hypophosphatemia can depress levels of calcium and magnesium [21], and hypomagnesemia is common in the initial presentation of DKA. Ionized calcium, however, usually is normal.

Hypomagnesemia can be extreme in DKA and can inhibit parathyroid hormone response to hypocalcemia.

Management of diabetic ketoacidosis

- Assess airway, breathing, and circulation (ABCs) and level of consciousness [1,2]. In patients who have a Glasgow coma scale score below 8 [22], one may want to consider intubation to secure the airway and prevent aspiration pneumonia. A nasogastric tube may be indicated to empty the stomach and reduce the risk of aspiration. Assess circulatory status in terms of heart rate, blood pressure, skin turgor, capillary refill, peripheral pulses, renal and cerebral perfusion, and pulse oximetry. Administer oxygen if patient is in shock or pulse oximetry is low.
- Weigh the patient and obtain intravenous access.
- Obtain a blood sample for laboratory determination of blood glucose, electrolytes, bicarbonate, lactate, BUN, creatinine, osmolality, pH, partial pressure of carbon dioxide (pCO_2), arterial partial pressure of oxygen (if pulse oximetry is low or unobtainable), hemoglobin and hematocrit, complete blood cell count, calcium and ionized calcium, magnesium, phosphorus, hemoglobin A1c, and blood beta-hydroxybutyrate.
- Obtain a urinalysis and urine for ketones.
- If there is evidence of infection, obtain appropriate specimens for culture: blood, urine, throat, wound.
- Obtain an EKG for baseline evaluation of intracellular potassium status.
- Assess clinical severity of dehydration:
  - 5%: reduced skin turgor, dry mucous membranes, tachycardia

- 10%: capillary refill time longer than 3 seconds, sunken eyes
- >10%: weak or impalpable peripheral pulses, hypotension, shock, oliguria
- Fluid resuscitate to restore peripheral circulation with 10 to 20 mL/kg boluses of normal saline or Ringer's lactate until perfusion is reestablished.
- Calculate fluid deficit based on severity of dehydration and maintenance fluid requirements and plan to replace fluid deficit (less fluid given for resuscitation) over 24 to 48 hours in addition to maintenance fluid requirements.
- Initiate continuous low-dose insulin infusion of regular insulin at 0.1 units/kg/h and continue insulin infusion until resolution of DKA (pH > 7.30, bicarbonate > 18 mEq/L), which usually takes longer than normalization of blood glucose concentration.
- Commence replacement and maintenance fluids with normal saline with 20 mEq/L of potassium acetate and 20 mEq/L of potassium phosphate.
- Assess vital signs and neurologic status hourly (or more frequently if indicated).
- Assess accurate fluid input and output hourly.
- Measure blood glucose hourly.
- Reassess serum electrolytes, glucose, calcium, magnesium, phosphorus, and blood gases every 2 to 4 hours (or more frequently if indicated), and BUN, creatinine, and hemoglobin every 6 to 8 hours until they are normal. Calculate and follow the anion gap:

$$\text{Anion gap} = (\text{Na} + \text{K}) - (\text{Cl} + \text{HCO}_3)$$
$$(\text{normal anion gap is } 8 \pm 2)$$

- Follow urine ketones every void or every 4 hours until cleared.
- When blood glucose decreases to less than 300 mg/dL, change intravenous fluids to D51/2 normal saline with 20 mEq/L potassium chloride or potassium acetate plus 20 mEq/L of potassium phosphate to keep blood sugar between 250 and 300 mg/dL. It may be necessary to use 10% or even 12.5% dextrose to maintain the blood sugar between 250 and 300 mg/dL while continuing the insulin infusion to correct the metabolic acidosis.
- If biochemical parameters of DKA (pH, anion gap) do not improve, reassess the patient, review insulin therapy, and consider other possible causes of impaired response to insulin such as infection or errors in insulin preparation.
- After 36 to 48 hours, the insulin drip should be adjusted to bring the blood glucose down to the range of 150 to 200 mg/dL, and the patient can be transitioned to oral fluids and subcutaneous insulin.
- Oral fluids should be introduced only when substantial clinical improvement has occurred and the patient indicates a desire to eat. When oral fluid is tolerated, intravenous fluid should be reduced.

- In patients who have established diabetes, the patient's usual insulin regimen may be resumed. The most convenient time to change to subcutaneous insulin is just before a meal. To prevent rebound hyperglycemia, the first subcutaneous injection should be given 15 to 60 minutes (for rapid-acting insulin) or 1 to 2 hours (for regular insulin) before stopping the insulin infusion. For newly diagnosed diabetics, the recommended total daily dose (TDD) of insulin for prepubertal children is 0.75 to 1.0 units/kg and for pubertal patients is 1.0 to 1.2 units/kg. There are two recommended regimens for administering the subcutaneous insulin [2]:
  1. Thrice-daily administration
     Before breakfast: two thirds of TDD (one third as rapid-acting insulin; two thirds intermediate-acting insulin)
     Before dinner: one third to one half of the remainder of the TDD as rapid-acting insulin
     Before bedtime: one half to two thirds of the remainder of the TDD as intermediate-acting insulin
  2. An alternative approach, called the basal-bolus method consists of administering
     One half of the TDD as basal insulin (using insulin glargine) AND
     One half of the TDD as rapid-acting insulin divided equally before each meal.
- Blood sugars should be monitored frequently to prevent hypoglycemia or hyperglycemia. Supplemental rapid-acting insulin is given at about 4-hour intervals to correct blood glucose levels that exceed 200 mg/dL.

Cerebral edema

Symptomatic cerebral edema occurs in 0.5% to 1% of pediatric DKA episodes and has a high mortality rate (21%–24%) with a substantial proportion of survivors (15%–26%) left with permanent neurologic sequelae [2]. It is one of the most dreaded complications of DKA. Its pathophysiology and etiology are poorly understood, but it is believed that various aspects of DKA treatment may cause or exacerbate the development of cerebral edema [22].

The signs and symptoms of cerebral edema in DKA are:

Headache
New-onset vomiting
Cushing's signs of slowing of heart rate and hypertension
Changes in respiratory pattern: hyperpnea, apnea, bradypnea
Change in neurologic status: restlessness, irritability, stupor
Development of pathologic neurologic signs: cranial nerve palsies, abnormal pupillary reflexes, posturing

Mild, asymptomatic cerebral edema probably is present in most children who have DKA at the time of presentation and during therapy. Typically, symptomatic cerebral edema occurs 4 to 12 hours after the initiation of treatment for DKA, but cases have occurred before initiation of therapy and as late as 24 to 28 hours after initiating therapy [23]. Cerebral imaging studies have shown focal or diffuse cerebral edema, but as many as 40% of initial CT scans in children who have DKA and clinical signs of cerebral edema are normal [23]. Subsequent scans in these patients often demonstrate edema, hemorrhage, or infarction. Recent MRI findings have suggested that the cerebral edema in DKA is vasogenic, and not cytotoxic [24]. Animal studies have suggested that activation of ion transporters in the endothelial cells of the blood–brain barrier from ketosis, inflammatory cytokines, or hypoperfusion may be responsible for fluid influx into the brain [25]. Fluid influx into the brain from rapid declines in serum osmolality and overly vigorous fluid resuscitation has been blamed for the development of cerebral edema in DKA, but clinical studies do not support these hypotheses. Associations between the rate of fluid administration and risk for cerebral edema have been found in some studies, but not in others, and none of the studies have found an association between the rate of change in blood glucose values or change in osmolality and the risk for cerebral edema [26,27]. Bicarbonate treatment of metabolic acidosis has been implicated in causing cerebral edema in some studies.

The children at greatest risk for developing symptomatic cerebral edema are those who present with the greatest degree of dehydration, as reflected by high BUN concentrations, and those who have the most profound acidosis and hypocapnia [26,27]. An association also has been described with a lesser rise in serum sodium concentration as the blood glucose decreases with treatment [28].

The treatment of symptomatic cerebral edema is mannitol, 0.25 to 1.0 g/kg as a bolus, or 5 to 10 mL/kg of 3% hypertonic saline over 30 minutes [2]. Intubation may be necessary to protect the airway and ensure adequate ventilation, but hyperventilation to a pCO_2 less than 22 mm Hg should be avoided, because one study found poorer neurologic outcome in intubated patients who had DKA with cerebral edema who were excessively hyperventilated [29]. Hyperventilation to a pCO_2 of 25 to 30 mm Hg still can be used to treat spikes in intracranial pressure.

The Fencl-Stewart approach to acid–base disturbances in diabetic ketoacidosis

Hyperchloremic metabolic acidosis may be present on admission for DKA but is extremely common during treatment of DKA [12,30]. A recent study found that the incidence of hyperchloremia, as documented by a ratio of plasma chloride to sodium greater than 0.79, increased from 6% on admission to 94% after 20 hours of treatment. After 20 hours of treatment the mean base deficit had decreased from 24.7 mmol/L to 10.0 mmol/L, but the proportion that was caused by hyperchloremia had increased from 2% to 98% [12]. These authors estimated plasma ketonemia using the albumin-corrected anion gap:

$$\text{Anion gap} = (Na + K) - (Cl + TCO_2) + 0.25 \times [40 - \text{albumin}(g/L)]$$

One then can measure the unmeasured ion effect and the chloride effect from the following equations:

$$\text{Unmeasured ion effect}(mEq/L) = \text{standard base excess}$$
$$- (\text{sodium/chloride effect})$$
$$- (\text{albumin effect})$$

where standard base excess is measured from a blood gas machine.

$$\text{Sodium/chloride effect}(mEq/L) = [Na] - [Cl] - 38$$

and

$$\text{Albumin effect}(mEq/L) = 0.25 \times [42 - \text{albumin}(g/L)]$$

and

$$\text{Chloride effect}(mEq/L) = 102 - ([Cl] \times 140/[Na])$$

Summary

DKA is a common, life-threatening complication of DM in children. Central nervous system changes seen in DKA include the altered sensorium seen commonly in DKA and loosely characterized as diabetic coma and the uncommon but worrisome progressively deepening coma caused by cerebral edema, which has both a high morbidity and mortality.

References

[1] Dunger DB, Sperling MA, Acerini CL, et al. European Society for Paediatric Endocrinology/Lawson Wilkins Pediatric Endocrine Society consensus statement on diabetic ketoacidosis in children and adolescents. Pediatrics 2004;113:e133–40.
[2] Wolfsdorf J, Glaser N, Sperling MA. Diabetic ketoacidosis in infants, children, and adolescents. A consensus statement from the American Diabetes Association. Diabetes Care 2006; 29:1150–9.
[3] Rewers A, Klingensmith G, Davis C, et al. Diabetic ketoacidosis at onset of diabetes: the SEARCH for diabetes in youth study [abstract]. Diabetes 2005;54(Suppl 1):A63.

[4] Edge JA, Hawkins MM, Winter DL, et al. The risk and outcome of cerebral oedema developing during diabetic ketoacidosis. Arch Dis Child 2001;85:16–22.

[5] Rewers A, Chase HP, Mackenzie T, et al. Predictors of acute complications in children with type 1 diabetes. JAMA 2002;287:2511–8.

[6] Schade DS, Eaton RP. Dose response to insulin in man: differential effects on glucose and ketone body regulation. J Clin Endocrinol Metab 1977;44:1038–53.

[7] Miles JM, Gerich JE. Glucose and ketone body kinetics in diabetic ketoacidosis. Clin Endocrinol Metab 1983;12:303–19.

[8] Cryer PE. Glucose counterregulation in man. Diabetes 1981;30:261–4.

[9] Sperling MA. Diabetic ketoacidosis. Pediatr Clin North Am 1984;31:591–610.

[10] Halperin ML, Bear RA, Hannaford MC, et al. Selected aspects of the pathophysiology of metabolic acidosis in diabetes mellitus. Diabetes 1981;30:781–7.

[11] Owen OE, Trapp VE, Skutches CL, et al. Acetone metabolism during diabetic ketoacidosis. Diabetes 1982;31:242–8.

[12] Taylor D, Durward A, Tibby SM, et al. The influence of hyperchloraemia on acid base interpretation in diabetic ketoacidosis. Intensive Care Med 2006;32:295–301.

[13] Rose KL, Pin CL, Wang R, et al. Combined insulin and bicarbonate therapy elicits cerebral edema in a juvenile mouse model of diabetic ketoacidosis. Pediatr Res 2007;61:301–6.

[14] Tsalikian E, Becker DJ, Crumrine PK, et al. Electroencephalographic changes in diabetic ketosis in children with newly and previously diagnosed insulin-dependent diabetes mellitus. J Pediatr 1981;98:355–9.

[15] Goldman MH, Kashani M. Spurious hyponatremia in diabetic ketoacidosis with massive lipid elevations. J Med Soc N J 1982;79:591–2.

[16] Fulop M. Serum potassium in lactic acidosis and ketoacidosis. N Engl J Med 1979;300: 1087–90.

[17] Malone JI, Brodsky SJ. The value of electrocardiogram monitoring in diabetic ketoacidosis. Diabetes Care 1980;3:543–7.

[18] Gibby OM, Veale KE, Hayes TM, et al. Oxygen availability from the blood and the effect of phosphate replacement on erythrocyte 2,3-diphosphoglycerate and haemoglobin-oxygen affinity in diabetic ketoacidosis. Diabetologia 1978;15:381–5.

[19] Clerbaux T, Reynaert M, Willems E, et al. Effect of phosphate on oxygen-hemoglobin affinity, diphosphoglycerate and blood gases during recovery from diabetic ketoacidosis. Intensive Care Med 1989;15:495–8.

[20] Keller U, Berger W. Prevention of hypophosphatemia by phosphate infusion during treatment of diabetic ketoacidosis and hyperosmolar coma. Diabetes 1980;29:87–95.

[21] Becker DJ, Brown DR, Steranka BH, et al. Phosphate replacement during treatment of diabetic ketoacidosis: effects on calcium and phosphorus homeostasis. Am J Dis Child 1983;137:241–6.

[22] Fiordalisi I, Novotny WE, Holber D, et al. An 18-yr prospective study of diabetic ketoacidosis: an approach to minimizing the risk of brain herniation during treatment. Pediatr Diabetes 2007;8:142–9.

[23] Krane EJ, Rockoff MA, Wallman JK, et al. Subclinical brain swelling in children during treatment of diabetic ketoacidosis. N Engl J Med 1985;312:1147–51.

[24] Roberts JS, Vavilala MS, Schenkman KA, et al. Cerebral hyperemia and impaired cerebral autoregulation associated with diabetic ketoacidosis in critically ill children. Crit Care Med 2006;34:2217–23.

[25] Lam TI, Anderson SE, Glaser N, et al. Bumetanide reduces cerebral edema formation in rats with diabetic ketoacidosis. Diabetes 2005;54:510–6.

[26] Glaser NS, Wootton-Gorges SL, Marcin JP, et al. Mechanism of cerebral edema in children with diabetic ketoacidosis. J Pediatr 2004;145:164–71.

[27] Glaser N, Barnett P, McCaslin I, et al. Risk factors for cerebral edema in children with diabetic ketoacidosis: the Pediatric Emergency Medicine Collaborative Research Committee of the American Academy of Pediatrics. N Engl J Med 2001;344:264–9.

[28] Hoorn EJ, Carlotti AP, Costa LA, et al. Preventing a drop in effective plasma osmolality to minimize the likelihood of cerebral edema during treatment of children with diabetic ketoacidosis. J Pediatr 2007;150:467–73.
[29] Marcin JP, Glaser N, Barnett P, et al. Factors associated with adverse outcomes in children with diabetic ketoacidosis-related cerebral edema. J Pediatr 2002;141:793–7.
[30] Story DA, Morimatsu H, Bellomo R. Strong ions, weak acids and base excess: a simplified Fencl-Stewart approach to clinical acid-base disorders. Br J Anaesth 2004;92:54–60.

PEDIATRIC CLINICS
OF NORTH AMERICA

ELSEVIER
SAUNDERS
Pediatr Clin N Am 55 (2008) 589–604

In-Hospital Pediatric Cardiac Arrest

Marc D. Berg, MD[a],*, Vinay M. Nadkarni, MD[b,c,d],
Mathias Zuercher, MD[e,f], Robert A. Berg, MD[a]

[a]Division of Pediatric Critical Care Medicine, Department of Pediatrics, Steele Memorial
Research Center and Sarver Heart Center, The University of Arizona College of Medicine,
PO Box 245073, 1501 North Campbell Avenue, Tucson, AZ 85724, USA
[b]Department of Anesthesiology and Critical Care Medicine, The Children's Hospital
of Philadelphia, 34th Street and Civic Center Boulevard, Philadelphia,
PA 19104-4399, USA
[c]Center for Simulation, Advanced Education, and Innovation, The Children's Hospital
of Philadelphia, 34th Street and Civic Center Boulevard, Philadelphia,
PA 19104-4399, USA
[d]Center for Resuscitation Science, University of Pennsylvania School of Medicine,
Philadelphia, PA, USA
[e]Department of Anaesthesia and Intensive Care, University Hospital, Spitalstrasse 31,
CH–4031 Basel, Switzerland
[f]Sarver Heart Center, The University of Arizona College of Medicine,
1501 North Campbell Avenue, Tucson, AZ 85724, USA

Cardiac arrest is not rare in pediatric patients, occurring in 2% to 6% of children admitted to pediatric intensive care units (PICUs) [1,2]. The estimated frequency of pediatric out-of-hospital arrests is approximately 8 to 20 per 100,000 children per year [3,4]. Therefore, the rate of pediatric in-hospital cardiac arrests is approximately 100-fold higher than pediatric out-of-hospital arrests [5]. Although outcomes from pediatric cardiac arrests once were considered dismal [6,7], more recent data indicate that pediatric cardiopulmonary resuscitation (CPR) and advanced life support are saving many lives (Table 1). As many as two thirds of in-hospital pediatric cardiac arrest patients can be initially and successfully resuscitated [8–12] and more than 25% survive to hospital discharge.

* Corresponding author. Division of Pediatric Critical Care Medicine, Department of Pediatrics, Steele Children's Research Center and Sarver Heart Center, The University of Arizona College of Medicine, PO Box 245073, 1501 North Campbell Avenue, Tucson, AZ 85724.

E-mail address: marcb@peds.arizona.edu (M.D. Berg).

0031-3955/08/$ - see front matter © 2008 Elsevier Inc. All rights reserved.
doi:10.1016/j.pcl.2008.02.005
pediatric.theclinics.com

Table 1
Summary of representative studies of outcome after in-hospital pediatric cardiac arrest

Author, year	Setting	No. of patients	Return of spontaneous circulation	Survival to discharge	Good neurologic survival
Thiagarajan 2007 [69]	In-hospital, ECMO	682	N/A	(38%)	Not reported
Tibballs 2006 [70]	In-hospital	111	(73%)	(36%)	Not reported
Meaney 2006 [8]	All ICU patients <21	464	(50%)	(22%)	(14%)
Samson 2006 [12]	In-hospital CA (initial VF/VT rhythm)	272 (104)	(70%)	(35%)	(33%)
Nadkarni 2006 [9]	In-hospital CA	880	459 (52%)	236 (27%)	154 (18%)
Reis 2002 [11]	In-hospital CA	129	83 (64%)	21 (16%)	19 (15%)
Suominen 2000 [2]	In-hospital CA	118	74 (63%)	1-Year survival 21 (18%)	Not reported
Parra 2000 [10]	Ped CICU CA	32	24 (63%)	14 (44%)	8 (25%)
Rhodes 1999 [19]	In-hospital CA	34	23 (4%)	14 (2%)	Not reported
Young 1999 [3]	Meta-analysis in-hospital CA	544	Not reported	129 (24%)	Not reported
Slonim 1997 [1]	In-hospital PICU CA	205	Not reported	28 (14%)	Not reported
Torres 1997 [71]	In-hospital CA	92	Not reported	1-Year survival 9 (10%)	7 (8%)
Zaritsky 1987 [61]	In-hospital CA	CA 53	Not reported	CA 5 (9%)	Not reported
Hintz 2005 [72]	In-hospital CA resuscitation by ECMO	232	N/A all needed ECMO	88 (38%)	Not reported

Abbreviations: CA, cardiac arrest; N/A, not applicable; Ped CICU, pediatric cardiac intensive care unit.

Epidemiology of pediatric in-hospital cardiac arrest

The true incidence of pediatric pulseless arrest is difficult to estimate, because of inconsistent definitions and difficulty assessing pulselessness in children. The international Utstein guidelines for reporting cardiac arrest and CPR data were developed to provide consistent definitions and encourage standardized data acquisition. According to these guidelines, pulseless cardiac arrest is defined as the cessation of cardiac mechanical activity, determined by the absence of a palpable central pulse, unresponsiveness, and apnea.

Distinguishing severe hypoxic-ischemic shock with poor perfusion from the nonpulsatile state of cardiac arrest can be challenging in patients of any age. A rescuer's ability to make this determination by pulse check is neither sensitive nor specific in adults [13,14] and is more problematic in infants and children because of their smaller size and lower normal blood pressure [15–17]. In adults, pulses typically can be palpated until the systolic pressure is less than 50 mm Hg. Because the normal systolic blood pressure in neonates generally is in the 60s, a decrease in blood pressure to "nonpalpable pulse" may occur earlier in the continuum from hypotensive shock to nonpulsatile cardiac arrest. Nevertheless, children who are unresponsive, apneic, and pulseless as a result of severe hypotensive shock or cardiac arrest should be treated with prompt CPR.

Cardiac arrests are reported in 2% to 6% of all children admitted to PICUs [1,2,18] and in approximately 4% to 6% of children admitted to a cardiac PICU after cardiac surgery [10,19]. The most common causes of in-hospital cardiac arrests are respiratory failure (asphyxia) and circulatory shock (ischemia) [2,8,9,11,12,20,21]. Treatment of in-hospital pediatric cardiac arrest with CPR resulted in return of spontaneous circulation (ROSC) in approximately 43% to 64% of patients, and approximately 25% to 33% survived to hospital discharge (see Table 1) [2,8,9,11,12]. Almost three quarters of those who survived to hospital discharge have favorable neurologic outcomes.

More recently published reports of in-hospital pediatric cardiac arrests are derived from the American Heart Association's multicenter National Registry of Cardiopulmonary Resuscitation (NRCPR) [8,9,12,20]. The NRCPR is a prospective, multicenter observational registry of in-hospital cardiac arrests and resuscitations. The large size, scope, and quality of the NRCPR distinguish this North American data, which characterize the process and outcome of pediatric in-hospital CPR events. Summaries of these important characteristics are presented in Tables 2 and 3. Of NRCPR pediatric cardiac arrests, 95% were witnessed or monitored, 83% were monitored, and only 14% occurred on a general pediatric ward [9].

Outcomes after pediatric in-hospital cardiac arrests are superior to those after adult in-hospital cardiac arrests. Even though pediatric arrests less commonly are arrhythmogenic arrests resulting from ventricular tachycardia (VT)/ventricular fibrillation (VF) (14% of pediatric arrests versus 23% of adult arrests), 27% of the children survived to hospital discharge compared with 18% of the adults (odds ratio [OR] 2.29; 95% CI, 1.95–2.68) [9]. The superior overall pediatric survival rate reflected a substantially superior survival rate among children who had asystole or pulseless electrical activity (PEA) compared with adults who had asystole or PEA (24% versus 11%). Further investigations have shown that the superior survival rate among children predominantly is the result of better survival among infants and preschool children compared with older children or adults [8]. Perhaps the superior outcomes in the younger children in part are related to CPR resulting in better myocardial and cerebral blood flows in small children, who have compliant chest walls. In addition, survival from pediatric in-hospital CPR is more likely in hospitals staffed with pediatric physicians [20].

Table 2
Characteristics of pediatric in-hospital cardiac arrests (N = 880)

Age, year	
Mean (SD)	5.6 (6.4)
Median (range)	1.8 (0–17.0)
Gender	
Male	473 (54)
Female	407 (46)
Race/ethnicity (%)	
White	447 (51)
Black	226 (26)
Hispanic	105 (12)
Other/unknown	102 (12)
Patient type (%)	
In-patient	750 (85)
Emergency department	121 (14)
Other	9 (1)
Illness category	
Medical, noncardiac	402 (46)
Medical, cardiac	158 (18)
Surgical, cardiac	150 (17)
Trauma	91 (10)
Surgical, noncardiac	62 (7)
Other	17 (2)
Pre-existing conditions (%)	
Respiratory insufficiency	511 (58)
Hypotension/hypoperfusion	319 (36)
Congestive heart failure	273 (31)
Pneumonia/septicemia/other	259 (29)
Metabolic/electrolyte abnormality	178 (20)
Baseline depression in central nervous system function	151 (17)
Renal insufficiency	104 (12)
Major trauma	97 (11)
Acute central nervous system nonstroke event	94 (11)
None	69 (8)
Hepatic insufficiency	55 (6)
Metastatic or hematologic malignancy	43 (5)

Etiologic and pathophysiologic categories of cardiac arrest

Cardiac arrests can result from a multitude of pathophysiologic processes. The three most common causes and pathophysiologic categories of cardiac arrests are asphyxial arrests, ischemic arrests, and arrhythmogenic arrests. Asphyxial cardiac arrests are precipitated by acute hypoxia or hypercarbia. Ischemic arrests are precipitated by inadequate myocardial blood flow. For children, ischemic cardiac arrests most commonly are the result of systemic circulatory shock from hypovolemia, sepsis, or myocardial dysfunction (cardiogenic shock). Although coronary artery problems, such as aberrant left coronary artery, can lead to myocardial ischemia in children, they are less common causes of pediatric ischemic cardiac arrests than

Table 3
Event characteristics of pediatric in-hospital cardiac arrests

Characteristic	Pediatric cardiac arrest (N = 880)
Event location	
ICU	570 (65)
Emergency department	116 (13)
General inpatient	123 (14)
Diagnostic area	21 (2)
Outpatient, other, or unknown	20 (2)
Operating department or postanesthesia care unit	30 (3)
First-documented pulseless rhythm	
Asystole	350 (40)
VF and pulseless VT	120 (14)
VF	71 (8)
Pulseless VT	49 (6)
PEA	213 (24)
Unknown by documentation	197 (22)
Discovery status at time of event[a]	
Witnessed or monitored	834 (95)
Witnessed and monitored	727 (83)
Witnessed and not monitored	73 (8)
Monitored and not witnessed	34 (4)
Not monitored and not witnessed	46 (5)
Immediate causes of event	
Arrhythmia	392 (49)
Acute respiratory insufficiency	455 (57)
Hypotension	483 (61)
Metabolic/electrolyte disturbance	95 (12)
Acute pulmonary edema	33 (4)
Airway obstruction	41 (5)

Data are expressed as no. (%). Because of rounding, percentages may not all total 100. Totals do not sum to total number of pediatric patients for discovery status at time of event and immediate causes of event characteristics because patients have more than one characteristic.

[a] Monitored includes electrocardiogram, apnea or bradycardia, or pulse oximeter.

systemic circulatory shock. Finally, arrhythmogenic arrests are precipitated by VF or VT. In the NRCPR database, the immediate cause of the arrest was arrhythmogenic for 10%, asphyxial for 67%, and ischemic for 61% (some had both asphyxia and ischemia as immediate causes) [9,12].

Pediatric ventricular fibrillation and ventricular tachycardia

Although the rhythms during most in-hospital cardiac arrests (in children and adults) are asystole and PEA, in many arrests the rhythms are VF or pulseless VT [9]. Recent studies indicate that VF and VT (shockable rhythms) occur in 27% of in-hospital cardiac arrests at some time during the arrest and resuscitation [12]. Among pediatric cardiac ICU patients, as many as 41% of the arrests were associated with VF or VT [19]. Among the first 1005 pediatric in-hospital cardiac arrests in the American Heart Association's NRCPR, 10% had an initial rhythm of VF/VT, an additional 15% had subsequent VF/VT (ie, some time later during the resuscitation effort), and another 2% had VF/VT but the timing of the arrhythmia was not clear [12].

Arrhythmogenic ("electrical") cardiac arrests resulting from VF or pulseless VT occur most commonly in the setting of pre-existing heart disease, especially in the postoperative setting. Arrhythmogenic arrests can result from a multitude of congenital cardiac abnormalities and channelopathies associated with prolonged QT syndrome, familial cardiomyopathies (eg, hypertrophic, dilated, or arrhythmogenic right ventricle dysplasia), and mitochondrial diseases. In addition, VF and VT occur in the setting of acquired cardiomyopathies from drugs, toxins (eg, doxorubin cardiomyopathy), infections/myocarditis, electrolyte disturbances (eg, hyperkalemia), and commotio cordis or other mechanically induced VF.

In contrast to arrhythmogenic arrests, VF or VT can occur during resuscitation as subsequent VF/VT. For example, piglet animal models of asphyxial arrests demonstrate that VF often occurs during resuscitation even though the arrest initially was not arrhythmogenic and the first rhythm almost always is asystole or PEA. Asphyxia-associated VF also is well documented among pediatric drowning patients [22].

Traditionally, VF and VT have been considered "good" cardiac arrest rhythms, resulting in better outcomes than asystole and PEA. NRCPR data established, however, that survival to discharge was more common among children who had initial VF/VT than among children who had subsequent VF/VT (35% versus 11%; OR 2.6, 95% CI, 1.2–5.8) [12]. Surprisingly, the subsequent VF/VT group had worse outcomes than children who had asystole/PEA who never developed VF/VT during the resuscitation: 11% of children who had subsequent VF/VT (initial asystole/PEA followed by VF/VT during resuscitation) survived to hospital discharge versus 27% who had asystole/PEA alone. These data suggest that outcomes after initial VF/VT (an arrhythmogenic arrest) are "good," but outcomes after subsequent VF/VT (ie, VF/VT in the setting of an asphyxial or ischemic arrest) are substantially worse when compared with asystole/PEA rhythms.

Why was the outcome so poor in the subsequent VF/VT group? We do not yet know. Plausible explanations include (1) a delay in the diagnosis of subsequent VF/VT during the resuscitative effort, (2) adverse effects of resuscitative interventions (eg, too much epinephrine), or (3) subsequent VF/VT is an epiphenomenon (eg, a marker of severe underlying myocardial pathology).

Defibrillation (defined as termination of VF) is necessary for successful resuscitation from VF cardiac arrest. The goal of defibrillation is return of an organized electrical rhythm with a palpable pulse. When prompt defibrillation is provided soon after the induction of VF in a cardiac catheterization laboratory, the rates of successful defibrillation and survival approach 100%. When automated external defibrillators are used within 3 minutes of adult-witnessed VF, long-term survival can occur in more than 70% [23,24]. In general, mortality increases by 5% to 10% per minute of delay to defibrillation [25]. Early and effective chest compressions with minimal interruptions can maintain adequate coronary perfusion and slow the incremental increase in mortality with delayed defibrillation. Provision of high-quality CPR can improve outcome and save lives. Because pediatric cardiac arrests are commonly the result of progressive asphyxia or shock, the initial treatment of choice is prompt CPR, not defibrillation. Therefore, rhythm recognition has been de-emphasized compared with adult cardiac arrests. This historical emphasis must be counterbalanced by evidence that VF is not rare, outcomes from arrhythmogenic VF arrests are superior to other types of cardiac arrests, and early rhythm diagnosis is necessary for optimal care.

The four phases of cardiac arrest

Cardiac arrest may be categorized into four phases, each with unique physiology and treatment strategies: (1) prearrest, (2) no flow (untreated cardiac arrest), (3) low flow (CPR), and (4) post resuscitation.

The prearrest phase

The prearrest phase is the period before the arrest. The BRESUS study in the United Kingdom and the NRCPR data demonstrate that most in-hospital cardiac arrests are asphyxial or ischemic rather than sudden arrhythmia [9,26,27]. Many of these arrests could have been prevented by early recognition and treatment of respiratory failure and shock. This information has fueled interest in the development of medical emergency teams (or rapid response teams) to recognize and treat respiratory failure and circulatory shock before progression to cardiac arrest [28]. These issues were appreciated by the founders of the pediatric advanced life support course, designed to prevent cardiac arrests by early recognition and treatment of respiratory failure and shock in children [7]. In the prearrest phase, hospitalized children at high risk for a cardiac arrest should be in a monitored unit, where prompt diagnosis and treatment is available for respiratory failure, circulatory shock, and life-threatening arrhythmias.

The no-flow phase (untreated cardiac arrest)

Interventions during the no-flow phase of untreated pulseless cardiac arrest focus on early recognition of cardiac arrest and initiation of basic and advanced life support. To assure prompt diagnosis of cardiac arrest, children must be in a monitored unit with immediate health care provider availability. According to NRCPR data, 83% of pediatric in-hospital arrests were witnessed and the children were on monitors [9]. It is becoming increasingly clear that any in-hospital pediatric cardiac arrest that does not occur in a monitored unit should be evaluated as a potentially avoidable death.

The low-flow phase (cardiopulmonary resuscitation)

The goal of effective CPR is to optimize coronary and cerebral perfusion pressure and blood flow to critical organs during the low flow phase. Excellent quality basic life support with continuous effective chest compressions (ie, push hard, push fast, allow full chest recoil, and minimize interruptions) is the emphasis in this low-flow phase. During this phase, the only source of coronary and cerebral perfusion comes from the blood pressure generated by good chest compressions. Providing adequate coronary and cerebral perfusion pressure is critical for successful resuscitation. Any interruption, to perform procedures, analyze rhythms, check for pulses, or change rescuer position for ventilation, is potentially harmful [29]. For VF and pulseless VT, rapid determination of electrocardiographic rhythm and prompt defibrillation when appropriate are important. For cardiac arrests resulting from asphyxia or ischemia, provision of adequate myocardial perfusion and myocardial oxygen delivery with ventilation to match blood flow is important.

Despite evidence-based guidelines, extensive provider training, and provider credentialing in resuscitation medicine, the quality of CPR typically is poor. Slow compression rates, inadequate depth of compression, and substantial pauses are the norm [30–32]. Moreover, observed ventilation rates during professional rescuer CPR often are too high, potentially leading to deleterious effects on venous return and outcome [32,33]. The mantra must be, "Push hard, push fast, minimize interruptions, allow full chest recoil, and do not over-ventilate." This approach can markedly improve myocardial, cerebral, and systemic perfusion and likely will improve outcomes [34].

Although animal studies indicate that epinephrine can improve initial resuscitation success after asphyxial and VF cardiac arrests, no single medication is shown to improve survival to hospital discharge outcome from pediatric cardiac arrests. Medications commonly used for CPR in children are vasopressors (epinephrine or vasopressin), calcium chloride, sodium bicarbonate, and antiarrhythmics (amiodarone or lidocaine). During CPR, epinephrine's α-adrenergic effect increases systemic vascular resistance, increasing diastolic blood pressure, which in turn increases coronary perfusion pressure and blood flow and the likelihood of ROSC. Epinephrine also increases cerebral blood flow during CPR because peripheral vasoconstriction directs a greater proportion of flow to the cerebral circulation. The β-adrenergic effect increases myocardial contractility and heart rate and relaxes smooth muscle in the skeletal muscle vascular bed and bronchi although this effect is of less importance. Epinephrine also changes the character of VF (ie, higher amplitude, more "coarse"), increasing the likelihood of successful defibrillation.

High-dose epinephrine (0.05–0.2 mg/kg) improves myocardial and cerebral blood flow during CPR more than standard-dose epinephrine (0.01–0.02 mg/kg) and may increase the incidence of initial ROSC [35,36]. Prospective and retrospective studies indicate, however, that use of high-dose epinephrine in adults or children does not improve survival and may be associated with a worse neurologic outcome [37,38]. A randomized, blinded, controlled trial of rescue high-dose epinephrine after failed initial standard-dose epinephrine versus standard dose epinephrine for pediatric in-hospital cardiac arrest demonstrated a worse 24-hour survival in the high-dose epinephrine group (1/27 versus 6/23, $P < .05$) [39]. High-dose epinephrine cannot be recommended for routine use during CPR.

The postresuscitation phase

The post–cardiac arrest syndrome is a unique and complex combination of pathophysiologic processes that occurs after successful resuscitation. This post–cardiac arrest syndrome includes (1) post–cardiac arrest brain injury, (2) post–cardiac arrest myocardial dysfunction, (3) systemic ischemia/reperfusion response, and (4) the unresolved pathologic process that caused the cardiac arrest.

Clinical manifestations of post–cardiac arrest brain injury include coma, seizures, myoclonus, varying degrees of neurocognitive dysfunction (ranging from memory deficits to persistent vegetative state), and brain death. Mild induced hypothermia is the most well-established postresuscitation therapy for adult post–cardiac arrest brain injury. Two seminal articles established that induced hypothermia (32°C–34°C) could improve outcome for comatose adults after resuscitation from VF cardiac arrest [40,41]. In both randomized controlled trials, the inclusion criteria were patients older than 18 years who were persistently comatose after successful resuscitation from nontraumatic VF. Interpretation and extrapolation of these studies to children is difficult. Fever after cardiac arrest, brain trauma, stroke, and other ischemic conditions is associated with poor neurologic outcome. Hyperthermia after cardiac arrest is common in children [42]. It is reasonable to believe that mild induced systemic hypothermia may benefit children resuscitated from nontraumatic cardiac arrest. Benefit from this treatment, however, has not been rigorously studied and reported in children or in any patients who have had non-VF arrests. Emerging neonatal trials of selective brain cooling and systemic cooling show promise for this therapy in neonatal hypoxic-ischemic encephalopathy, suggesting that induced hypothermia may improve outcomes [43].

Post–cardiac arrest myocardial dysfunction and hypotensive shock are common among human survivors of cardiac arrest. For example, Laurent and colleagues [44] reported that 90 of 165 consecutive patients admitted to an ICU after successful resuscitation after an out-of-hospital cardiac arrest needed vasoactive infusions for hypotensive shock. Other studies have similarly demonstrated that LV dysfunction and hypotension are common among adult and pediatric survivors after cardiac arrests and generally are reversible among long-term survivors [40,41,45–49]. Postarrest myocardial dysfunction seems pathophysiologically similar to sepsis-related myocardial dysfunction, including increases in inflammatory mediators and nitric oxide production [44,46,47,50]. Although the optimal management of post–cardiac arrest hypotension and myocardial dysfunction are not defined, data suggest that aggressive hemodynamic support may improve outcomes. Controlled trials in animal models show that dobutamine, milrinone, or levosimendan can effectively ameliorate post–cardiac arrest myocardial dysfunction [51–55]. In clinical observational studies, fluid resuscitation has been provided for patients who have hypotension and concomitant low central venous pressure, and various vasoactive infusions, including epinephrine, dobutamine, and dopamine, have been provided for the myocardial dysfunction [40,41,45–49].

How should patients be managed in the postarrest setting? An organized multidisciplinary postresuscitation protocol that includes hemodynamic support, induced hypothermia, and percutaneous coronary intervention where indicated seems to improve outcomes in adults [49]. Post–cardiac arrest myocardial dysfunction and hemodynamic instability are common and should be anticipated. Therefore, continuous electrocardiographic and hemodynamic monitoring should be provided for all patients after successful resuscitation from a cardiac arrest. Furthermore, postarrest echocardiography should be considered for monitoring myocardial function. General critical care principles suggest that appropriate therapeutic goals are adequate blood pressure and adequate myocardial, cerebral, and systemic blood flows and oxygen delivery. The definition of "adequate" is elusive, however. Reasonable interventions for vasodilatory shock with low central venous pressure include fluid resuscitation and vasoactive infusions. Appropriate considerations for left ventricular myocardial dysfunction include euvolemia, inotropic infusions, and afterload reduction. The available evidence for many of these recommendations is taken from the adult critical care literature; the entire field of postresuscitation care, in adult and pediatric patients, is ripe for further study.

Extracorporeal membrane oxygenation cardiopulmonary resuscitation

The use of venoarterial extracorporeal membrane oxygenation (ECMO) to re-establish circulation and provide controlled reperfusion after cardiac arrest has been published, but prospective, controlled studies are lacking. Nevertheless, these series have reported extraordinary results with the use of ECMO as a rescue therapy for pediatric cardiac arrests, especially from potentially reversible acute postoperative myocardial dysfunction or arrhythmia [10,56–59]. In one study, 11 children who suffered cardiac arrest in the PICU after cardiac surgery were placed on ECMO during CPR after 20 to 110 minutes of CPR. Prolonged CPR was continued until ECMO cannulae, circuits, and personnel were available. Six of these 11 children were long-term survivors who had no apparent neurologic sequelae. Most remarkably, Morris and coworkers reported 66 children who were placed on ECMO during CPR over 7 years [59]. In this single institution study, the median duration of CPR before establishment of ECMO was 50 minutes, and 35% (23/66) of these children survived to hospital discharge. These children had brief periods of "no flow," excellent CPR during the "low flow" period, and a well-controlled postresuscitation phase. CPR and ECMO are not curative treatments. They simply are cardiopulmonary supportive measures that may allow tissue perfusion and viability until recovery from the precipitating disease process.

When should cardiopulmonary resuscitation be discontinued?

Several factors determine the likelihood of survival after cardiac arrest, including the mechanism of the arrest (eg, traumatic or asphyxial), location (eg, out-of-hospital versus in-hospital or ward versus PICU), response (eg, monitored versus unmonitored or witnessed versus unwitnessed), and underlying pathophysiology (eg, cardiomyopathy, congenital defect, single ventricle physiology, drug toxicity, or metabolic derangement). Additionally, discontinuation of resuscitation in the prehospital setting is further complicated as the environment may not be conducive to making such an important decision. A study of emergency medical system providers found most to be uncomfortable discontinuing CPR of pediatric patients in cardiac arrest before transport to the hospital [60]. These factors all should be considered before deciding to terminate resuscitative efforts. Continuation of CPR has been considered futile beyond 15 to 20 minutes of CPR or when more than two doses of epinephrine are needed [61–63]. Monitoring children in the prearrest phase, prompt CPR to minimize the no-flow phase, excellent CPR quality during the low-flow phase, and excellent critical care management in the postresuscitation phase seem to have improved outcomes from cardiac arrests. Survival with good outcomes is increasingly common despite greater than 15 minutes of CPR and more than two doses of epinephrine [9–11,56–59,64–68]. The age-old question, "When should we stop?" does not seem to have an easy answer.

Summary

In many ways this is the Golden Age of CPR research. Through the work of several CPR pioneers, most of whom still are actively involved in CPR research, a greater understanding has been gained in many areas. In the past, the concept of evidence-based pediatric cardiac arrest recommendations seemed fanciful. Recommendations were based on extrapolated animal and adult data. These approaches no longer are acceptable. The past 2 decades have brought advances in understanding the pathophysiology of cardiac arrest and VF, better treatment strategies (eg, emphasis on chest compressions before defibrillation for prolonged out-of-hospital cardiac arrests), and a more robust standard for CPR research reporting with the development and acceptance of the Utstein criteria. Moreover, rigorous methodology is improving outcomes at the intersection of CPR science and practical application with the advent of public access defibrillation and a greater emphasis on teaching techniques and CPR performance. Evolving understanding of the pathophysiology of events and titration of the interventions to the timing, etiology, duration, and intensity of the cardiac arrest event can improve resuscitation outcomes. Interventions increasingly are tailored to the phase of cardiac arrest and the etiopathophysiology (ie, arrhythmogenic versus asphyxial versus ischemic arrests). Outcomes from pediatric cardiac arrest and CPR seem to be improving from less than 10% survival in the 1970s to 27% survival in the NRCPR data in the twenty-first century.

Exciting discoveries in basic and applied science are on the immediate horizon for study in specific populations of cardiac arrest victims. By strategically focusing therapies to specific phases of cardiac arrest and resuscitation and to evolving pathophysiology, there is great promise that critical care interventions will lead the way to more successful CPR and cerebral resuscitation in children. Treatment of sudden death in children in the future requires more evidence-based and less anecdotal interventions. Emerging technology interfaced with evolving teams and systems of postresuscitative care likely will facilitate high quality interventions and ensure optimal odds for survival.

New epidemiologic initiatives, such as the NRCPR for in-hospital cardiac arrests and the large-scale, multicenter National Heart, Lung, and Blood Institute Resuscitation Outcome Consortium for out-of-hospital arrests, are providing new data to guide resuscitation practices and generate hypotheses for new approaches to improve outcomes. Excellent basic life support often is not provided. Innovative technical advances, such as directive and corrective real-time feedback, can increase the likelihood of effective basic life support. In addition, team dynamic training and debriefing can improve self-efficacy and operational performance substantially. Mechanical interventions, such as ECMO or other cardiopulmonary bypass systems, already are used in many centers during prolonged in-hospital pediatric cardiac arrests.

Clinical trials are necessary for appropriate evidence-based recommendations for the treatment of pediatric cardiac arrest. The first successful randomized, controlled, blinded trial of any pediatric cardiac arrest intervention was completed and published in the twenty-first century [39]. Evidence-based pediatric cardiac arrest therapeutics will be based on randomized controlled trails of important interventions. It is likely that the evolution of systems, such as cardiac arrest centers, similar to trauma, stroke, and myocardial infarction centers, will help direct children who require specialized postresuscitation care to centers best able to provide this.

References

[1] Slonim AD, Patel KM, Ruttimann UE, et al. Cardiopulmonary resuscitation in pediatric intensive care units. Crit Care Med 1951;25:1997.

[2] Suominen P, Olkkola KT, Voipio V, et al. Utstein style reporting of in-hospital paediatric cardiopulmonary resuscitation. Resuscitation 2000;45:17.

[3] Young KD, Seidel JS. Pediatric cardiopulmonary resuscitation: a collective review. Ann Emerg Med 1999;33:195.

[4] Donoghue AJ, Nadkarni V, Berg RA, et al. Out-of-hospital pediatric cardiac arrest: an epidemiologic review and assessment of current knowledge. Ann Emerg Med 2005;46:512.

[5] Morris MC, Nadkarni VM. Pediatric cardiopulmonary-cerebral resuscitation: an overview and future directions. Crit Care Clin 2003;19:337.

[6] Guidelines for cardiopulmonary resuscitation and emergency cardiac care. Emergency Cardiac Care Committee and Subcommittees, American Heart Association. Part VI. Pediatric advanced life support. JAMA 1992;268:2262.

[7] Callas PW. Textbook of pediatric advanced life support. Dallas (TX): American Heart Association; 1988.

[8] Meaney PA, Nadkarni VM, Cook EF, et al. Higher survival rates among younger patients after pediatric intensive care unit cardiac arrests. Pediatrics 2006;118:2424.

[9] Nadkarni VM, Larkin GL, Peberdy MA, et al. First documented rhythm and clinical outcome from in-hospital cardiac arrest among children and adults. JAMA 2006;295:50.

[10] Parra DA, Totapally BR, Zahn E, et al. Outcome of cardiopulmonary resuscitation in a pediatric cardiac intensive care unit. Crit Care Med 2000;28:3296.

[11] Reis AG, Nadkarni V, Perondi MB, et al. A prospective investigation into the epidemiology of in-hospital pediatric cardiopulmonary resuscitation using the international Utstein reporting style. Pediatrics 2002;109:200.

[12] Samson RA, Nadkarni VM, Meaney PA, et al. Outcomes of in-hospital ventricular fibrillation in children. N Engl J Med 2006;354:2328.

[13] Eberle B, Dick WF, Schneider T, et al. Checking the carotid pulse check: diagnostic accuracy of first responders in patients with and without a pulse. Resuscitation 1996;33:107.

[14] Moule P. Checking the carotid pulse: diagnostic accuracy in students of the healthcare professions. Resuscitation 2000;44:195.

[15] Cavallaro DL, Melker RJ. Comparison of two techniques for detecting cardiac activity in infants. Crit Care Med 1983;11:189.

[16] Inagawa G, Morimura N, Miwa T, et al. A comparison of five techniques for detecting cardiac activity in infants. Paediatr Anaesth 2003;13:141.

[17] Lee CJ, Bullock LJ. Determining the pulse for infant CPR: time for a change? Mil Med 1991; 156:190.

[18] Kuisma M, Suominen P, Korpela R. Paediatric out-of-hospital cardiac arrests: epidemiology and outcome. Resuscitation 1995;30:141.

[19] Rhodes JF, Blaufox AD, Seiden HS, et al. Cardiac arrest in infants after congenital heart surgery. Circulation 1999;100:II194.

[20] Donoghue AJ, Nadkarni VM, Elliott M, et al. Effect of hospital characteristics on outcomes from pediatric cardiopulmonary resuscitation: a report from the national registry of cardiopulmonary resuscitation. Pediatrics 2006;118:995.

[21] Skrifvars MB, Saarinen K, Ikola K, et al. Improved survival after in-hospital cardiac arrest outside critical care areas. Acta Anaesthesiol Scand 2005;49:1534.

[22] Graf WD, Cummings P, Quan L, et al. Predicting outcome in pediatric submersion victims. Ann Emerg Med 1995;26:312.

[23] Caffrey SL, Willoughby PJ, Pepe PE, et al. Public use of automated external defibrillators. N Engl J Med 2002;347:1242.

[24] Valenzuela TD, Roe DJ, Nichol G, et al. Outcomes of rapid defibrillation by security officers after cardiac arrest in casinos [see comments]. N Engl J Med 2000;343:1206.

[25] Larsen MP, Eisenberg MS, Cummins RO, et al. Predicting survival from out-of-hospital cardiac arrest: a graphic model. Ann Emerg Med 1993;22:1652.

[26] Peberdy MA, Kaye W, Ornato JP, et al. Cardiopulmonary resuscitation of adults in the hospital: a report of 14720 cardiac arrests from the National Registry of Cardiopulmonary Resuscitation. Resuscitation 2003;58:297.

[27] Tunstall-Pedoe H, Bailey L, Chamberlain DA, et al. Survey of 3765 cardiopulmonary resuscitations in British hospitals (the BRESUS Study): methods and overall results. BMJ 1992; 304:1347.

[28] Brilli RJ, Gibson R, Luria JW, et al. Implementation of a medical emergency team in a large pediatric teaching hospital prevents respiratory and cardiopulmonary arrests outside the intensive care unit. Pediatr Crit Care Med 2007;8:236.

[29] Berg RA, Sanders AB, Kern KB, et al. Adverse hemodynamic effects of interrupting chest compressions for rescue breathing during cardiopulmonary resuscitation for ventricular fibrillation cardiac arrest. Circulation 2001;104:2465.

[30] Abella BS, Alvarado JP, Myklebust H, et al. Quality of cardiopulmonary resuscitation during in-hospital cardiac arrest. JAMA 2005;293:305.

[31] Berg RA, Sanders AB, Milander M, et al. Efficacy of audio-prompted rate guidance in improving resuscitator performance of cardiopulmonary resuscitation on children. Acad Emerg Med 1994;1:35.

[32] Milander MM, Hiscok PS, Sanders AB, et al. Chest compression and ventilation rates during cardiopulmonary resuscitation: the effects of audible tone guidance. Acad Emerg Med 1995; 2:708.

[33] Aufderheide TP, Sigurdsson G, Pirrallo RG, et al. Hyperventilation-induced hypotension during cardiopulmonary resuscitation. Circulation 2004;109:1960.

[34] Edelson DP, Abella BS, Kramer-Johansen J, et al. Effects of compression depth and pre-shock pauses predict defibrillation failure during cardiac arrest. Resuscitation 2006;71:137.

[35] Brown CG, Martin DR, Pepe PE, et al. A comparison of standard-dose and high-dose epinephrine in cardiac arrest outside the hospital. The Multicenter High-Dose Epinephrine Study Group. N Engl J Med 1992;327:1051.

[36] Lindner KH, Ahnefeld FW, Bowdler IM. Comparison of different doses of epinephrine on myocardial perfusion and resuscitation success during cardiopulmonary resuscitation in a pig model. Am J Emerg Med 1991;9:27.

[37] Behringer W, Kittler H, Sterz F, et al. Cumulative epinephrine dose during cardiopulmonary resuscitation and neurologic outcome. Ann Intern Med 1998;129:450.

[38] Callaham M, Madsen C, Barton C, et al. A randomized clinical trial of high-dose epinephrine and norepinephrine versus standard-dose epinephrine in prehospital cardiac arrest. JAMA 1992;268:2667.

[39] Perondi MB, Reis AG, Paiva EF, et al. A comparison of high-dose and standard-dose epinephrine in children with cardiac arrest. N Engl J Med 2004;350:1722.

[40] (HACA) HACASG. Mild therapeutic hypothermia to improve the neurologic outcome after cardiac arrest. N Engl J Med 2002;346:549.

[41] Bernard SA, Gray TW, Buist MD, et al. Treatment of comatose survivors of out-of-hospital cardiac arrest with induced hypothermia. N Engl J Med 2002;346:557.

[42] Hickey RW, Kochanek PM, Ferimer H, et al. Hypothermia and hyperthermia in children after resuscitation from cardiac arrest. Pediatrics 2000;106(pt 1):118.

[43] Gluckman PD, Wyatt JS, Azzopardi D, et al. Selective head cooling with mild systemic hypothermia after neonatal encephalopathy: multicentre randomised trial. Lancet 2005; 365:663.

[44] Laurent I, Monchi M, Chiche JD, et al. Reversible myocardial dysfunction in survivors of out-of-hospital cardiac arrest. J Am Coll Cardiol 2002;40:2110.

[45] Mullner M, Domanovits H, Sterz F, et al. Measurement of myocardial contractility following successful resuscitation: quantitated left ventricular systolic function utilising non-invasive wall stress analysis. Resuscitation 1998;39:51.

[46] Adrie C, Adib-Conquy M, Laurent I, et al. Successful cardiopulmonary resuscitation after cardiac arrest as a "sepsis-like" syndrome. Circulation 2002;106:562.

[47] Laurent I, Adrie C, Vinsonneau C, et al. High-volume hemofiltration after out-of-hospital cardiac arrest: a randomized study. J Am Coll Cardiol 2005;46:432.

[48] Ruiz-Bailen M, Aguayo de Hoyos E, Ruiz-Navarro S, et al. Reversible myocardial dysfunction after cardiopulmonary resuscitation. Resuscitation 2005;66:175.

[49] Sunde K, Pytte M, Jacobsen D, et al. Implementation of a standardised treatment protocol for post resuscitation care after out-of-hospital cardiac arrest. Resuscitation 2007;73:29.

[50] Niemann JT, Garner D, Lewis RJ. Tumor necrosis factor-alpha is associated with early postresuscitation myocardial dysfunction. Crit Care Med 2004;32:1753.

[51] Kern KB, Hilwig RW, Berg RA, et al. Postresuscitation left ventricular systolic and diastolic dysfunction. Treatment with dobutamine. Circulation 1997;95:2610.

[52] Meyer RJ, Kern KB, Berg RA, et al. Post-resuscitation right ventricular dysfunction: delineation and treatment with dobutamine. Resuscitation 2002;55:187.

[53] Niemann JT, Garner D, Khaleeli E, et al. Milrinone facilitates resuscitation from cardiac arrest and attenuates postresuscitation myocardial dysfunction. Circulation 2003;108:3031.

[54] Vasquez A, Kern KB, Hilwig RW, et al. Optimal dosing of dobutamine for treating post-resuscitation left ventricular dysfunction. Resuscitation 2004;61:199.

[55] Huang L, Weil MH, Tang W, et al. Comparison between dobutamine and levosimendan for management of postresuscitation myocardial dysfunction. Crit Care Med 2005;33:487.

[56] Dalton HJ, Siewers RD, Fuhrman BP, et al. Extracorporeal membrane oxygenation for cardiac rescue in children with severe myocardial dysfunction. Crit Care Med 1993;21: 1020.

[57] del Nido PJ, Dalton HJ, Thompson AE, et al. Extracorporeal membrane oxygenator rescue in children during cardiac arrest after cardiac surgery. Circulation 1992;86(Suppl):II300.

[58] Thalmann M, Trampitsch E, Haberfellner N, et al. Resuscitation in near drowning with extracorporeal membrane oxygenation. Ann Thorac Surg 2001;72:607.

[59] Morris MC, Wernovsky G, Nadkarni VM. Survival outcomes after extracorporeal cardio-pulmonary resuscitation instituted during active chest compressions following refractory in-hospital pediatric cardiac arrest. Pediatr Crit Care Med 2004;5:440.

[60] Hall WL 2nd, Myers JH, Pepe PE, et al. The perspective of paramedics about on-scene termination of resuscitation efforts for pediatric patients. Resuscitation 2004;60:175.

[61] Zaritsky A. Cardiopulmonary resuscitation in children. Clin Chest Med 1987;8:561.

[62] Innes PA, Summers CA, Boyd IM, et al. Audit of paediatric cardiopulmonary resuscitation. Arch Dis Child 1993;68:487.

[63] Schindler MB, Bohn D, Cox PN, et al. Outcome of out-of-hospital cardiac or respiratory arrest in children. N Engl J Med 1996;335:1473.

[64] Athanasuleas CL, Buckberg GD, Allen BS, et al. Sudden cardiac death: directing the scope of resuscitation towards the heart and brain. Resuscitation 2006;70:44.

[65] Yu HY, Yeh HL, Wang SS, et al. Ultra long cardiopulmonary resuscitation with intact cerebral performance for an asystolic patient with acute myocarditis. Resuscitation 2007; 73:307.

[66] Chen YS, Chao A, Yu HY, et al. Analysis and results of prolonged resuscitation in cardiac arrest patients rescued by extracorporeal membrane oxygenation. J Am Coll Cardiol 2003; 41:197.

[67] Grogaard HK, Wik L, Eriksen M, et al. Continuous mechanical chest compressions during cardiac arrest to facilitate restoration of coronary circulation with percutaneous coronary intervention. J Am Coll Cardiol 2007;50:1093.

[68] Lopez-Herce J, Garcia C, Dominguez P, et al. Characteristics and outcome of cardiorespiratory arrest in children. Resuscitation 2004;63:311.

[69] Thiagarajan RR, Laussen PC, Rycus PT, et al. Extracorporeal membrane oxygenation to aid cardiopulmonary resuscitation in infants and children. Circulation 2007;116:1693.

[70] Tibballs J, Kinney S. A prospective study of outcome of in-patient paediatric cardiopulmonary arrest. Resuscitation 2006;71:310.

[71] Torres A Jr, Pickert CB, Firestone J, et al. Long-term functional outcome of inpatient pediatric cardiopulmonary resuscitation. Pediatr Emerg Care 1997;13:369.

[72] Hintz SR, Benitz WE, Colby CE, et al. Utilization and outcomes of neonatal cardiac extracorporeal life support: 1996–2000. Pediatr Crit Care Med 2005;6:33.

ELSEVIER
SAUNDERS

PEDIATRIC CLINICS
OF NORTH AMERICA

Pediatr Clin N Am 55 (2008) 605–616

The Psychologic Impact on Children of Admission to Intensive Care

Gillian Colville, MPhil[a,b,*]

[a]*St. George's University of London, London, UK*
[b]*Paediatric Psychology Service, St. Georges Hospital, 2nd Floor Clare House,
Blackshaw Road, London SW17 0QT, UK*

In the first issue of the *Pediatric Clinics of North America* to cover the topic of pediatric intensive care, Rothstein [1] described our knowledge of the psychologic impact of critical illness on the child and family as "still quite rudimentary." Nearly 3 decades later we have a much better understanding of the impact on the family [2–4] yet relatively little is known about children's understanding of what happens to them or their longer-term psychologic recovery, despite the increasing numbers of children going through this experience (estimated at more than 200,000 annually in the United States, on the basis of recent admission rates [5]). In this article the current evidence on the psychologic impact on children of admission to the pediatric intensive care unit (PICU) is reviewed.

Literature review

Following consideration of the methodologic difficulties inherent in this field, the available evidence relating to the following questions is examined:

What do children remember about their time on the PICU?
What is the evidence that they suffer short-term distress?
What is the evidence that they suffer long-term distress?
Which variables are associated with poorer psychologic outcome?

Summaries of the main characteristics of the most recent studies discussed are provided in Tables 1 and 2. Other studies of heterogeneous PICU samples, performed before 2000, are also referred to as appropriate,

_____

* Paediatric Psychology Service, St. Georges Hospital, 2nd Floor Clare House, Blackshaw Road, London SW17 0QT, UK.
E-mail address: g.colville@sgul.ac.uk

0031-3955/08/$ - see front matter © 2008 Elsevier Inc. All rights reserved.
doi:10.1016/j.pcl.2008.02.006   *pediatric.theclinics.com*

Table 1
Recent studies of children's memories of the pediatric intensive care unit

First author	Date	n	Country	Age range	Length of follow-up	Informant	Main findings
Playfor [10]	2000	38	United Kingdom	4–16 y	2 d to 4 mo	Child	66% remembered PICU; recollections predominantly neutral; two reports of strange dreams
Colville [11]	2004	15	United Kingdom	7–15 y	8 mo	Child	13/15 had some memory; 2 children recalled nightmares
Karande [12]	2005	50	India	5–12 y	<5 d	Child	100% remembered PICU; 74% reported pain; 26% saw dead body
Board [13]	2005	21	United States	7–12 y	24 h	Child	67% remembered something; 33% remembered invasive procedures
Colville [14]	2006	102	United Kingdom	7–17 y	3 mo	Child	63% report factual memory; 32% report delusional memory; delusional memory associated with duration of sedation

Table 2
Recent studies of children's behavior and distress after pediatric intensive care

First author	Date	n	Country	Age range	Length of follow-up	Informant	Main findings
Rennick [19]	2002	60 + 60 controls	Canada	6–17 y	6 wk; 6 mo	Child	No differences between groups
Colville [24]	2004	48	United Kingdom	0–15 y	8 mo	Parent	No evidence of elevated behavior problems but 60% mothers reported change in relationship
Colville [11]	2004	15	United Kingdom	6–15 y	8 mo	Child	27% children report significant PTS but also report fewer fears
Rees [17]	2004	19 + 27 controls	United Kingdom	5–18 y	7 mo	Child	21% PICU children reporting PTS versus 0% general patients
Rennick [18]	2004	60	Canada	6–17 y	6 wk; 6 mo	Child	Invasiveness of treatment associated with PTS
Board [13]	2005	21	United States	7–12 y	24 h	Child	Intubated children used fewer coping strategies; anxiety associated with lack of memory
Small [21]	2006	163	United States	2–7 y	3 mo; 6 mo	Parent	Negative behavior associated with maternal anxiety, marital status, previous behavior, and child age
Colville [14]	2006	102	United Kingdom	7–17 y	3 mo	Child	27% reporting significant levels of PTS; main predictors were emergency admission and delusional memory

Abbreviation: PTS, posttraumatic stress.

but research relating to specific subgroups of PICU patients (eg, cardiac patients) is not included.

Methodologic difficulties

Truog [6] has emphasized the need for more research on the child's experience of critical care but this work is difficult to do for several reasons. By definition, children in the PICU are critically ill. It is therefore not usually possible to talk to them acutely because they are unconscious or heavily sedated. Also, although the age range of patients treated in the PICU is 0 to 18 years, most children admitted are younger than 2 years of age [7], which has implications for direct communication with children and the assessment of their psychologic distress.

Furthermore, there are clearly ethical issues about approaching families to take part in research while they are still in the PICU, when they are easiest to locate, because the child may die during admission and also has an elevated risk of death after discharge. Ethics committees are also traditionally reluctant for families to be approached after traumatic events, although there is mounting evidence that people taking part in such research do not regret it later and may even find it therapeutic [8,9]. Even when the child is out of immediate danger, parents' ability to give informed consent could be questioned on the grounds of their high levels of anxiety. They are also understandably protective of their children and consequently not always prepared to involve them in research, particularly if they realize this will involve discussion of traumatic events.

Longitudinal follow-up work is especially difficult because PICUs tend to be sited in large hospitals in urban centers, with the result that the distances families live from units are sometimes substantial. Many families have limited means [2,7] and so have limited access to resources, such as private transport; therefore it is not easy for some families to attend regular follow-up appointments at the base hospital.

What do children remember about their time in the pediatric intensive care unit?

Four recent cross-sectional studies have looked specifically at what children remember about their time in the PICU. Playfor and colleagues [10] interviewed 38 children about what they remembered and found that two thirds remembered something about their admission. However, although a third remembered being in pain and a couple reported having had nightmares at the time, few remembered being intubated. Given their findings that most children's recollections were neutral, the authors propose that their lack of recall for negative experiences in the PICU may protect against development of posttraumatic stress, citing the specific amnesic effect of benzodiazepines in this context. Colville [11], however, in interviews with

15 children 8 months after discharge, found that several did not fully understand what had happened to them and were not, as the authors of the previous study had supposed, reassured by their lack of memory. In fact 6 children said they would like to revisit the unit to try to see if they could remember more:

> "I think I lost about 2 or 3 weeks." (13-year-old girl, spinal surgery)

> "Most of the time, it felt like I was going asleep for two minutes, then waking up—it felt like—days later. When I woke up, I asked my mum if I was dead—all I could see was white." (15-year-old girl, epilepsy)

It was also striking how clearly some children remembered disturbing dreams so many months later:

> "I had this really horrible dream, ...there was these three men ...and they put this ladder up and they got into our room and they gave us all this glue stuff ... and I went and I told daddy and he said 'Don't be silly, they are just repair men' ... but they had poisoned us." (9-year-old girl, cancer)

> "I fell asleep and dad was holding my hand, and then I saw these people getting their heads chopped off." (11-year-old boy, asthma)

In another study of children's recollections of the PICU performed in a unit in India [12] with a much higher mortality rate ($>30\%$), children's reports of being disturbed by pain and by witnessing the fate of other patients led to changes in the unit's protocols regarding sedation and analgesia. In contrast, and possibly reflecting different sedation practices, Board [13] found in interviews with 21 children the day after discharge that although most children remembered something about the PICU, only a third remembered invasive procedures and many had positive recollections of staff and family.

Finally, in a larger study (n = 102) in the United Kingdom, Colville and colleagues [14] found that 1 in 3 reported delusional memories, such as nightmares or hallucinations, which they could still vividly recall 3 months after discharge. Although most children in this study (63%) remembered something factual of their PICU stay (see Fig. 1 for an example of what one child remembered of his stay), their memories were fragmented, with only 20% remembering being intubated.

What is the evidence that they suffer short-term distress?

The largest study to date of children's behavior while still in the PICU remains that of Cataldo and colleagues [15], who made a series of 708 structured behavioral observations of 99 patients. Although more than half of this sample were asleep or heavily sedated, one third were awake and alert, but for the most part disengaged with their environment. A subsequent, and often quoted, observational study by Jones and Fiser [16] in 1992 found that PICU patients (n = 18) exhibited higher levels of distress than other pediatric patients in the days immediately following extubation. Board [13], in

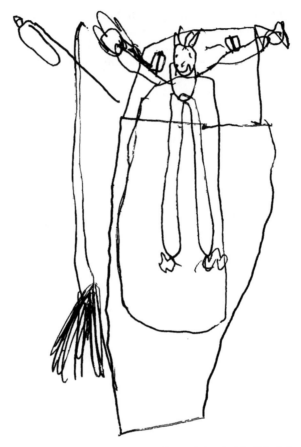

Fig. 1. Drawing of the PICU by a 7-year-old boy admitted with diabetic ketoacidosis.

contrast, reporting more recently on direct interviews with 21 children inter-viewed the day after discharge, did not find high levels of anxiety in the chil-dren in her sample but noted that they were still spending long periods asleep at this stage.

What evidence is there that they suffer long-term distress?

Rees and colleagues [17] in a cross-sectional cohort study 7 months after discharge found significant rates of posttraumatic stress in 19 PICU patients in clinical interviews. One in 5 children reported clinically significant levels of posttraumatic stress and, in particular, elevated rates of avoidance. Colville and colleagues found similar rates of posttraumatic stress in two separate in-terview studies at 3 and 8 months after discharge [11,14]. Another group fol-lowing a sample (n = 60) at two separate time points by postal survey found, worryingly, that most children who had significant levels of posttraumatic stress at 6 weeks were still reporting high levels at 6 months [18].

There are mixed findings regarding comparisons with rates of distress in control samples of pediatric patients. Rees and colleagues [17] found a significant difference between groups, with no child in the control group meeting criteria for a diagnosis of posttraumatic stress disorder. Rennick and colleagues [19] found no differences between groups, however, echoing the earlier work by Youngblut and Shiao [20] who found, 2 to 4 weeks after discharge from the PICU, that parental report of behavior problems was similar to that reported in other studies of other hospitalized children.

Finally, there is also evidence that some patients believe they have changed in positive as well as negative ways as a result of their experiences. In particular, children in one study reported lower numbers of childhood fears than age- and sex-matched peers [11] and this quantitative finding was reinforced by their comments:

"I am a bit more grown up." (9-year-old girl, cancer)

"Now when I get a cut, it is just nothing. I am not as scared as I was." (13-year-old girl, abdominal surgery)

Which variables are associated with poorer child psychologic outcome?

Several authors have found an association between premorbid behavior problems and the development of distress after being in the PICU [16,21], but for the most part studies have not found a clear relationship between the severity of illness, whether measured by length of stay or standardized mortality risk. The degree of life threat perceived by either the child or the parent has, however, been found to be associated with later distress in the child [17], just as the parent's perception of the likelihood of the child dying is significantly correlated with their own stress at long-term follow up [22].

Rennick and colleagues [18] found younger children and those who had undergone more invasive procedures reported more distress at follow-up at 6 weeks. The effect of age had diminished by 6 months postdischarge, but the effect of the number of invasive procedures had not. However, the authors did not demonstrate that the children remembered these invasive procedures and the evidence from studies of children's memories would suggest that many do not, so a simple association between memory for PICU procedures and subsequent development of posttraumatic stress cannot be assumed.

Despite previous anecdotal reports of a link between emergency intubation and posttraumatic stress [23], no such association has been found in more systematic studies, not least because of the small numbers of children actually remembering being intubated, although Board [13] did find that children intubated for longer time reported using fewer coping strategies on the general ward after discharge. Perhaps counterintuitively this study also found that children who did not remember their admission were more anxious than those who did. This finding was echoed by the observation that two of the four children who had clinically significant levels of posttraumatic stress at follow-up in another study reported no factual memories of the PICU at all [11].

The evidence for a link with delusional memory is stronger. An interview study of 102 children [14] found a significant independent association between duration of sedation/analgesia and child's report of delusional memories, including hallucinations. The presence of delusional memory was in turn related to posttraumatic stress symptoms, and in particular intrusive thoughts, at 3 months. This last finding is consistent with earlier work demonstrating higher rates of observable anxiety in children receiving more sedative agents [16].

Another finding reported in several studies is that of a relationship between child and parent distress, although the direction of this relationship and the mechanisms underlying it are not well understood. Rees and colleagues [17] found an association between child and parent posttraumatic stress scores and Small and Melnyk [21], in a secondary analysis of a longitudinal intervention study, found that maternal anxiety within the first 24 hours predicted negative behavioral outcome in children at 3 and at 6 months. These findings suggest that parents' own emotional state during admission may impact negatively on the child's psychologic recovery. This possibility was acknowledged in a follow-up study, in which 48 mothers were surveyed about the long-term impact of admission [24]. Although for the most part they did not believe their child had changed, 60% believed their relationship with their child continued to be affected by the stress they had experienced on the PICU, 8 months after the child's discharge:

> "I just feel my whole life revolves around just making sure (child) is OK." (Mother of 1-month-old girl, bowel surgery)

> "I don't let him to go to sleep on his own and I think that is definitely from intensive care. I wake up the second he makes a noise." (Mother of 1-year-old boy, meningitis)

Discussion

In summary there is mounting evidence that a significant minority of children suffer lasting psychologic problems following their treatment in the PICU. The recent evidence is particularly compelling because, in the past 10 years, greater research effort has been directed at eliciting information directly from the children themselves, rather than relying solely on either observed behavior or parent report. Also there is now a growing evidence base on the long-term psychologic reactions of these children, quantified using standardized psychologic measures, with less reliance being placed on anecdotal report in this field. Reports of children's recollections have not usually been combined with follow-up measures of distress in the longer term, however, making it difficult to determine what it is about the child's subjective experience of the PICU that puts them at most risk for a poor psychologic outcome. Another significant gap in the literature remains the description of the behavior of children aged less than 5 years, which is especially important given the high proportion of infants on the PICU [7].

The levels of posttraumatic stress symptoms reported by older children suggest that this is a population at risk that should be more routinely screened and monitored, given that there are established treatments available [25]. In this context, the importance of asking children directly about their symptoms has been stressed by researchers who have found a tendency for parents' own levels of posttraumatic stress to affect their estimations of their child's distress [26–28].

The association between parental and child psychologic state also warrants further investigation. The seminal work of Carter and Miles [29] has shown that it is the interpersonal aspects of the PICU experience, such as the impact on parent's role, that are experienced as most stressful by parents during admission, and we now know that parents exhibit elevated distress levels in relation to their experiences for many months after their child is discharged [17,22,30,31]. More generally the tendency for parents to be overprotective in caring for their child after life-threatening events is a phenomenon that is well known to pediatricians [32] and that has been shown to lead to problematic family functioning [33].

Several children described disturbing nightmares and hallucinations, which were similar in content to those described by adult intensive care survivors [34], suggesting that this is another aspect of their experience that merits further systematic exploration, especially given the association, found in adults, between delusional memories and the development of posttraumatic stress [35].

The finding, in one study, that children reported positive as well as negative changes [11] may simply reflect that the convenience sample used was atypically resilient. It may, however, be evidence of a phenomenon that is currently attracting a great deal of interest in the traumatic stress literature, namely posttraumatic growth [36], which commonly coexists with posttraumatic stress. To date, only a couple of studies in the wider pediatric traumatic stress literature have described this in children [37,38].

Implications for future research

More longitudinal studies are needed to clarify the natural history of psychologic adaptation of children in this situation [39] and to clarify which aspects of the child's experience related to injury, illness, or treatment are associated with poorer psychologic outcome [40]. Specifically there is a need to develop tools for use across the pediatric age range to assess delirium and withdrawal [41,42], and to investigate associations with these aspects of experience and long-term psychologic well being. More information is also needed on the interactions, over time, between the parent's symptoms and the child's psychologic state.

A better understanding of the mechanisms underlying the development and maintenance of psychologic distress in these children will inform the design of future interventions, such as the promising COPE package [43]. This intervention, in which timely advice is provided to parents on how to facilitate their child's adaptation to PICU treatment and its aftermath, seems to improve long-term psychologic outcomes for children and parents alike, by reducing mothers' anxiety and increasing their participation in care [44].

Clinical implications

The literature has uncovered several aspects of the PICU experience that could theoretically give rise to adverse psychologic effects in child patients and that have the potential to be addressed clinically, even while the child is still in hospital. The possibility that the child may be troubled by disturbing factual or delusional memories should be acknowledged, as should the child's confusion about what has happened to him or her. Age-appropriate explanations about the child's injuries, treatment, and side effects of treatment should be provided when the child is in a position to take this information on board. Written information in diary form has been well received by adult intensive care survivors [45], many of whom report being troubled by their inability to remember their admission. Case reports of individually tailored interventions with children highlight the importance of finding creative ways to impart information, reduce anxiety, facilitate communication, and prepare them for procedures during admission, along with helping them to process all that has happened, after discharge [46]. The high prevalence of anxiety in parents, when considered with the evidence that this is associated with the child's psychologic outcome, indicates the need to provide support for relatives during and after admission, when required.

Summary

The literature on the psychologic impact of the PICU on children shows a mixed picture of resilience and distress. Children report disturbing nightmares and hallucinations associated with their admission and a significant minority have elevated levels of posttraumatic stress many months after discharge, indicating that there is a need for (a) more support for this group of patients, and (b) further longitudinal research into risk factors associated with distress. By understanding more about the range of psychologic reactions of children in this situation, workers in this field will be better placed to identify those families most in need of support and to design appropriate interventions for them.

References

[1] Rothstein P. Psychological stress in families of children in a pediatric intensive care unit. Pediatr Clin North Am 1980;27(3):613–20.

[2] Shudy M, de Almeida ML, Ly S, et al. Impact of pediatric illness and injury on families: a systematic literature review. Pediatrics 2006;118(S3):S203–18.

[3] Noyes JA. Critique of studies exploring the experiences and needs of parents of children admitted to paediatric intensive care units. J Adv Nurs 1998;28:134–42.

[4] Board R, Ryan-Wenger N. State of the science on parental stress and family functioning in pediatric intensive care units. Am J Crit Care 2000;9(2):106–22.

[5] Odetola FO, Clark SJ, Freed GL, et al. A national survey of pediatric critical care resources in the United States. Pediatrics 2005;115(4):e382–6.

[6] Truog RD. Increasing the participation of children in clinical research. Intensive Care Med 2005;31:760–1.

[7] Paediatric Intensive Care Audit Network. Annual Report 2003–2004. Sheffield (UK): Universities of Leeds, Leicester and Sheffield; 2005.

[8] Newman E, Kaloupek DG. The risks and benefits of participating in trauma-focused research studies. J Trauma Stress 2004;17:383–94.

[9] Kassam-Adams N, Newman E. Child and parent reactions to participation in clinical research. Gen Hosp Psychiatry 2005;27(1):29–35.

[10] Playfor S, Thomas D, Choonara I. Recollection of children following intensive care. Arch Dis Child 2000;83:445–8.

[11] Colville GA. Children's views on the psychological impact of admission to PICU. European Psychotherapy 2004;4:80.

[12] Karande S, Kelkar A, Kulkarni M. Recollections of Indian children after discharge from an intensive care unit. Pediatr Crit Care Med 2005;6:303–7.

[13] Board R. School–age children's perceptions of their PICU hospitalization. Pediatr Nurs 2005;31:166–75.

[14] Colville G, Kerry S, Pierce C. Children's factual and delusional memories of intensive care. Am J Respir Crit Care Med 2008;177(9):976–82.

[15] Cataldo M, Bessman CA, Parker LH, et al. Behavioral assessment for pediatric intensive care units. J Appl Behav Anal 1979;12:83–97.

[16] Jones S, Fiser DH. Behavioral changes in pediatric intensive care units. Am J Dis Child 1992;14:375–9.

[17] Rees G, Gledhill J, Garralda ME, et al. Psychiatric outcome following paediatric intensive care unit (PICU) admission: a cohort study. Intensive Care Med 2004;30:1607–14.

[18] Rennick JE, Monin I, Kim D, et al. Identifying children at high risk for psychological sequelae after pediatric intensive care unit hospitalization. Pediatr Crit Care Med 2004;5:358–63.

[19] Rennick JE, Johnston CC, Dougherty G, et al. Children's psychological responses after critical illness and exposure to invasive technology. J Dev Behav Pediatr 2002;23(3):133–44.

[20] Youngblut JM, Shiao SP. Child and family reactions during and after pediatric ICU hospitalization: a pilot study. Heart Lung 1993;22(1):46–54.

[21] Small L, Melnyk BM. Early predictors of post-hospital adjustment problems in critically ill young children. Res Nurs Health 2006;29:622–35.

[22] Balluffi A, Kassam-Adams N, Kazak A, et al. Traumatic stress in parents admitted to the pediatric intensive care unit. Pediatr Crit Care Med 2004;5:547–53.

[23] Gavin LA, Roesler TA. Posttraumatic distress in children and families after intubation. Pediatr Emerg Care 1997;13:222–4.

[24] Colville GA. Parents' views on the psychological impact of admission to PICU. European Psychotherapy 2004;4:81.

[25] Cohen JA, Berliner L, March JS. Treatment of children and adolescents. In: Foa E, Matthew J, Keane T, editors. Effective treatments for PTSD: practice guidelines from the International Society for Traumatic Stress Studies. New York: Guilford Press; 2000. p. 106–38.

[26] Kassam-Adams N, Garcia-Espana JF, Miller VA, et al. Parent-child agreement regarding children's acute stress: the role of parent acute stress reactions. J Am Acad Child Adolesc Psychiatry 2006;45(12):1485–93.

[27] Shemesh E, Newcorn JH, Rockmore L, et al. Comparison of parent and child reports of emotional trauma symptoms in pediatric outpatient settings. Pediatrics 2005;115:582–9.

[28] Koplewicz HS, Vogel JM, Solanto MV, et al. Child and parent response to the 1993 World Trade Center bombing. J Trauma Stress 2002;15:77–85.

[29] Carter MC, Miles MS. The parental stressor scale: pediatric intensive care unit. Matern Child Nurs J 1989;18:187–98.

[30] Board R, Ryan-Wenger N. Stressors and stress symptoms of mothers with children in the PICU. J Pediatr Nurs 2003;18:195–202.

[31] Colville GA, Gracey D. Mothers' recollections of PICU: psychopathology and views on follow up. Intensive Crit Care Nurs 2006;22:49–55.

[32] Green M, Solnit AJ. Reactions to the threatened loss of a child: a vulnerable child syndrome. Pediatrics 1964;34:58–66.

[33] McFarlane AC. Family functioning and over-protection following a natural disaster: the longitudinal effects of post-traumatic morbidity. Aust N Z J Psychiatry 1987;21:210–8.

[34] Magarey JM, McCutcheon HH. "Fishing with the dead"—recall of memories from the ICU. Intensive Crit Care Nurs 2005;21:344–54.

[35] Jones C, Griffiths RD, Humphris G, et al. Memory, delusions and the development of acute post traumatic stress disorder-related symptoms after intensive care. Crit Care Med 2001;29:573–80.

[36] Linley P, Joseph S. Positive change following trauma and adversity. J Trauma Stress 2004;17:11–21.

[37] Salter E, Stallard P. Posttraumatic growth in child survivors of a road traffic accident. J Trauma Stress 2004;17:335–40.

[38] Barakat LP, Alderfer MA, Kazak AE. Posttraumatic growth in adolescent survivors of cancer and their mothers and fathers. J Pediatr Psychol 2006;31(4):413–9.

[39] Ehlers A, Clark DM. Early psychological interventions for adult survivors of trauma: a review. Biol Psychiatry 2003;53:817–26.

[40] Ward-Begnoche W. Posttraumatic stress symptoms in the pediatric intensive care unit. J Spec Pediatr Nurs 2007;12(2):84–92.

[41] Schieveld JN, Leroy PL, van Os J, et al. Pediatric delirium in critical illness: phenomenology, clinical correlates and treatment response in 40 cases in the pediatric intensive care unit. Intensive Care Med 2007;33:1033–40.

[42] Ista E, van Dijk M, Gamel C, et al. Withdrawal symptoms in children after long-term sedatives and/or analgesics: a literature review. "Assessment remains troublesome." Intensive Care Med 2007;33:1396–406.

[43] Melnyk BM, Alpert-Gillis L, Feinstein NF, et al. Creating opportunities for parent empowerment: program effects on the mental health/coping outcomes of critically ill young children and their mothers. Pediatrics 2004;113:597–607.

[44] Melnyk BM, Crean HF, Feinstein NF, et al. Testing the theoretical framework of the COPE program for mothers of critically ill children: an integrative model of young children's posthospital adjustment behaviors. J Pediatr Psychol 2007;32(4):463–74.

[45] Bäckman CG, Walther SM. Use of a personal diary written on the ICU during critical illness. Intensive Care Med 2001;27(2):426–9.

[46] Colville G. The role of a psychologist on the paediatric intensive care unit. Child Psychology and Psychiatry Review 2001;6(3):102–9.

PEDIATRIC CLINICS

OF NORTH AMERICA

Pediatr Clin N Am 55 (2008) 617–646

Multiple Organ System Extracorporeal Support in Critically Ill Children

Joseph A. Carcillo, MD

Pediatric Critical Care, Children's Hospital of Pittsburgh,
3705 Fifth Ave., Pittsburgh, PA 15213, USA

Multiple organ system extracorporeal support is becoming commonplace in the care of critically ill children who have multiple organ failures (Fig. 1). Unlike the adult experience, contemporary outcomes in children who have multiple-system organ failure are cause for optimism. In a recent survey of United States children's hospitals a survival rate of 90% was observed in children who had multiple-system organ failure [1]. This better outcome in children may occur in part because the majority of children have multiple organ failure at the time of presentation, whereas adults commonly develop multiple organ failure over time in the ICU. With notable exceptions, patients who present to the ICU with multiple organ failure are more likely to have an underlying condition that can be reversed compared with those who develop multiple organ failure despite therapies in the ICU. It also is possible that this better outcome could result from "tricks of the trade" learned in pediatric medicine. This article is organized to help the pediatric critical care practitioner understand (1) the mechanics of individual extracorporeal support devices alone, in tandem, and in circuit; (2) the indications for use of these techniques in children who have multiple organ failure; and (3) the practical specifications and therapeutic goals necessary for optimal outcomes with the use of multiple machine modes.

Keys to success

In the use of multiple organ system extracorporeal support, there are three keys to successful patient outcomes.

First, the practitioner must be willing to implement a change in the plan of care for a patient before implementing extracorporeal support. This

E-mail address: carcilloja@ccm.upmc.edu

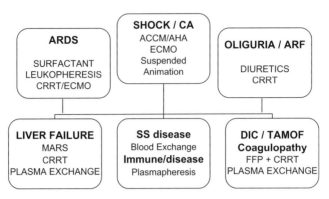

Fig. 1. Multiple organ system extracorporeal support systems are used to support brain, cardiac, pulmonary, liver, kidney, coagulation, blood, and immune cell function in children who have multiple organ failure syndromes. ACCM, American College of Critical Care Medicine; ARDS, acute respiratory distress syndrome; ARF, acute renal failure; CA; cardiac arrest; CRRT, continuous renal replacement therapy; DIC, disseminated intravascular coagulation; ECMO, extracorporeal membrane oxygenator; FFP, fresh frozen plasma; MARS, molecular absorbent reactivation system; SS, sickle S; TAMOF, thrombocytopenia associated mulitple organ failure.

requirement is obvious and intuitive for patients who arrive in extremis to the pediatric ICU after being previously healthy at home. These children who have trauma, aspiration pneumonia/acute respiratory distress syndrome (ARDS), sepsis/inflammation, or toxin-induced multiple organ failure receive new therapies that they were not receiving at home. It is reasonable to hope that these new therapies will reverse the underlying pathologic process while extracorporeal support facilitates recovery. This requirement is less obvious and commonly is not intuitive for patients who have been previously ill. For example a bone marrow transplant recipient being treated with immunosuppressive therapies who presents with sepsis-induced multiple organ failure while treated with antibiotics/antifungals/antivirals is unlikely to survive, even with extracorporeal support, unless immune suppression is withheld and then substantially tapered so that the infection can be killed and cleared by the child. It makes little sense to press on with a treatment plan that is not working, in the hope that it will work if extracorporeal support is used to "buy time"; the extra time usually confirms that the treatment does not work. On the other hand, if the treatment plan is reversed and substantially changed, extracorporeal support can be the answer for this patient.

Second, extracorporeal support must be administered according to proper specifications. For example, appropriately sized catheters, flow rates, and equipment are needed. Troubleshooting is the norm in successful extracorporeal support and can be attained with protocolized standard procedure manuals and practices and a dedicated extracorporeal support team interested in doing whatever is needed to attain optimal machine performance.

Third, the enemy of all extra corporeal support therapy is hemolysis. Free hemoglobin must be monitored and prevented to the greatest degree possible in all patients. The target is a measured free hemoglobin less than 10 μg/L or spun plasma that is clear yellow to visual inspection. Clinical knowledge of this key element for success has been lost from collective consciousness in the past 20 years, in part because extracorporeal machines are better than they used to be. In the early days of extracorporeal support technology, patients developed multiple organ failure caused by hemolysis and free hemoglobin induced and released by the extracorporeal support machines. Bubble oxygenators produced so much hemolysis that multiple organ failure was seen within 1 hour of cardiopulmonary bypass, and dialysis membranes were so unfriendly to erythrocytes and white blood cells that ARDS/multiple organ failure could be seen immediately following an intermittent dialysis session in sick patients. Although present membrane technology is vastly improved, hemolysis still can be induced with the longer runs or with inadequate techniques commonly observed with multiple organ system extracorporeal support. Today, science has explained the link between hemolysis and multiple organ failure [2–4]. Free hemoglobin scavenges nitric oxide, adenosine, and a disentigrin-like and metalloproteinase with thrombospondin type 1 repeats-13 (ADAMTS 13), leading to microvascular vasoconstriction and platelet thrombi that result in multiple organ failure. Recognition of the problem and reversal of hemolysis by changing lines, circuits, or flow rates can prevent and reverse organ failure in these patients.

Modes of extracorporeal support

Extracorporeal membrane oxygenation

The extracorporeal membrane oxygenator (EMCO), also known as "extracorporeal life support," is used for support of intractable cardiac or pulmonary failure (Appendix 1; Fig. 2) [5–25]. Cannulation can be performed through arterio-venous vessels, the best support system for cardiac failure, or through veno-venous vessels, the best support system for respiratory failure. The Extracorporeal Life Support Organization has maintained a registry for 20 years. ECMO can be provided with systemic anticoagulation, predominantly achieved with heparin, or without systemic anticoagulation when using the heparin-bonded circuit (circuit life approximately 48 hours). The duration of ECMO support generally runs from 7 days or less in children who have isolated acute cardiac failure (unless listed for transplantation) and newborns who have meconium aspiration or secondary persistent pulmonary hypertension of the newborn, to up to 2 months in children who have pulmonary failure. Survival in children who have refractory cardiopulmonary failure is approximately 50%. Survival for newborns who have intractable cardiopulmonary failure is approximately 80%. A number of trials have found improved outcomes with ECMO use in these populations [5–9].

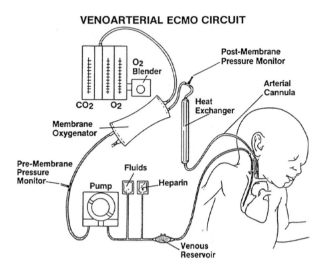

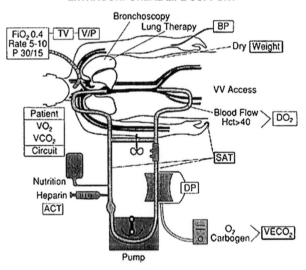

Fig. 2. ECMO can be applied by veno-arterial or veno-venous access and can be used as a platform for provision of any and all extracorporeal support therapy, particularly in babies and infants. ACT, activated clotting time; BP, blood pressure; DO$_2$, oxygen delivery; DP, diastolic pressure; Hct, hematocrit; TV, tidal volume; VCO$_2$, carbon dioxide production; VO$_2$, oxygen consumption; V/P, volume/pressure.

Continuous renal replacement therapy

Continuous renal replacement therapy (CRRT) provides continuous veno-venous hemofiltration and/or continuous veno-venous hemodialysis or hemodiafiltration and allows gentle fluid removal or dialysis in hemodynamically compromised patients (Appendix 2, Fig. 3, and Table 1) [22–42].

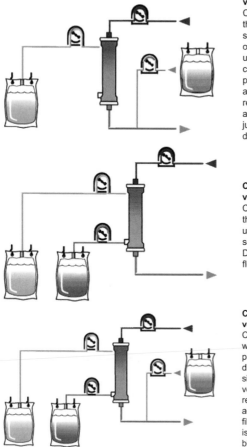

CVVH(Continuous venovenous hemofiltration)
Continuous hemofiltration with the aid of a blood pump provides solute removal by convection. It offers high volume ultrafiltration using replacement fluid, which can be administered pre-filter or post-filter. The pump guarantees adequate blood flow to maintain required UF rates. Venous blood access is usually femoral, jugular or subclavian using a double lumen cannula.

CVVHD(Continuous venovenous hemodialysis)
Continuous hemodialysis with the aid of a blood pump and using venous access. It provides solute removal by diffusion. Dialysate is pumped in counter flow to the blood.

CVVHDF(Continuous venovenous hemodiafiltration)
Continuous hemodiafiltration with the aid of a blood pump provides solute removal by diffusion and convection simultaneously. It offers high volume ultrafiltration using replacement fluid, which can be administered pre-filter or post-filter. Simultaneously, dialysate is pumped in counter flow to blood.

Fig. 3. CRRT can be performed on the ECMO circuit without an additional machine or by using a separate machine in patients who do not require ECMO. (*Courtesy of* Gambro Inc., Lakewood, CO; with permission.)

Access usually is attained through a large central vein but can be successful with arterio-venous (the historical method) or veno-venous access as well. The circuit can be run with anticoagulation using citrate or heparin or without systemic anticoagulation using frequent filter changes (although using no anticoagulation in pediatric patients leads to significant filter loss because of the smaller access size than in adults). A recent randomized trial found better outcomes in patients who received citrate-based systemic anticoagulation than in patients who received heparin-based anticoagulation [32]. The mechanism of this effect remains unclear; however, citrate is a known substrate for the Krebs cycle, which could contribute to energy production, whereas heparin is not. CRRT is used most commonly for fluid removal. In this

Table 1
Troubleshooting alarms in hemofiltration

Alarm	Possible problem	Action required
High venous pressure	Kinked line	Unkink
	Clamped line	Unclamp
	Clotted access	Remove clot or replace access
	Clot in bubble trap	Replace circuit
Low venous pressure	Venous line disconnected	Reconnect
	Blood pump stopped because of another alarm	Resolve problem that caused initial alarm
Arterial pressure alarm	Kinked line	Unkink
	Clamped line	Unclamp
	Clotted access	Remove clot or replace access
	Arterial line disconnected	Reattach line
	Catheter against wall	Reposition catheter or swap over venous and arterial lines
Blood leak alarm	Ruptured membrane	Stop treatment and change circuit
	Cloudy filtrate	Replace chamber with one full of saline
	Chamber out of housing	Reposition chamber in the detector
	Dirty mirror in detector	Remove mirror, clean, and replace
Blood pump will not run	Air detected	Clear air in circuit
	Blood pump door open	Ensure blood pump door closed
Air detector alarm	Air in venous line	Draw air into bubble trap with syringe
	Low blood level in bubble trap	Draw blood into bubble trap with syringe
	Venous line not positioned between sensors	Reposition venous line
Transmembrane pressure (TMP) alarm	Rapid rise: filtrate line clamped	Unclamp
	Slow rise: filter clotted	Change circuit
	High from start: program too high for filter performance	Reduce fluid loss and replacement rate
Temperature alarm	Constant alarm: heater plate > 41°C	Remove heater bag. Needs repair.
	Flashing alarm: heater plate < 33°C	Remove heater bag. Needs repair.
Bag change alarm	Filtrate bag full	Change bag
	Replacement bag empty	Change bag
Balance alarm	Bags swinging on scales	Stop bags swinging
	Clamp on replacement or filtrate line	Unclamp lines
	Airlock in heater bag	Disconnect line and purge air by gravity
	Weighing scales need calibration	Stop treatment and change machine, which needs recalibration.

Courtesy of Q. Mok, Great Ormond Street, London.

regard, a pediatric CRRT registry supports the use of CRRT before the patient who has multiple organ failure develops a fluid overload greater than 10% (weight $>$ 10% of baseline or positive fluid balance of 100 mL/kg), because patients who received CRRT before reaching this point had better outcomes than those who received CRRT after this time [27,29]. High-flux CRRT (>35 mL/kg/h) is used in cancer-associated ARDS and in sepsis. A small series found improved outcome compared with historical controls in patients who had ARDS after bone marrow transplantation who received CRRT [34]. The treatment volumes of 60 mL/kg/h allowed nearly complete turnover of total body water (600 mL/kg). The authors suggested that clearance of chemotherapy and cancer toxins and stimulation of lymphatic flow contributed to improved outcomes in this patient population. In randomized trials in patients who had sepsis with shock and multiple organ failure, investigators have shown a dose-dependent improvement in outcome and shock resolution when providing treatment volumes higher than 35 mL/kg/h [30,41,42]. Experimental models show that high-flux CRRT reverses shock, immunoparalysis (restores the tumor necrosis factor-alpha response), and apoptosis (prevents caspase activation) [40]. The mechanism remains unclear. A five-center study is underway to address the effectiveness of convective compared with diffusive methods in cytokine clearance.

Molecular absorbents recirculation system/albumin dialysis

A molecular absorbents recirculation system (MARS) or albumin dialysis can be performed through the same vascular access as ECMO or CRRT (Fig. 4) [22–25]. The MARS machine provides in tandem (1) a continuous albumin dialysis circuit to remove protein-bound toxins; (2) a column that removes these albumin-bound toxins and reactivates and recycles the albumin for further use, preventing the need for large volumes of albumin; and (3) a continuous renal replacement circuit that then can be used to perform traditional hemofiltration/dialysis. Traditional hemodialysis removes only toxins that are not bound to albumin; however, the newer generation of high-flux dialyzers with high flow rates now clears protein-bound drugs [43]. Albumin dialysis/MARS is most effective in improving outcomes in patients who have acute or chronic liver disease or liver failure–associated hepatorenal syndrome, encephalopathy, or multiple organ failure [44–48]. The MARS cartridge usually is used once daily for approximately 8 hours.

Pheresis and exchange therapies

"Exchange" is the term used to describe a procedure during which a component of the patient's blood is removed by the machine and then a component of donor blood is returned to the patient in exchange (Fig. 5) [49–65]. For example, during whole blood exchange, whole blood is removed, and fresh donor packed cells and platelets are returned. During plasma exchange, plasma is removed, and thawed fresh-frozen plasma is returned.

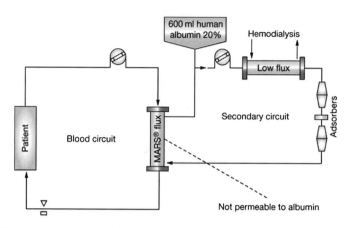

Fig. 4. Liver support therapy can be provided in addition by the molecular adsorbents recirculating system (MARS), which is based on the principles of albumin dialysis and adsorption, using a secondary circuit prefilled with 20% albumin solution. The free fraction of albumin-bound toxins passes by diffusion through the albumin-impermeable membrane to the secondary circuit, where it transiently binds to albumin and is adsorbed when albumin–toxin complexes pass through two sequential columns. Water-dissolved substances, after diffusing through the first dialyzer, are removed by additional low-flux hemodialysis in the secondary circuit.

"Pheresis" is the term used to describe a procedure during which a component of the patient's blood is removed by the machine, but the component is not returned to the patient. For example, during leukopheresis white blood cells are removed but are not returned to the patient, and, during plasmapheresis, plasma is removed, but plasma is not returned to the patient. These therapeutic procedures can be performed through the same cannulae used in ECMO, CRRT, or MARS. Anticoagulation of blood products usually is achieved by the citrate provided by these procedures. Two different machine approaches may be used. The centrifugation machine spins the blood, separating its components by weight and removing the desired component according to sedimentation during the spin. The filtration method can be performed using the CRRT and/or MARS machines simply by replacing the CRRT hemofilter (which allows the removal of everything < 70 kd) with the plasma filtration filter (which allows removal of everything < 1 million kd).

Whole blood exchange is considered the treatment of choice for ABO-induced hemolytic disease of the newborn, sickle cell crisis syndromes including stroke, multiple organ failure, chest syndrome, and severe malarial anemia associated with cerebral edema. During newborn ABO incompatibility, whole blood exchange is performed manually because of the large extracorporeal blood volume of plasmapheresis machines. In older children the procedure is performed by machine, but a blood prime is used, particularly in children weighing less than 15 kg. Leukopheresis is considered standard therapy for reducing white blood cell counts in patients who have leukemia with leukosequestration lung syndromes and ARDS. Several

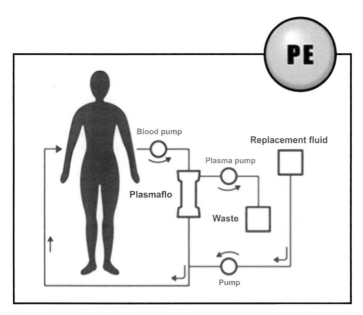

Fig. 5. Blood, plasma, or white blood cell pheresis can also be added to ECMO, CRRT, and MARS to support coagulation, blood, and immune cell functions using a filtration or centrifugation machine. When plasma exchange is performed with a centrifugal cell separator, the University of Pittsburgh uses a whole blood/anticoagulant ratio of 14:1. The inlet flow rate (whole blood removal rate) ranges between 10 and 50 mL/min depending on patient weight, tolerance of volume changes, and citrate load. Ionized calcium levels are monitored at 15-minute intervals. Calcium chloride 10% solution (20 mg/kg) is given for citrate-mediated hypocalcemia symptoms or ionized calcium levels less than 0.9 mmol/L. To maintain a total extracorporeal volume less than 10% of total blood volume, a red blood cell prime consisting of one unit of leuko-reduced packed red blood cells is diluted with normal saline to a hematocrit no less than 30% for patients who have a total blood volume between 500 and 1750 mL (weight, 5–22 kg). Intensive plasma exchange is performed for thrombocytopenia-associated multiple organ failure using a 1.5 plasma volume exchange on day 1 followed by a 1.0 plasma volume exchange daily until resolution of multiple organ failure or thrombocytopenia. Increases in inotrope and sedation dosages also are commonly needed during the procedure. Therefore bedside vigilance is recommended for the 1- to 2-hour sessions.

case reports support the use of leukopheresis or whole blood exchange to reverse leukostasis in critical pertussis syndrome with ARDS and pulmonary hypertension [57–59]. At autopsy, these patients have leukocyte plugging of the pulmonary vasculature. Plasmapheresis also is considered standard therapy in many immune complex–mediated diseases, including antibody-mediated rejection of solid organ transplants, vasculitic disorders, and immune-complex mediated diseases [49].

Several randomized trials have demonstrated that plasma exchange for a mean of 2 to 18 days improves outcomes compared with plasma infusion alone in patients who have complex coagulopathies caused by autoimmune disease, sepsis, and liver disease [52–55]. The patients most likely to benefit are those who have new-onset thrombocytopenia and multiple organ failure. These patients have coagulopathies that span a spectrum ranging from disseminated intravascular coagulation (DIC) to thrombotic thrombocytopenic purpura (TTP). Plasma exchange removes the prothrombotic/antifibrinolytic factors, including tissue factor, ultra-large von Willibrand factor (vWF) multimers, plasminogen activator inhibitor type 1, and ADAMTS 13 inhibitors, while restoring antithrombotic/profibrinolytic factors including protein C, antithrombin III, ADAMTS 13, and tissue plasminogen activator. In patients who have liver failure, plasma exchange similarly restores an evenly balanced pro- and anticoagulant state without the costly side effect of fluid overload.

Indications for multiple organ system extracorporeal support

Cardiac arrest

The most rapidly increasing indication for ECMO therapy recorded in the Extracorporeal Life Support Organization registry is extracorporeal cardiopulmonary resuscitation (ECPR) (Table 2). Patients undergoing ECPR have a 45% survival rate. Restoration of circulation after cardiopulmonary resuscitation is complicated by secondary cardiac dysfunction and prolonged states of inadequate perfusion. Extracorporeal support should be considered in any patient who suffers a cardiac arrest, who has inadequate restoration of circulation to prevent secondary organ ischemia, and who is thought to have a chance of recovery if adequate cardiac support is provided. Hypothermia, if present, should be maintained during the cannulation period to reduce cardiac demands. Effective ECPR requires an institutional commitment [11–13]. The ECPR circuit may be maintained in a crystalloid-primed fashion or be a short, hollow-fiber circuit that can be primed with crystalloid within a few minutes. A rapidly responding team should be maintained to initiate ECMO cannulation and to initiate and maintain ECPR. Percutaneous cannulae also should be available to facilitate faster femoral cannulation and the placement of ECMO cannulae over guide wires through already existing central venous and arterial catheters. The transcutaneous approach through the femoral vein-femoral artery can provide rapid partial support while more definitive cut-down techniques are performed. Percutaneous techniques are very difficult to perform successfully in newborns, so open surgical placement remains the approach of choice for this population, even in ECPR. Cannulation also may be performed via the mediastinum, especially in patients who have a recent sternotomy for cardiac surgery.

"Suspended animation" was proposed by Safar and Tisherman [14] for hemorrhagic cardiac arrest. In this setting, the patient in cardiac arrest caused by hemorrhagic shock is cannulated transcutaneously and then cooled on ECMO with circulating crystalloid to 8°C. This technique allows up to 3 hours for surgical repair of wounds. The patient then is rewarmed

Table 2
Indications for multiple organ system extracorporeal support

Type of support	Indications
Extracorporeal cardiopulmonary resuscitation	Inability to restore adequate circulation after cardiac arrest despite use of American Heart Association guidelines Likelihood of good outcome if perfusion is restored
Extracorporeal membrane oxygenator	Inability to restore adequate circulation during shock despite use of American College of Critical Care Medicine/American Heart Association guidelines Inability to maintain oxygenation and ventilation with nontoxic ventilatory setting; oxygenation index > 40 in newborn, high airway pressures or inspired oxygen content for less than 7 days in a child
Continuous renal replacement therapy	Fluid overload > 10% body weight despite use of diuretics and maintenance of adequate perfusion pressures Refractory hyperammonemia or hyperlactatemia Bone marrow transplantation–associated acute respiratory distress syndrome High-flux hemofiltration with high-volume plasma infusion to reverse disseminated intravascular coagulation /purpura fulminans
Molecular absorbents recirculation system	Acute-on-chronic liver failure with hyperbilirubinemia or encephalopathy Bridge to liver transplantation
Plasma exchange	Coagulopathy unresponsive to fresh-frozen plasma infusion without volume overload New-onset thrombocytopenia and three-organ failure Hemolytic thrombotic microangiopathy Hemophagocytic syndrome Severe rhabdomyolysis
Blood exchange	Hemolytic disease of newborn associated with ABO incompatibility Sickle cell disease with organ failure Severe malarial anemia with cerebral malaria
Leukopheresis	Leukosequestration-associated acute respiratory distress syndrome Critical pertussis-associated acute respiratory distress syndrome
Plasmapheresis	Immune complex–mediated diseases unresponsive to steroids/ intravenous immunoglobulin Humoral organ rejection Antiphospholipid antibody crisis

slowly. Human field-testing of suspended animation is in the planning stage (S. Tisherman, personal communication, 2008).

Other forms of extracorporeal support also have a role after cardiac arrest. A group of French investigators showed improved outcome with the addition of one treatment session of high-flux CRRT to the management of patients after cardiac arrest [26]. Plasma exchange also has a role in treating patients who have cardiac arrest and subsequent coagulopathy or thrombocytopenia-associated multiple organ failure.

Shock

The consideration and use of extracorporeal support is recommended in patients who have shock that is refractory despite the use of other goal-directed therapies. Therapies should be directed to maintaining central venous oxygen saturation ($ScvO_2$) above 70%, normal perfusion pressure for age, capillary refill time of less than 2 seconds, and cardiac index above 3.3 L/min/m^2 and below 6.0 L/min/m^2. Some recommend strong consideration of extracorporeal support when patients have undergone proper volume resuscitation and still require more than 1 μg/kg/min of norepinephrine or epinephrine. A cardiac index below 2.0 L/min/m^2 or a $ScvO_2$ below 50% is another indication for strong consideration [8]. Strong consideration also should be given to the concomitant use of type III phosphodiesterase inhibitors (milrinone, enoximone) and/or a calcium-binding sensitizer (levosimendan) and, in the face of normotension and normovolemia, to the use of vasodilators (nitroglycerin, nitroprusside, prostacyclin). This approach may rescue low cardiac output syndromes before the need to proceed to ECMO.

ECMO is equally effective in cardiogenic and septic shock, although septic shock can be associated with a greater incidence of bleeding or thrombotic complications. Coagulopathy during ECMO in children who have septic shock often can be reversed with fresh-frozen plasma. Low cardiac output shock (septic or cardiogenic) responds well to arterio-venous ECMO because improved oxygen delivery and decreased cardiac preload may improve overall cardiac and secondary organ performance. Venovenous ECMO also has been used effectively in shock, particularly if the need for inotropic support of the heart is caused by pulmonary hypertension or by associated high levels of ventilatory support that reduce venous return or cause cardiac compromise.

Acute respiratory distress syndrome

ARDS in the newborn is treated with inhaled nitric oxide for pulmonary hypertension, whereas surfactant often is used in respiratory distress syndrome. Older infants and children who have respiratory failure receive lung-protective ventilation and surfactant. The pathophysiology of ARDS in the first 24 hours includes both surfactant inactivation and massive leukosequestration, with a more than 10-fold increase in polymorphonuclear neutrophil sequestration in the pulmonary microvasculature. Patients who have ARDS and severe leukocytosis are treated with leukopheresis. The indication usually used is more than 100,000 cells/mm^3, but this indication can be practiced more liberally or conservatively. The number of treatments also varies.

CRRT should be considered early as a fluid-management tool in the child who has total body edema and who is approaching fulfillment of the clinical criteria for ARDS, regardless of serum creatinine level. In newborns with an oxygen index higher than 40 despite inhaled nitric oxide and lung recruitment maneuvers, and in children receiving high airway pressures and/or oxygen (peak inspiratory pressure > 35; fraction of inspired oxygen of 1.00) for less than 7 to 14 days, ECMO is recommended to preserve lung function. Beyond 7 days of toxic oxygen and pressure settings, ECMO seems to be less efficacious [7].

Hepatic failure

Acute hepatic failure is treated with adequate glucose delivery to prevent hypoglycemia, with fresh-frozen plasma to correct coagulopathy, with albumin to correct hypoalbuminemia, and with lactulose/neomycin to remove hyperammonemia. Extracorporeal support is indicated in patients who develop encephalopathy and or hepatorenal syndrome. Randomized trials have shown that MARS can reverse encephalopathy and hepatorenal syndrome in patients who have acute or chronic liver failure [44–48]. In centers without access to MARS, a combination of CRRT with fresh-frozen plasma infusion or use of daily plasma exchange is also effective. MARS or albumin dialysis is most effective in removing bilirubin, CRRT is most effective in removing ammonia, and plasma exchange is most effective for reversing coagulopathy. An occasional patient who has fulminant hepatic failure will exhibit a tendency toward hypercoagulability (from DIC) manifested by almost immediate clotting of the CRRT circuit. A single plasma exchange before CRRT will improve the viability of the hemofiltration circuit.

Oliguria/anuria

CRRT is recommended for patients who have multiple organ dysfunction and more than 10% fluid overload despite diuretic management [27,29]. Although the exact timing of CRRT following fluid resuscitation of shock is unknown, prolonging the time to initiation of CRRT is associated with worse outcomes, possibly because body and tissue edema contributes to secondary organ dysfunction.

Disseminated intravascular coagulation and purpura fulminans

DIC and purpura fulminans occur when circulating tissue factor initiates consumptive coagulation with depletion of the anticoagulant proteins antithrombin III and protein C. The prothrombin time (PT) and partial thromboplastin time (PTT) increase when prothrombotic factors are reduced to less than 20% of normal, because they are rapidly consumed in thrombi. The treatment of choice is fresh-frozen plasma. If a transfusion of 20 mL/kg is not effective in attaining a nearly normal PT/PTT, this finding suggests a consumptive coagulopathy. These patients may require 50 to 200 mL/kg/d of fresh-frozen plasma to meet these needs [63]. This plasma can be provided without causing harmful fluid overload by performing plasma infusion with CRRT or daily plasma exchange until maintenance of a normal PT/PTT is attained.

Thrombocytopenia-associated multiple organ failure

Patients who have failure of three or more organs and new-onset thrombocytopenia probably have thrombotic microangiopathy mediated in part by high levels of thrombogenic ultra-large vWF multimers and low ADAMTS 13 activity. Randomized trials have shown that outcomes can be improved in these patients with daily centrifugation-based plasma exchange therapy until the resolution of thrombocytopenia-associated multiple organ failure [52–55] Plasma exchange removes ultra-large vWF multimers and ADAMTS 13 inhibitors while replacing ADAMTS13. Plasma infusion replaces only ADAMTS 13. The effects of filtration-based plasma exchange on outcome in these patients are not known.

Autoimmune-induced organ failure

Plasmapheresis with albumin replacement is recommended for autoimmune diseases including Guillain-Barre syndrome, anti-phospholipid crisis, Goodpasture's disease, acute disseminated encephalomyelitis, and antibody-mediated organ rejection. Most suggest that this procedure is indicated if steroids and intravenous immunoglobulin therapy are unsuccessful.

Hemolytic anemia, sickle cell disease, severe malarial anemia, and newborn ABO incompatibility

Whole blood exchange is recommended for sickle cell anemia–related stroke, chest syndrome, and multiple organ failure, for severe malarial anemia–associated encephalopathy, and for newborn ABO incompatibility–induced hemolytic anemia with rising bilirubin unresponsive to phototherapy.

Hemophagocytic syndrome and other disorders of hyperlactatemia

Hemophagocytic syndromes can be associated with overwhelming lactatemia and lactic acidosis. CRRT is very effective in removing lactate, but quite high clearance rates are required. These clearance rates can be achieved by using hemofiltration and dialysis rates to attain flux treatments of 60 mL/kg/h or more. Daily plasma exchange also can be helpful in patients who have not responded to intravenous immunoglobulin therapy.

Specifications for extracorporeal support: alone, in tandem, and in circuit

Each multiple organ system extracorporeal support team should have predetermined specifications and protocols for the use of extracorporeal support therapies. This article includes protocols from several institutions. Whole blood exchange can be performed manually in newborns. Although plasmapheresis and CRRT can be accomplished in infants weighing less than 10 kg, both techniques require blood priming of the circuit and very careful attention to detail, particularly in the neonatal period [66]. The ECMO machine can be used as the platform of choice for instituting multiple organ support in infants weighing less than 5 kg because the ECMO circuit is secured by surgical exposure, allowing placement of a large cannula and a machine flow of 110 mL/kg/min. Plasma exchange, CRRT, and/or albumin dialysis can be performed while on the ECMO circuit [22–25]. The centrifugation-based plasmapheresis/exchange machine can be connected in line, using a set of low-resistance stopcocks. Plasma exchange, CRRT, and albumin dialysis also can be done using the ECMO circuit alone [22–25]. Plasma filters are secured into the circuit for plasma exchange, and CRRT filters are secured into the circuit for continuous hemofiltration and/or dialysis. The ECMO circuit must be preprimed with 250 mL of priming fluid (blood, albumin, and calcium) to fill the extracorporeal volume of the circuit. By necessity, this priming volume increases with the larger tubing and oxygenator requirements for larger patients with each extra machine added to the circuit.

Infants and children can have tandem extracorporeal support without the use of ECMO. In this setting access usually is attained percutaneously. Newer CRRT technology allows tandem placement of pheresis machines in line with the CRRT device. For infants weighing less than 10 kg, blood priming often is used to initiate CRRT. Alternately, if a centrifugation-based plasma exchange/pheresis machine is used, one volume exchange is done per day over 1 to 2 hours; when the exchange session is completed, the patient again is attached to the CRRT machine for continuous hemofiltration and/or dialysis. In centers where plasma exchange is performed by the same filtration machine as CRRT, there is no need to change machines. Instead filters are changed when the patient changes from a plasma exchange session to a continuous hemofiltration/dialysis. Caution must be used when using the filtration-based pheresis technique in patients weighing less than 10 kg because of the blood flow required. The manufacturers' recommendations should be reviewed in detail.

Choosing and troubleshooting extracorporeal support

Extracorporeal membrane oxygenator

Circuit choice
The ECMO circuit should be chosen and prepared before the call occurs. The two most popular oxygenators are the membrane oxygenator and the hollow fiber oxygenator. The hollow fiber oxygenator provides less resistance to blood flow and therefore is less prone to cause hemolysis [20]. It also can be heparin bonded and allow less use of heparin anticoagulation. The two most popular pumps are the centrifugal vortex pump and the roller pump. When used properly in experimental settings, the vortex pump can

cause less shear stress and hemolysis; however, with improper clinical use it can cause more hemolysis than the roller pump [21]. The roller pump has an in-line bladder that is set to collapse when negative pressure generated on the venous side by the pump falls below 20 cm H_2O. The vortex pump has no bladder and no alarm, so negative pressures below 20 cm H_2O can go unnoticed for some time, unless the circuit inlet pressures are monitored and an alarm attached. In the absence of the chatter from the bladder, dangerously low pressures may be ignored. Newer versions of centrifugal pumps now have integrated monitoring and alarm systems that are intended to minimize hemolysis.

Access choice

Age-specific and appropriately sized cannula and circuit tubing should already be specified and available at the time of call. Newborns should be cannulated by surgical exposure. Older children can be cannulated by percutaneous exposure over a guidewire. Veno-venous cannulation can be effective in patients who have isolated respiratory failure and good cardiac function. The internal jugular vein remains the site of choice for veno-venous ECMO. Arterio-venous cannulation is indicated for patients who have inadequate cardiac function; the right common carotid artery is the site of choice. In older and larger children, a combination of femoral and internal jugular vessels may be needed to meet increased flow requirements. The need for increased venous drainage may require three cannulae (two for drainage and one for return). The femoral vessels usually are large enough to support patients older than 3 years, although care must be taken to ensure adequate drainage and perfusion of the ipsilateral extremity. In the setting of cardiac arrest the femoral artery and vein can be the first vessels accessed while maintaining CPR.

Troubleshooting

The most common adverse event noted when a patient is first placed on ECMO is hypotension. Hypotension can occur as ionized calcium levels decrease when the citrated blood used to prime the circuit chelates calcium. The treatment is provision of calcium to normalize calcium concentration. Another cause is hypovolemia that occurs as the extracorporeal circuit is added to the corporeal circuit. This problem becomes more important with smaller babies with small corporeal volumes. The remedy is volume resuscitation until the central venous blood pressure is restored. The next common problem encountered is inadequate flow. Properly sized and placed cannulae should afford ECMO flow at 110 mL/kg/min with a negative pressure of 0 to −20 cm H_2O. When this flow is not attained, one first should check to make sure the cannulae are placed properly. One should obtain radiographic and echocardiographic images to demonstrate that the arterial cannula is above the aortic arch and that the venous cannula is in the right atrium. Next, one should document that cannulae of the proper size are being used. At times, technical difficulties preclude the use of appropriately sized cannulae. Under these circumstances, one should calculate the expected flow volumes for the size cannula that is in place and subsequently scale back the flow parameters on the pump to attain only these values. For example, if the cannula size used in a 10-kg infant is appropriate for a 5-kg infant, the flow should be scaled back to 550 mL/kg/min (appropriate for the 5-kg infant). Use of a cannula that cannot provide adequate flow (when there is no reasonable option to upsize or provide additional access) may require the use of cardiovascular therapies such as epinephrine, milrinone, and nitroprusside to augment native cardiac output. Another problem is extreme negative pressure (below -20 cm H_2O) despite adequate cannula size and placement. In this circumstance flow should be reduced until the negative pressure improves; if negative pressure does not improve, a second venous cannula should be placed. In patients who have very poor left heart function, the left ventricle may not empty. The left atrial pressure may be so high that it bows into the right atrium, collapsing it. In some patients the use of afterload reduction (vasodilators) with volume loading can overcome severe ventricular dysfunction. In other patients, an atrial septostomy may be needed to allow blood to get to the venous cannula until left ventricular cardiac function returns (usually after 7 days of ECMO). In other patients left atrial drainage may be attained with a transseptal femoral vein catheter.

Careful attention to maintaining free hemoglobin to less than 10 μg/L may help prevent the onset of new renal and multiple organ failure during prolonged pump runs. If all these suggestions have been followed, and the circuit has been in place for some time, a circuit change can be considered, because acquired clots within the circuit may have developed.

Continuous renal replacement therapy

Anticoagulation choice

The first decision when beginning CRRT is whether to use anticoagulants [28]. Some change filters every 8 hours and use no anticoagulants; however, in smaller children (<10 kg) requiring blood priming, this approach can lead to very high exposure to multiple blood antigens. Others use continuous anticoagulation and tend to change filters less frequently. Systemic anticoagulation generally is performed, as is the case with ECMO, using heparin. In this procedure, heparin is infused before the filter with the goal of reaching higher PTT and activated coagulation time in the filter. This procedure involves a simple anticoagulation process but carries the risk of increased bleeding when systemic anticoagulation is high. Others use local citrate anticoagulation. In this procedure, citrate is infused before the filter, and calcium is infused after the filter. The amount of citrate infused prefilter is calculated to be enough to chelate calcium from the blood, rendering it unable to coagulate in the filter. The amount of calcium infused postfilter is the amount needed to saturate citrate so that it can no longer chelate any systemic calcium and therefore cannot act as a systemic anticoagulant. The advantage of this approach is that local anticoagulation is attained without systemic anticoagulation [67,68]. The risk of this procedure is citrate lock syndrome, in which systemic citrate levels become high. After metabolism by liver mitochondria, citrate is transformed from a weak acid to a weak base, and systemic alkalosis occurs. When alkalosis is too great, the patient is exposed to alkali syndrome.

The choice of anticoagulant may be driven in part by the underlying disease process. Systemic heparin anticoagulation can be risky in children already at risk of bleeding, such as patients who have cancer with thrombocytopenia. On the other hand local citrate anticoagulation can be risky in children who have liver failure, particularly in infants. Poor liver metabolic function leads to increased citrate loads and hypocalcemia. The relative inability of infants to mobilize calcium from bone stores makes this hypocalcemia more life threatening. An infant receiving citrate/calcium infusions (especially for more than 10 days) may manifest the consequences of excess calcium, with calcifications observed on heart valves and other tissues. Hence one can consider using citrate-based CRRT in patients who have cancer and minimum heparin-based CRRT or CRRT without anticoagulation in babies who have liver failure. If citrate is used in babies who have liver failure, the dose should be reduced to 70% of normal, and calcium levels must be monitored more frequently.

Choosing hemofiltration and/or hemodialysis

The choice of dialysis or filtration is becoming less important because high-flux therapy is becoming the norm, and both are used simultaneously. Solute clearance in dialysis is attained by diffusion; hence, smaller molecules are cleared, and maintaining a concentration gradient is important. Solute clearance in filtration is by convection and solvent drag associated with fluid clearance; hence, middle-sized molecules are cleared, and higher ultrafiltration rates lead to higher solute clearance. Filtration is simpler and is effective in removing fluid and middle-sized molecules that may potentiate systemic inflammatory response syndrome. The flux rate is set, and ultrafiltrate is removed accordingly as it passes through the filter pores by hydrostatic pressure. Pressure differences are generated by the hemofiltration machine, and ultrafiltration rates are set manually on the machines. Dialysis uses diffusion as its predominant clearance method, and molecules pass from higher to lower concentrations as dialysate is run countercurrent to blood flow through the hemofilters. The choice depends on the patient. If the child is 10% fluid overloaded, hemofiltration may be the most efficient way to remove fluid and solute. If the child is not fluid overloaded but requires detoxification for urea, lactate, or ammonia, one can begin with hemofiltration with fluid replacement for fluid removed (net even). One also can begin hemodialysis and remove urea, lactate, or ammonia by increasing the dialysate flow rate. Commonly, children requiring multiple organ system extracorporeal support require both hemofiltration and dialysis, also known as "hemodiafiltration," to keep up with the need for massive clearance required during liver failure or hemophagocytosis.

Choosing treatment dose and duration

Many routinely use a rate of more than 35 mL/kg/h as the rate of ultra-filtrate production during continuous hemofiltration or dialysis related to multiple organ system failure, as opposed to the rate of 20 mL/kg/h used in stable non-ICU patients who have renal failure. Increasing dosage should be titrated to achieving normal ammonia or lactate levels. Achieving these levels can require a great deal of fluid filtration and dialysate clearance. Total body water is 600 mL/kg. It generally takes three exchanges of fluid to reduce the body load by 85%. Therefore up to 1800 mL/kg of hemofiltration/dialysis clearance is required to reduce the toxin to 15% of its initial level. At a rate of 60 mL/kg/h, this process takes 30 hours. Many suggest that the treatment flux should be increased until stable normal levels are attained for several days and/or until the resolution of organ failure.

Troubleshooting

Despite blood priming of CRRT circuits, hypotension has been noted, particularly in infants weighing less than 10 kg when a PAN filter is used [69]. Increasing the infusion rates of any inotropes and maintaining even fluid balance without fluid removal can help prevent initiation-associated hypotension. Low flows and very negative pressures can be observed and usually require adjustment of access, sometimes requiring placement of larger venous access (www.pcrrt.com) and at other times requiring a different site of access. For example, femoral access may not be effective in a fluid-overloaded patient who has abdominal compartment syndrome, but internal jugular access could be ideal. If access is not the problem, filter clotting might be. Hypercoagulation is common in patients who have multiple organ failure and sepsis, and several filter changes can be required in the first day or two. A single plasma exchange can obviate the problem of hypercoagulability.

Hemofiltration requires careful attention to electrolyte levels. Phosphorous replacement often is required. In addition to electrolyte imbalance, fluid balance must be monitored carefully. Errors in electrolyte management may be minimized with use of commercially available solutions [70]. Hypotension commonly is associated with rapid intravascular fluid removal and less rapid intravascular fluid replacement. Hypotension should be treated with fluid replacement while reviewing the machinery set-up to ensure no lines are inadvertently clamped and that replacement fluid is running into the patient. Hypothermia also can be a side effect if the circuit is not thermally controlled with a heater; convective heat loss can be minimized in larger children by using a space blanket wrapped around the circuit and hemofilter.

Molecular absorbents recirculation system

In patients who have liver failure, MARS should also be added to CRRT, with placement of the MARS cartridge to perform albumin dialysis. The commencement of therapy should be strongly considered in patients who have acute liver failure and who fulfill criteria for transplantation and should be considered in patients who have acute decompensation of chronic liver disease who do not respond to several days of other therapies. The MARS treatment generally lasts up to 8 hours, after which CRRT is resumed. Alternatively, continuous MARS treatment is possible and sometimes is preferred in patients who have acute liver failure. The number of MARS treatments given is based on experience. Most treat at least every 3 days. Therapy should be directed to normalizing bilirubin in the same manner as CRRT dosage and to normalizing ammonia and lactate. Fresh-frozen plasma should be given also to reverse coagulopathy.

Troubleshooting

The complication most commonly observed when using MARS in patients who have liver failure is bleeding, which occurs when platelet counts are below $50,000/mm^3$ and the international normalized ratio is above 2.3. Little or no heparin/citrate should be used when this degree of coagulopathy is present. Plasma and platelet infusion with fluid removal through CRRT or plasma exchange may be used to reverse coagulopathy.

Exchange and pheresis

Choosing exchange and pheresis machines

Exchange therapies should be chosen when a patient's disease can be improved by removing a diseased blood component and replacing it with healthy blood. Pheresis should be chosen when the patient's disease can be improved by removing the diseased blood component. A disease with high levels of pathogenic circulating immune complexes or white blood cells can respond to removal or pheresis (leukopheresis or plasmapheresis). Albumin usually is used to replace the volume lost during this procedure. In diseases treated with daily pheresis, albumin infusion may dilute out factors and require occasional replacement with fresh-frozen plasma as well. Complex diseases such as coagulopathies or hemoglobinopathies require both removal and replenishment (plasma exchange or whole blood exchange). In diseases treated with daily exchange, an experienced and expert blood bank is required.

When the decision to perform pheresis or exchange is made, the next question is which machine to use: manual, filtration based, or centrifugation based. Although time-consuming, the manual technique is effective for whole blood exchange. Whole blood exchange performed for newborn-associated hemolytic anemia and recalcitrant hyperbilirubinemia usually is performed with a one- to two-volume exchange. Calcium is given to reverse hypocalcemia caused by chelation by citrate in donor blood; fresh-frozen plasma is given for prolonged PT/PTT, and platelets are given for thrombocytopenia. Manual exchange is cumbersome in older children and is not effective when removal and replacement of an isolated blood component is required. These procedures can be performed using the filtration or centrifugation machine. The filtration machine is the same machine used for CRRT. Depending on the pore size of the filtration filter used, whole blood, white blood cells, or plasma can be removed. The centrifugation machine is a different machine that separates out blood components based on size and can be used to remove whole blood, white blood cells, platelets, or plasma. So how does one choose between machines? The pore size of the filtration filter for plasma is 1 million kd; however, the size of ultra-large vWF multimers, which need to be removed for TTP, is over 2 million kd. Therefore centrifugation-based plasma exchange should be more effective than filtration-based exchange, because it will remove the ultra-large vWF multimers more effectively. Nevertheless, many use filtration in the treatment of TTP. One study suggests that the plasma filtration filter can absorb ultra-large vWF multimers and remove them in this way [60]. The only randomized clinical trial that did not show a benefit in the treatment of infection- or sepsis-associated thrombotic microangiopathy used continuous plasma filtration for more than 24 hours with only partial replacement of plasma [61]. This approach is not recommended, because two other randomized trials showed benefit with the use of daily centrifugation-based plasma exchange therapy [52,53].

Choosing the length of therapy

Although regimens for exchange and pheresis therapy sometimes are arbitrary, if the treatment effect is measurable, it seems prudent to continue daily therapy until multiple organ system failure is resolved. Furthermore, if, after stopping therapy, organ failure recrudesces, it seems reasonable to resume therapy. For example plasma exchange therapy requires a median of 18 days for TTP [54], a median of 9 days for other thrombotic microangiopathies [53], and a median of 3 days for DIC [52].

Troubleshooting exchange and pheresis therapies

All exchange therapies can be associated with hypotension, and, similar to ECMO and CRRT circuits, the plasma exchange circuit should be blood and calcium primed. Nevertheless, hypotension still may occur because of fluid removal before fluid is replaced by the machine. Also the chelation of calcium by the citrate used to preserve the blood or plasma replaced during exchange can cause hypocalcemia and hypotension. A calcium bolus of 20 to 30 mg/kg followed by an infusion of 20 mg/kg/h can be used to reduce the risk. Patients also can experience hypotension caused by the removal of any inotrope, vasopressor, or hydrocortisone infusion being administered at the time. It is prudent to titrate these infusions as needed during the

Table 3
Goal-directed extracorporeal support therapy

Type of support	Goal-directed extracorporeal support
Extracorporeal cardiopulmonary resuscitation	Central venous oxygen saturation $> 70\%$, cardiac index (CI) > 2.0 L/min/m^2 If unable to attain flow of 110 mL/kg/min with negative pressure -20 cm H$_2$O, check cannula placement, sizes; rule out tamponade or left atrium dilation, consider second or third cannula. Use therapeutic hypothermia (suspended animation), inotropes to facilitate these goals.
Extracorporeal membrane oxygenator	(a) Central venous oxygen saturation $> 70\%$ (ateriovenous O$_2$ saturation difference $< 25\%$), CI > 2.0 L/min/m^2 If unable to attain flow of 110 mL/kg/min with negative pressure -20 cm H$_2$O, check cannula placement, sizes; rule out tamponade or LA dilation, consider second or third cannula. Use therapeutic hypothermia (suspended animation), inotropes and vasodilators to facilitate these goals. (b) Minimal airway pressures and oxygen concentration through mechanical ventilator (open lung strategy for children) Accept arterial oxygen saturation $> 85\%$
Continuous renal replacement therapy	(a) $<10\%$ body weight fluid overload Use hemofiltration to attain this goal. (b) Normalization of ammonia, lactate, and pH levels May require addition of dialysis for high-flux continuous renal replacement therapy to attain clearance (c) Increase in Pao$_2$/fraction of inspired oxygen to > 200 in bone marrow transplantation–associated acute respiratory distress syndrome Requires continuous veno-venous hemodialysis to attain 60 mL/kg/h clearance
Molecular absorbents recirculation system	(a) Normalization of bilirubin levels (b) Recovery of Glasgow coma score to > 8
Plasma exchange	(a) Normalization of prothrombin time and partial thromboplastin time (b) Normalization of platelet count (c) Resolution of organ failure
Blood exchange	(a) Normalization of bilirubin in newborn ABO incompatibility hemolytic anemia (b) Normalization of hemoglobin levels to > 10 g/dL in patients who have severe sickle cell anemia or severe malarial anemia
Leukopheresis	(a) Improvement in PaO$_2$/fraction of inspired oxygen ratio to > 200 in critical pertussis and leukocytosis-associated acute respiratory distress syndrome
All forms of support	(a) Maintain free hemoglobin concentrations < 10 μg/L. Normal portal vein resistive indices. This measure requires attention to proper-sized cannula, changing circuits, appropriate anticoagulation, and reducing blood flows to levels that prevent the use of too much negative pressure in the venous cannulae. Long-term circuit change for microthrombi.

procedure. Awakening also can be observed as sedatives, analgesics, and, in the case of patients who have liver failure, endogenous benzodiazepines are removed. Titration of sedatives also is prudent during this procedure. Bedside vigilance is recommended during the procedure.

Summary

Multiple organ system extracorporeal support effectively supports brain, heart, lung, liver, kidney, coagulation, red blood cell, and immune cell function in the sickest infants and children who have multiple organ system failure. These therapies have optimum benefit if (1) the underlying disease is reversible; (2) the therapies are performed expertly and are monitored to prevent and minimize systemic hemolysis, the major side effect of extracorporeal circuits; and (3) the therapies are provided in a goal-directed manner (Table 3). These therapies represent a significant advance in pediatric critical care medicine. This article provides a framework for this multidisciplinary team approach for implementing these therapies.

Acknowledgments

Dr. Carcillo thanks the MOSES investigators for offering their expert suggestions: Patrick Brophy, Tim Bunchman, Warwick Butt, Billy Casey, Heidi Dalton, Joseph V. Dicarlo, Geoffrey Fleming, James Fortenberry, Barbara Gaines, Yong Y. Han, Joseph Kiss, Paddy McMaster, Steffen Mitzner, Quen Mok, Michael Moritz, Mark Peters, and Peter Wearden.

Appendix 1

Successful use of ECMO requires specifications for initiation and troubleshooting. The following is an example of a checklist used by Eggleston Children's Hospital, Atlanta, Georgia

	2–5 kg	6–10 kg	10–16 kg	16–40 kg	>40 kg
Circuit	1/4″	1/4″	3/8″	3/8″	1/2″
Raceway	1/4″	3/8″	3/8″	1/2″	1/2″
Oxygenator	0.8	1.5	2.5	4.5	4.5 × 2
Maximum blood flow	1.2 liters per minute	1.8 liters per minute	4.5 liters per minute	6.5 liters per minute	10 liters per minute
Occlusion flow					
Plasma-Lyte needs	1 L	1 L	2 L	3 L	4 L
Prime packed red blood cells	2 units	3 units	4 units	5 units	5 units
Albumin to circuit	10 cm³	10 cm³	20 cm³	30 cm³	50 cm³
On-bypass platelets	1 unit	1/4 pheresis	1/2 pheresis	1/2 pheresis	1 pheresis

(continued on next page)

Appendix 1 (*continued*)

	2–5 kg	6–10 kg	10–16 kg	16–40 kg	>40 kg
Cannulas: veno-arterial					
Arterial	8–12	12–15	12–15	17–19	21
Venous	10–14	12–17	14–23	21–25	23, 27, 29
Cannulas: veno-venous					
Arterial return	8–10	12–15	14–21	19–21	21
Venous	10–14	14–15	15–19	21–25	25+
Double lumen	12 French ≤ 3.0	14 French ≤ 5 kg	15 French ≤ 6 kg	18 French ≤ 12 kg	18 French 12–20 add second cannula
Cannulas: cephalad	One to two sizes smaller than the right internal jugular cannula				

Prime drugs per unit packed red blood cells
  100 units heparin diluted in 1 cm^3 normal saline
  40 cm^3 25% albumin
  25 cm^3 THAM
  10 cm^3 sodium bicarbonate
  300 mg calcium gluconate (100 mg/cm)
Once circulating, give 300 mg calcium gluconate to 1/4" circuit or 100 mg/unit blood for 3/8" or 1/2" circuit

Problem	Cause	Treatment
High CO_2 (normal, 35–40)	Insufficient time on gas or inadequate amount of blended gas. Loose occlusion	Allow more time, decrease amount of carbogen, increase blended gas.
Low CO_2	Excessive amount of blended gas in sweep gas	Reduce blended gas flow, increase carbogen flow
Low ionized Ca (normal, 3.5–4.5)	Insufficient amount in prime	< 3.5: add 200 mg calcium gluconate < 2.5: add 300 mg. calcium gluconate Check anticoagulant therapy in 5 minutes
High ionized Ca	Excessive amount in prime	Alkalinize with Tham or sodium bicarbonate
Low potassium + (normal, 3.5–5.5)	Washed cells in prime	< 2.0: add 1mEq potassium chloride < 3.0: add 0.5mEq potassium chloride
High potassium +	Old blood in prime	Alkalinize with sodium bicarbonate, calcium, Tham
Low hemoglobin (range desired, 14–16)	Excessive dilution during prime	Consider exchange transfusion of circuit if < 10
Low anticoagulant therapy (range desired, 500–1000)	Inadequate heparin dose at prime	<350: add 50 units 250–350: add 100 units <250: add 100 units

Appendix 2

Successful use of CRRT therapies requires institution-based specifications for initiation and troubleshooting for heparin and for citrate-based CRRT

1) Dialysis Access_____Location_____Lumen Vols: Red_____Blue_____

2) Baseline laboratory studies:

☐ Chemistry 10 plus albumin
☐ Ionized calcium
☐ CBC
☐ Art. Blood Gas

3)

Circuit	Pt Size	Cannula	Filter	XCV	Pump Blood Flow	Predilution Flow
Neonatal	2.7-5.0 kg	6.5 Fr	M10	50 mL	25 mL/min	100-200 ml/h
Pediatric	5.0-8.5 kg	6.5 Fr	M60	90 mL	50 mL/min	200-400 mL/hr
Pediatric	8.5-14 kg	8.0 Fr	M60	90 mL	70 mL/min	300-500 mL/hr
Pediatric	14-21 kg	8.0Fr	M60	90 mL	110 mL/min	450-900 mL/hr
Adult	21-35 kg	10Fr,12cm	M100	107 mL	150 mL/min	600-1000 mL/hr
Adult	35+ kg	11.5 Fr, 13.5cm	M100	107 mL	200 mL/min+	800-1400 mL/hr+

4) Priming Solution (check selection, add 5,000 u heparin per liter)

☐ Normal Saline

☐ 5% Albumin

☐ Normalized blood (when circuit volume exceeds 10% estimated blood volume; estimated blood volume = 80 cc/kg)

PRBC < 5 days old	80 ml
5% Albumin	55 ml
Heparin	150 units
NaHCO$_3$	12 mEq
Calcium Gluconate 10%	2 ml

Additives mixed with PRBC's in above order to prevent clotting. Obtain ionized calcium and pH on normalized prime before using to prime circuit: Ionized Calcium must be >1.0 mmol/L; pH must be 7.3-7.5.

☐ Other _____

5) Modality   ☐ CVVH
                    CVVHD
                    ☐ CVVHDF

6) Replacement/Predilution Fluid (use commercially prepared fluid other wise consider formulation)

☐ Yes   ☐ No

☐ LPCH Pharmacy to formulate   _____,_____ liter bags:

Sodium	_____mEq/L	(130-145 mEq/L)
Potassium	_____mEq/L	(0-5 mEq/L)
Chloride	_____mEq/L	(To Balance)
Bicarbonate	_____mEq/L	(25-40 mEq/L)
Calcium	_____mEq/L	(2-3 mEq/L) * Remove if citrate
anticoagulation		
Magnesium	_____mEq/L	(1-2 mEq/L)
Phosphate	_____mmol/L	(0.5 – 1.0 mmol/L)
Dextrose	_____mg/dL	(80 - 100 mg/dl)

Replacement Infusion Rate = _____ml/hr.

Na Phosphate 15 mmol to 50 mL with ___% saline ___% glucose @ ___ mL/hr (1 mL/hr = 0.3 mmol PO$_4$)

7) Dialysis Fluid   ☐ Yes   ☐ No

☐ 0 K$^+$ Commercial Hemodiafiltration solution (0.1% Dextrose, with lactate as a base) send _____, 3 liter bags.

☐ 2 K$^+$ Commercial Hemodiafiltration solution (0.1% Dextrose, with lactate as a base) send _____, 3 liter bags.

Normocarb

☐ LPCH Pharmacy to formulate_____,_____ liter bags:

Sodium	_____mEq/L	(130-145 mEq/L)
Potassium	_____mEq/L	(0-5 mEq/L)
Chloride	_____mEq/L	(To Balance)
Bicarbonate	_____mEq/L	(25-40 mEq/L)
Calcium	_____mEq/L	(2-3 mEq/L) *Remove if citrate
anticoagulation		
Magnesium	_____mEq/L	(1-2 mEq/L)
Dextrose	_____mg/dL	(80 - 100 mg/dl)

☐ Send a sample of each bag for sodium and potassium analysis if the patient is <10 kg. Sodium must be ± 8mEq of ordered sodium values, potassium must be ± 0.5 mEq/L of ordered potassium value.

Dialysate Infusion Rate =_____ml/hr countercurrent to blood flow.

8) Anticoagulation: ☐ Heparin   ☐ Citrate☐ None
    a.   Heparin
        i. Heparin concentration   ☐ 1 U/ml
                                          ☐ 10 U/ml
                                          ☐ 100 U/ml
                                          ☐ 1000 U/ml
        ii. Initial bolus = _____units (5-20 units/kg), followed by a continuous infusion of _____units/hour. Infuse pre-dialyzer, post-pump.
        iii. Titrate heparin drip to keep ACT-post-filter_____seconds (160-200 seconds)
        iv. Give heparin bolus of____units if ACT < _____seconds
        v. If use PTT Ratio (systemic sample not CVVH line) maintain PTTR between 2.0-2.5
             < 2.0 give bolus of heparin 5 u/kg and increase infusionrtae by 10%
             > 2.5 repeat in 1 hr, if still elevated decrease heparin infusion rate by 10%

    b.   Citrate
        i. 3% trisodium citrate, infuse at a rate of _____ml/hour (1.5 to 2.0 times the blood flow rate in ml/hr. [example: if BFR = 80 ml/min, citrate rate = 120 – 160 ml/hr]
        ii. Location of trisodium citrate infusion:
             ☐ Afferent limb take-off (stopcock)- 1 hour maximum volume of trisodium citrate in buretrol in patients < 10 kg.
        iii. 0.8% calcium chloride (1 gram $CaCl_2$ in 1000 ml normal saline), infuse at ____ _____ml hour (50% of citrate rate). Infuse into a separate central line.
        iv. Check patient and circuit ionized calcium q 1 hr until stable within target ranges for 2 hrs in a row, then q 4 hrs.
        v. Ionized calcium target ranges: see sliding scales.

Citrate Sliding Scale

Circuit ionized Ca++ (blue port)	Change citrate rate		
	<5 kg	5 – 30 kg	> 30 kg
<0.25	Down 3 ml/hr	Down 5 ml/hr	Down 10 ml/hr
0.25 – 0.35	No change	No change	No change
0.36 – 0.45	Up 3 ml/hr	Up 5 ml/hr	Up 10 ml/hr
>0.45	Up 5 ml/hr	Up 10 ml/hr	Up 20 ml/hr

Calcium Chloride Sliding Scale

Patient ionized calcium	Change $CaCl_2$ rate		
	<5kg	5 – 30 kg	>30 kg
<1.00	Up by 5 ml/hr	Up by 10 ml/hr	Up by 20 ml/hr
1.00 – 1.09	Up by 3ml/hr	Up by 5 ml/hr	Up by 10 ml/hr
1.10 – 1.30	No change	No change	No change
>1.30	Down by 3 ml/hr	Down by 5 ml/hr	Down by 10 ml/hr

9)   Replace the hemofiltration circuit every _____ days.
10) ☐ Place patient on a scale bed

HEMOFILTRATION

Clearance is achieved by convection (ultrafiltration), with the addition of diffusion (dialysate) if needed to control electrolyte balance (e.g., if patient has hyperkalemia due to renal insufficiency). Total clearance is the sum of the volumes of ultrafiltrate and dialysate solution.

Blood flow: 2 - 5 mL/kg/min [common range: 50 - 200 mL/minute]

Ultrafiltration: 50 ± 10 mL/kg/hr if used alone (CVVH)
                      40 ± 10 mL/kg/hr if used with dialysate (CVVHDF)

Dialysate: 20 ± 10 mL/kg/hr (if used)
Anticoagulation: citrate or heparin (citrate preferred but not required)
                    citrate: ionized calcium in circuit [0.25 – 0.35 mmol/L]
                    - or -
                    heparin: patient PTT [55 - 65 seconds]

References

[1] Mariscalco MM, et al. In submission.
[2] Yeo TW, Lampah DA, Gitawati R, et al. Impaired nitric oxide bioavailability and L-arginine reversible endothelial dysfunction in Falciparum malaria. J Exp Med 2007;204(11): 2693–704.
[3] Thachil J. Thrombotic thrombocytopenic purpura: is there more than ADAMTS13? J Thromb Haemost 2007;5(3):634–5.
[4] Gladwin MT. Role of the red blood cell in nitric oxide homeostasis and hypoxic vasodilation. Adv Exp Med Biol 2006;588:189–205.
[5] UK Collaborative ECMO Trial group. UK collaborative randomized trial of neonatal extracorporeal membrane oxygenationRole of the red blood cell in nitric oxide homeostasis and hypoxic vasodilation. Lancet 1996;348(9020):75–82.
[6] McNally H, Bennett CC, Elbourne D, et al. United Kingdom collaborative randomized trial of neonatal extracorporeal membrane oxygenation: follow up to age 7 years. Pediatrics 2006; 117(5):E845–54.
[7] Green TP, Timmons OD, Fackler JC, et al. The impact of extracorporeal membrane oxygenation on survival in pediatric patients with acute respiratory failure. Pediatric Critical Care Study Group. Crit Care Med 1996;24(2):323–9.
[8] Parr GV, Blackstone EH, Kirklin JW. Cardiac performance and mortality early after intracardiac surgery in infants and young children. Circulation 1975;51(5):867–74.
[9] Dalton HJ, Rycus PT, Conrad SA. Update on extracorporeal life support 2004. Semin Perinatol 2005;29(1):24–33.
[10] Pettignano R, Fortenberry JD, Heard ML, et al. Primary use of veno-venous approach for extracorporeal membrane oxygenation in pediatric acute respiratory failure. Pediatr Crit Care 2003;4(3):291–8.
[11] Alsoufi B, AlRadi OO, Nazer RI, et al. Survival outcomes after rescue extracorporeal cardiopulmonary resuscitation in pediatric patients with refractory cardiac arrest. J Thorac Cardiovasc Surg 2007;134(4):952–9.
[12] Thiagarajan RR, Laussen PC, Rycus PT, et al. Extracorporeal membrane oxygenation to aid cardiopulmonary resuscitation in infants and children. Circulation 2007;116(15): 1693–700.

[13] Hannan RL, Ojito JW, Ybarra MA, et al. Rapid cardiopulmonary support in children with heart disease: a nine year experience. Ann Thorac Surg 2006;82(5):11637–41.

[14] Safar PJ, Tisherman SA. Suspended animation for delayed resuscitation. Curr Opin Anaesthesiol 2002;15(2):203–10.

[15] Maclaren G, Butt W. Extracorporeal membrane oxygenation and sepsis. Crit Care Resusc 2007;9(1):76–80.

[16] Maclaren G, Butt W, Best S, et al. Extracorporeal membrane oxygenation for refractory septic shock in children: one institution's experience. Pediatr Crit Care Med 2007;8(5): 447–51.

[17] Goldman AP, Kerr SJ, Butt W, et al. Extracorporeal support for intractable cardiorespiratory failure due to meningococcal disease. Lancet 1997;349(9050):466–9.

[18] Davis MC, Anderson NE, Johansson P, et al. Use of thromboelastograph and factor VII for the treatment of postoperative bleeding in a pediatric patient on ECMO after cardiac surgery. J Extra Corpor Technol 2006;38(2):165–7.

[19] Drews T, Stiller B, Hubler M, et al. Coagulation management in pediatric mechanical circulatory support. ASAIO J 2007;53(5):640–5.

[20] Maeda T, Iwasaki A, Kawahito S, et al. Preclinical evaluation of hollow fiber silicone membrane oxygenator for ECMO application. ASAIO J 2000;46(4):426–30.

[21] Valeri CR, MacGregor H, Ragno G, et al. Effects of centrifugal and roller pumps on survival of autologous red cells in cardiopulmonary bypass surgery. Perfusion 2006;21(5):291–6.

[22] Fortenberry JD, Paden ML. Extracorporeal therapies in the treatment of sepsis: experience and promise. Semin Pediatr Infect Dis 2006;17(2):72–9.

[23] Shaheen IS, Harvey B, Watson AR, et al. Continuous venovenous hemofiltration with or without extracorporeal membrane oxygenation in children. Pediatr Crit Care Med 2007; 8(4):362–5.

[24] Bunchman TE. Extracorporeal therapies in pediatric organ dysfunction. Pediatr Crit Care Med 2007;8(4):405–6.

[25] Tiruvoipati R, Moorthy T, Balasubramanian SK, et al. Extracorporeal membrane oxygenation and extracorporeal albumin dialysis in pediatric patients with sepsis and multi-organ dysfunction syndrome. Int J Artif Organs 2007;30(3):227–34.

[26] Laurent I, Adrie C, Vinsonneau C, et al. High volume hemofiltration after out of hospital cardiac arrest: a randomized trial. J Am Coll Cardiol 2005;46(3):432–7.

[27] Foland JA, Fortenberry JD, Warshaw BL, et al. Fluid overload before continuous hemofiltration and survival in critically ill children: a retrospective study. Crit Care Med 2004;32(8):1771–6.

[28] Brophy PD, Somers MJ, Baum MA, et al. Multi centre evaluation of anticoagulation in patient receiving continuous renal replacement therapy. Nephrol Dial Transplant 2005; 20(7):1416–21.

[29] Goldstein SL, Somers MJ, Baum MA, et al. Pediatric patients with multiple organ dysfunction syndrome receiving continuous renal replacement therapy. Kidney Int 2005; 67(2):653–8.

[30] Ronco C, Bellomo R, Homel P, et al. Effects of different doses in continuous veno-venous haemofiltration on outcomes of acute renal failure: a prospective randomized trial. Lancet 2000;356(9223):26–30.

[31] Smith OP, White B, Caughn D, et al. Use of protein C concentrate, heparin, and hemofiltration in meningococcemia. Lancet 1997;350(9091):1590–3.

[32] Oudemans–van Stratten, et al. Submitted for publication.

[33] Karnad V, Thakar B. Continuous renal replacement therapy may aid recovery after cardiac arrest. Resuscitation 2006;68(3):417–9.

[34] DiCarlo JV, Alexander SR, Agarwal R, et al. Continuous veno-venous hemofiltration may improve survival from acute respiratory distress syndrome after bone marrow transplantation or chemotherapy. J Pediatr Hemtaol Oncol 2003;25(10):801–5.

[35] Saccente SL, Kohaut EC, Berkow RL. Prevention of tumor lysis syndrome using continuous veno-venous hemofiltration. Pediatr Nephrol 1995;9(5):569–73.

[36] DiCarlo JV, Auerbach SR, Alexander SR. Clinical review: alternative vascular access techniques for continuous hemofiltration. Crit Care 2006;10(5):230.

[37] DiCarlo JV, Dudley TE, Sherbotie JR, et al. Continuous arteriovenous hemofiltration/ dialysis improves pulmonary gas exchange in children with multiple organ system failure. Crit Care Med 1990;18(8):822–6.

[38] Harvey B, Hickman C, Hinson G, et al. Severe lactic acidosis complicating metformin overdose successfully treated with high volume venovenous hemofiltration and aggressive alkalinization. Pediatr Crit Care Med 2005;6(5):598–601.

[39] DiCarlo JV, Lui WY, Frankel L, et al. The hemophagocytic syndrome: titrating continuous hemofiltration to the degree of lactic acidosis. Pediatr Hematol Oncol 2006; 23(7):599–610.

[40] Du C, Fang G, Zhao W, et al. Impact of high volume hemofiltration on apoptosis of major inflammatory cells in experimental multiple organ dysfunction of pigs. Acta Biochimica et Biophysica Sinica, in press.

[41] Cole L, Bellomo R, Journois D, et al. High volume hemofiltration in septic shock. Intensive Care Med 2001;27:978–86.

[42] Bellomo R, Hart G, Journois D, et al. A phase II randomized controlled trial of continuous hemofiltration in sepsis. Crit Care Med 2002;30:100–6.

[43] Schuerer DH, Brophy PD, Maxvold NJ, et al. High efficiency dialysis for carbamazepine overdose. J Toxicol Clin Toxicol 2000;38:321–3.

[44] Sen S, Davies NA, Mookerkee RP, et al. Pathophysiological effects of albumin dialysis in acute on chronic liver failure: a randomized controlled study. Liver Transpl 2004;10(9): 1109–19.

[45] Laleman W, Wilmer A, Evenepoel P, et al. Effect of the molecular adsorbent recirculating system and Prometheus devices on systemic haemodynamics and vasoactive agents in patients with acute-on-chronic alcoholic liver failure. Crit Care 2006;10(4):R108.

[46] Mitzner SO, Stange J, Klammt S, et al. Improvement of hepatorenal syndrome with extracorporeal albumin dialysis MARS: results of a prospective, randomized, controlled clinical trial. Liver Transpl 2000;6(3):277–86.

[47] Issieres P, Sasbon JS, Devictor D. Liver support for fulminant hepatic failure: is it time to use the molecular adsorbents recycling system in children? Pediatr Crit Care Med 2005;6(5): 585–91.

[48] Fuhrman BP, Zimmerman JJ, editors. Pediatric critical care. 3rd edition. Philadelphia: Mosby; 2006.

[49] Bosch T. Therapeutic apheresis-state of the art in the year 2005. Ther Apher Dial 2005;9(6): 459–68.

[50] Nguyen TC, Stegmayr B, Busund R, et al. Plasma therapies in thrombotic syndromes. Int J Artif Organs 2005;28(5):459–65.

[51] Matsumoto Y, Nasniwa D, Banno S, et al. The efficacy of therapeutic plasmapheresis for the treatment of fatal hemophagocytic syndrome: two case reports. Ther Apher 1998;2(4):300–4.

[52] Busund R, Koukline V, Utrobin U, et al. Plasmapheresis in severe sepsis and septic shock: a prospective, randomized, controlled trial. Intensive Care Med 2002;28(10):1434–9.

[53] Darmon M, Azoulay E, Thiery G, et al. Time course of organ dysfunction in thrombotic microangiopathy patients receiving either plasma perfusion or plasma exchange. Crit Care Med 2006;34(8):2127–33.

[54] Rock GA, Shumak KH, Buskard NA, et al. Comparison of plasma exchange with plasma infusion in the treatment of thrombotic thrombocytopenic purpura. Canadian Apheresis Study Group. N Engl J Med 1991;325(6):393–7.

[55] Stegmayr BG, Banga R, Berggren L, et al. Plasma exchange as rescue therapy in multiple organ failure including acute renal failure. Crit Care Med 2003;31(6):1730–6.

[56] Pahl E, Crawford SE, Cohn RA, et al. Reversal of severe late left ventricular failure after pediatric heart transplantation and possible role of plasma pheresis. Am J Cardiol 2000; 85(6):735–9.

[57] Grzeszczak MJ, Churchwell KB, Edwards KM, et al. Leukopheresis therapy for severe infantile pertussis with myocardial and pulmonary failure. Pediatr Crit Care Med 2006; 7(6):580–2.

[58] Donoso AF, Cruces PI, Camacho JF, et al. Exchange transfusion to reverse severe pertussis induced cardiogenic shock. Pediatr Infect Dis J 2006;25(9):846–8.

[59] Romano MJ, Webber MD, Weisse ME, et al. Pertussis pneumonia, hypoxemia, hyperleuko-cytosis, and pulmonary hypertension: improvement in oxygenation after a double volume exchange transfusion. Pediatrics 2004;114(2):E264–6.

[60] Peng ZY, Kiss JE, Cortese Hasset A, et al. Plasma filtration on mediators of thrombotic microangiopathy: an in vitro study. Int J Artif Organs 2007;30(5):401–6.

[61] Reeves JH, Butt WW, Shann F, et al. Continuous plasmafiltration in sepsis syndrome. Crit Care Med 1999;27:2096–104.

[62] Kato Y, Ohnishi K, Sawada Y, et al. Purpura fulminans: an unusual manifestation of severe Falciparum malaria. Trans R Soc Trop Med Hyg 2007;101(10):1054–7.

[63] Churchwell KB, McManus ML, Kent P, et al. Intensive blood and plasma exchange for treatment of coagulopathy in meningococcemia. J Clin Apher 1995;10(4):171–7.

[64] Wilkinson RJ, Brown JL, Pasvol G, et al. Severe Falciparum malaria: predicting the effect of exchange transfusion. QJM 1994;87(9):553–7.

[65] Sarode R, Altunta F. Blood bank issues associated with red cell exchange in sickle cell disease. J Clin Apher 2006;21(4):271–3.

[66] Symons JM, Brophy PD, Gregory MJ, et al. Continuous renal replacement therapy in children up to 10 kg. Am J Kidney Dis 2003;41:984–9.

[67] Bunchman TE, Maxvold NJ, Brophy PD. Pediatric convective hemofiltration (CVVH): normocarb replacement and citrate anticoagulation. Am J Kidney Dis 2003;42:1248–52.

[68] Bunchman TE, Maxvold NJ, Barnett J, et al. Pediatric hemofiltration: normocarb dialysate with citrate anticoagulation. Pediatr Nephrol 2002;17:150–4.

[69] Brophy PD, Mottes TA, Kudelka TL, et al. AN-69 membrane reactions are pH dependent and preventable. Am J Kidney Dis 2001;38:173–8.

[70] Barletta JF, Ahrens CL, Tyburski JG, et al. Medication errors and patient complications with continuous renal replacement therapy. Pediatr Nephrol 2006;21:842–5.

ELSEVIER
SAUNDERS

PEDIATRIC CLINICS
OF NORTH AMERICA

Pediatr Clin N Am 55 (2008) 647–668

Immunoparalysis and Adverse Outcomes from Critical Illness

W. Joshua Frazier, MD[a,b,c], Mark W. Hall, MD[a,b,c],*

[a]Critical Care Medicine, Nationwide Children's Hospital, 700 Children's Drive,
Columbus, OH 43205, USA
[b]Department of Pediatrics, Section of Critical Care Medicine, The Ohio State University
College of Medicine, Columbus, OH, USA
[c]The Research Institute at Nationwide Children's Hospital, 700 Children's Drive,
Columbus, OH 43205, USA

Children can face a variety of inflammatory challenges ranging from the benign (otitis media) to the life threatening (severe trauma, open heart surgery, and septic shock). The immune system is of vital importance for the successful weathering of these challenges. A massive proinflammatory response without proper controls is pathologic and places patients at risk for organ dysfunction and death. Conversely, an underactive immune system that is unable to detect pathogens, mount an inflammatory response, destroy microbial invaders, or repair damaged tissue places patients at risk for death from secondary infection and persistent organ failure.

In the 1980s and 1990s, multiple therapies targeting proinflammatory mediators and aimed at reducing inflammation reached phase III clinical trials in adults who had severe sepsis and septic shock [1–12]. Nearly all of these studies failed to demonstrate a survival benefit, suggesting that reducing inflammation is not the appropriate therapeutic goal in all cases. Subsequent studies have suggested that late mortality from surgery, sepsis, or trauma can be associated with an acquired immune deficiency state. If prolonged and severe, this state has been termed immunoparalysis. Characterized by markedly impaired innate immune function, immunoparalysis now is recognized as a predictor of morbidity and mortality for children and adults [13–18]. Moreover, the phenomenon often is occult, is not heralded by

This work was supported by Grant No. K08HL085525 from the National Institutes of Health.

* Corresponding author. Critical Care Medicine, Nationwide Children's Hospital, 700 Children's Drive, Columbus, OH 43205.

E-mail address: mark.hall@nationwidechildrens.org (M.W. Hall).

any premorbid phenotype, and commonly occurs in patients previously believed immunocompetent. Although immunoparalysis cannot be detected by analysis of patients' complete blood count or white blood cell differential, methods of immune monitoring exist that can permit the diagnosis to be made in a same-day fashion. Recent investigations offer evidence that immunoparalysis can be reversed with benefit to patients.

To provide a biologic framework, this discussion begins with an overview of the immune system. After this, the phenomenon of immunoparalysis is reviewed in detail with attention to mechanisms of disease, clinical significance, and potential for therapeutic intervention. The overall goal of this review is to highlight the anti-inflammatory end of the spectrum of the immune response as an underappreciated yet highly relevant contributor to outcomes in critically ill patients.

The monocyte and the inflammatory response

The innate immune system

In general terms, the immune system can be divided into the innate and the adaptive arms (Table 1). The innate immune system is understood most easily as the body's first cellular line of defense. It includes members whose primary roles include phagocytosis and intracellular killing (polymorphonuclear cells), cytotoxic killing (natural killer cells), and antigen presentation (dendritic cells). Another innate immune cell, the monocyte, is believed a key determinant of the acute immune response. Its diverse roles (and those of its descendant, the tissue macrophage) include recognition and phagocytosis of pathogens, presentation of digested peptides on its cell surface to

Table 1
Elements of the innate and adaptive immune systems

Innate	Adaptive
Cellular elements	Cellular elements
Phagocytosis	Antibody production
Monocytes/macrophages	B cells/plasma cells
Polymorphonuclear leukocytes	Cytotoxic killing
Dendritic cells	CD8+ T cells
Antigen presentation	Cytokine/chemokine production
Monocytes/macrophages	CD4+ T cells
Dendritic cells	T_H1 cells (proinflammatory)
Cytotoxic killing	T_H2 cells (anti-inflammatory)
Natural killer cells	T_{reg} cells (anti-inflammatory)
Polymorphonuclear leukocytes	
Cytokine/chemokine production	
All of the above	
Noncellular elements	Noncellular elements
Cytokines	Immunoglobulins
Chemokines	Cytokines
Complement	Chemokines

activate the adaptive immune response, and secretion of mediators that modulate the overall immune response (Fig. 1). A characteristic feature of monocytes and other innate immune cells is their ability to consistently respond to pathogens regardless of prior exposure history. They do not require prior sensitization to mount a robust immune response. This is accomplished through the presence of constitutively expressed receptors present on the plasma membranes of innate immune effector cells. These receptors recognize broad classes of microbial constituents. For example, bacterial lipopolysaccharide (LPS) is recognized by monocytes through its interaction with the Toll-like receptor (TLR) 4 complex on the monocyte cell surface. A monocyte that encounters LPS should vigorously produce proinflammatory cytokines whether or not it has been exposed to LPS in the past.

Once stimulated, monocytes engulf and destroy microbes, which then are processed into antigenic peptides. These are presented on the external surfaces of innate immune cells in conjunction with class II major histocompatibility complex (MHC) molecules, such as HLA-DR. Antigens presented in this way, along with costimulatory input from the innate immune cells, activate the adaptive arm of the immune response. Additionally, innate immune cells secrete cytokines and chemokines, which modulate the inflammatory response by recruiting and activating other immune effector cells and activating noncellular aspects of the immune response, such as the complement and coagulation cascades. Local production of proinflammatory cytokines, such as tumor necrosis factor (TNF)-α, results in activation of nearby immune cells and proinflammatory changes in vascular endothelium promoting cellular migration into the periphery. It is when this modulation becomes systemic that the clinical signs and symptoms of

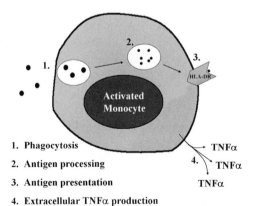

1. Phagocytosis

2. Antigen processing

3. Antigen presentation

4. Extracellular TNFα production

Fig. 1. Functions of the activated monocyte. A normal monocyte, on activation, is capable of ingesting pathogens; effecting intracellular killing and processing the foreign proteins into antigenic peptides; presenting these peptides on its cell surface in conjunction with HLA-DR molecules; and producing proinflammatory cytokines, such as TNF-α. An immunoparalyzed monocyte demonstrates reduced HLA-DR expression and impaired TNF-α production capacity.

hyperinflammation (fever, hemodynamic instability, and capillary leak) become evident.

The adaptive immune system

Although measures of immunoparalysis reflect primarily the innate immune response, the innate and adaptive immune systems do not act in isolation. Adaptive immune elements respond to, and in turn affect, the pro- and anti-inflammatory balance of the patient.

T and B lymphocytes are adaptive immune cells. In contrast to innate immunity, the adaptive immune system produces responses that are highly antigen specific. Adaptive immune responses typically require antigen presentation by innate immune cells. The initial lymphocyte response to a pathogen takes more time and is of smaller magnitude than the initial innate response. Repeat exposure to an antigen, however, provokes a more rapid and powerful adaptive immune response because of the presence of antigen-specific T- and B-cell clones that can be maintained for decades.

On stimulation, B cells mature into plasma cells, which produce antibodies that opsonize invaders, thus marking them for clearance by lymphoid organs and phagocytes. Activated T cells regulate the immune response through the production of cytokines (CD4+) and via cytotoxic killing (CD8+). Naïve CD4+ T cells can differentiate into one of several T-cell subtypes depending on the cytokine milieu in which they are activated. Although a detailed review of T-cell biology is beyond the scope of this review, three major classes of CD4+ T cells merit general discussion. These include the helper T (T_H)-1, T_H2, and regulatory T (T_{reg}) cells. In the presence of proinflammatory cytokines, naïve T cells differentiate into T_H1 cells. These cells in turn produce proinflammatory cytokines, such as interferon (IFN)-γ and serve to perpetuate the inflammatory response. T_H2 cells, by contrast, arise when naïve T cells are activated in an anti-inflammatory environment. They themselves produce anti-inflammatory cytokines, including interleukin (IL)-10 and transforming growth factor (TGF)-β, with a resultant inhibitory effect on the inflammatory response. T_{reg} cells represent a more recently described subgroup of CD4+ T cells. Often (but not always) characterized by cell surface expression of CD25 and the transcription factor FOXP3, these cells exert an even more powerful anti-inflammatory effect through contact-mediated direct inhibition of other immune cells and production of high levels of TGF-β and IL-10 (reviewed in Ref. [19]).

Cytokines and chemokines

To accomplish communication between cells of the innate and adaptive immune systems, a common language is needed. Cytokines and chemokines are the extracellular vocabulary of the immune system (Table 2). Certain cytokines (eg, TNF-α, IFN-γ, and IL-1β) have proinflammatory effects.

Table 2
Selected cytokines and their effects

	Cytokine	Primary producers	Actions
Proinflammatory	IL-1β	Monocytes/macrophages	Fever, vasodilation, activation of T cells, monocytes/ macrophages
	TNF-α	Monocytes/macrophages, T cells (T_H1), NK cells	Fever, vasodilation, apoptosis, activation of T cells, monocytes/macrophages
	IL-18	Macrophages	Activation of T cells and monocytes
	IL-12	Macrophages, DCs	Activation of NK cells
	IFN-γ	T cells (T_H1), NK cells	Activation of monocytes/ macrophages
	GM-CSF	T cells, macrophages	Increases production and promotes growth and activation of monocytes/ macrophages, PMNs, DCs
Mixed	IL-6	Monocytes, macrophages, Vascular endothelium	Promotes acute phase response (pro), activates adrenal axis (anti)
Anti-inflammatory	IL-10	Monocytes/macrophages, T cells (T_H2, T_{reg})	Inhibits monocyte/ macrophage activation
	TGF-β	Monocytes, T cells (T_H2, T_{reg})	Inhibits monocyte/ macrophage proliferation and activation
	IL-13	T cells (T_H2)	Inhibits monocyte/ macrophage cytokine production
	IL-1ra	Hepatocytes, monocytes/ macrophages, PMNs	Inhibits IL-1 action by blocking the IL-1 receptor

Abbreviations: DC, dendritic cell; NK, natural killer; PMN, polymorphonuclear cell.

Anti-inflammatory cytokines (eg, IL-10 and TGF-β) deactivate effector cells and inhibit the proinflammatory response. Chemokines, such as IL-8, are chemoattractants, which result in cellular migration into an inflamed area. When considering cytokines, it is important to appreciate that these molecules often have differing effects depending on the specific cell type being stimulated. Therefore, defining cytokines as purely pro- or anti-inflammatory can be misleading. An example of this can be found in IL-6. This cytokine is induced by proinflammatory stimuli and plasma IL-6 levels often are used as a marker of systemic inflammation [20–23]. Although IL-6 is known to stimulate the hepatic acute phase response, it also results in other, decidedly anti-inflammatory effects, including the induction of an adrenal glucocorticoid response [24,25]. It is in this setting of competing pro- and anti-inflammatory mediators that the concept of immunoparalysis becomes relevant.

Immunoparalysis

SIRS, CARS, and immunoparalysis in critical illness

When a sufficiently severe proinflammatory insult occurs, patients typically experience a constellation of vital sign and laboratory changes (tachycardia, tachypnea, abnormal temperature, and leukocytosis) termed the systemic inflammatory response syndrome (SIRS) [26]. In the most severe cases of hyperinflammation (eg, septic shock), the acute morbidity and mortality result not from overwhelming infection but from the systemic immune response to that infection. In short order (likely less than 24 hours later) compensatory mechanisms come into play and shut down the immune system's inflammatory response, often through the induction of anti-inflammatory cytokines. This phenomenon is referred to as the compensatory anti-inflammatory response syndrome (CARS). Although a transient CARS state is a necessary countermeasure to regulate and protect against inflammatory injury, like SIRS it also must be regulated. Immunoparalysis represents a persistent, severe form of a CARS state that has become pathologic (Fig. 2). Given the importance of the immune system in responding to pathogens and remodeling injured tissue, it is intuitive that patients recovering from septic shock or major surgery who develop immunoparalysis find themselves at increased risk for development of nosocomial infection and death.

Diagnosis and quantification of immunoparalysis

The concept of innate immune dysfunction associated with critical illness is hardly a new one. In the mid-1980s Polk and colleagues [16] investigated the behavior of the immune system in adults after trauma, with an interest in identifying the immunologic basis for late mortality and nosocomial infections in their patients. Their systematic examination of the immune response demonstrated an association between reduction in monocyte antigen-presenting capacity and development of secondary infections. Subsequent investigations have focused largely on two measures of innate immune competence in critical illness: monocyte class II MHC expression and whole blood ex vivo LPS-induced cytokine production capacity.

As discussed previously, monocytes activate the adaptive immune response through the presentation of antigens on cell-surface class II MHC molecules, such as HLA-DR. HLA-DR expression on circulating monocytes can be quantified by flow cytometry. Flow cytometric analysis involves the staining of whole blood with fluorochrome-tagged antibodies. Comparison of anti–HLA-DR fluorescence in CD14+ cells (monocytes) with that of a nonspecific control antibody enables the calculation of HLA-DR percent positivity. A monocyte HLA-DR expression level of less than 30%, for example, can be interpreted to mean that less than 30% of a subject's circulating monocytes have anti–HLA-DR fluorescence that is greater than

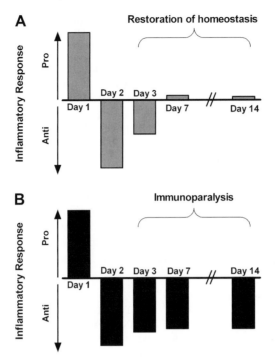

Fig. 2. Immunologic homeostasis versus immunoparalysis. A transient compensatory anti-inflammatory response typically follows a proinflammatory insult, but the immunologic balance between pro- and anti-inflammatory forces should be restored within a few days (*A*). If the anti-inflammatory response is severe and prolonged, it is termed immunoparalysis (*B*).

background fluorescence. Most of the literature on HLA-DR expression and immunoparalysis in ICUs uses this nomenclature. It is this threshold, less than 30% HLA-DR+ monocytes, that has become an accepted definition of immunoparalysis. In recent years, however, another option has become available that addresses the lack of standardization inherent in varying lots of antibodies and differences in cytometer calibration across centers. The Quantibrite system (Becton Dickinson, Franklin Lakes, New Jersey) is another flow cytometric tool for the quantification of monocyte HLA-DR expression. In this approach, a subject's monocyte anti–HLA-DR fluorescence is compared with that of a set of standard beads that express a known quantity of fluorescent antibodies on their surfaces. Using this technology the number of HLA-DR molecules per cell can be calculated in a way that is reproducible across centers. Although clinical investigators are beginning to use this method [27], it does not yet represent the standard approach in this field.

The other method commonly used for quantification of innate immune function in critical illness is measurement of the capacity of whole blood to produce proinflammatory cytokines when stimulated ex vivo. Although a normal monocyte produces copious amounts of TNF-α when exposed to LPS, an immunoparalyzed monocyte does not [28–33]. This approach suffers from a lack of standardization across investigators. There is no single protocol for defining immunoparalysis by ex vivo cytokine production capacity that has gained universal acceptance. The volume of blood used, the strain of bacteria from which the LPS originates, the method of LPS purification used, the incubation time, and the method of TNF-α measurement all are variables that must be held constant to define thresholds for diagnosis of immunoparalysis in a given patient. In the authors' laboratory, for example, a whole blood ex vivo LPS-induced TNF-α response less than 200 pg/mL after 4 hours of incubation at 37°C is the threshold for defining immunoparalysis [30]. This threshold value may be different in other laboratories if other reagents and experimental methods are used. This type of measurement does not reflect circulating TNF-α levels in the plasma; rather, it reflects the ability of a patient's blood to make TNF-α when it is needed.

Mechanisms of immunoparalysis

The underlying causes of immunoparalysis are, to date, poorly understood. Experimental and clinical evidence suggests, not surprisingly, that regulation of inflammation is not normal in innate immune cells that have an immunoparalyzed phenotype. The concept of "endotoxin tolerance" represents an experimental analog to the clinical entity of immunoparalysis. Culturing monocytes or monocytic cells lines in the presence of IL-10 or TGF-β, for example, induces a state of hyporesponsiveness to subsequent LPS challenge [34–36]. Perhaps the best inducer of experimental endotoxin tolerance is endotoxin itself. Pretreatment of cells or animals with a sublethal dose of LPS results in a long-lasting refractory period during which the innate immune cells respond weakly to a second dose of LPS [37–39]. As many patients have no known LPS exposure associated with the development of immunoparalysis, it seems unlikely that this accounts for most episodes of innate immune dysfunction in ICUs. Possible intracellular mechanisms associated with models of endotoxin tolerance include inhibition of the proinflammatory transcription factor, nuclear factor κB (NFκB), through alteration of its subunit composition [40,41] or up-regulation of its inhibitor, IκBα [42]; up-regulation of the NFκB pathway inhibitor, IRAK-M [43–45]; or impairment of TLR4 signaling [46–48].

Mechanistic data from human subjects who have immunoparalysis are rare, but Fumeaux and colleagues [49] demonstrated internalization of cell-surface HLA-DR molecules in normal human monocytes with co-incubation with serum from septic patients. This monocyte deactivation was partially reversed by the addition of anti–IL-10 neutralizing antibodies. Others have shown that septic adults who have impaired innate immune function demonstrate up-regulation of IRAK-M [44] and down-regulation of the receptor for granulocyte-macrophage colony-stimulating factor (GM-CSF) on monocytes [50]. Pachot and colleagues [51] examined the mRNA transcription characteristics of whole blood from 38 adult patients who had septic shock who survived at least 48 hours in an effort to identify differences in gene expression between survivors and nonsurvivors. The results of their analyses revealed 28 individual genes whose transcription levels predicted mortality. Survivors showed increased transcription of genes encoding chemokine receptors, cytokine receptors, and signal transducers, all involved in initiating and maintaining the innate immune response. Nonsurvivors did not demonstrate a similar up-regulation of proinflammatory gene transcription. These results suggest that preservation of the ability to mount a proinflammatory response may be an important determinant of survival. The authors' laboratory recently studied monocyte mRNA from 28 children who had multiple organ dysfunction syndrome (MODS) [52] and found that expression of mRNA coding for IL-10, IRAK-M, and pyrin (a putative inhibitor of intracellular inflammatory pathways) was elevated in nonsurvivors compared with survivors, with nonsurvivors demonstrating lower whole blood ex vivo LPS-induced TNF-α responses. These data suggest, therefore, that children dying from MODS are doing so with an anti-inflammatory innate immune phenotype.

Corticosteroids may play a role in the development or perpetuation of immunoparalysis. Le Tulzo and colleagues [53] in 2004 studied 48 septic patients and found an association between high levels of circulating cortisol and reductions in monocyte HLA-DR expression on day 6 of illness. They demonstrated in vitro that dexamethasone caused a down-regulation of a key transcription factor for HLA-DR in normal monocytes. The investigators suggest that glucocorticoid action may represent another mechanism for the development of innate immune dysfunction. Similarly, Volk and colleagues [54] demonstrated that the administration of methylprednisolone in the setting of cardiopulmonary bypass (CPB) resulted in an exacerbation of innate immunosuppression over that seen with bypass alone.

Acquired innate and adaptive immune dysfunction can coexist in critically ill patients. Monneret and others recently demonstrated associations between immunoparalysis and the subsequent development of a T_{reg}-dominant adaptive immune response [55,56]. It also has been shown in critically ill adults [57] and children [58] that lymphocyte apoptosis and lymphopenia are common in ICU nonsurvivors. The temporal and causal relationships between innate and adaptive immune dysfunction in critical illness remain incompletely understood.

It is likely that host genetic factors are important in determining who goes on to develop immunoparalysis after an inflammatory insult. To date, however, no single polymorphism (or group of polymorphisms) has been able to explain predisposition toward this phenotype. The importance of this issue was highlighted by the work of Westendorp and colleagues [59] who, in 1997, examined the ex-vivo LPS-induced cytokine production capacity of 190 first-degree relatives of patients who had invasive meningo-coccal disease. They found that family members of nonsurvivors produced less TNF-α and more IL-10 with ex vivo LPS stimulation than did the relatives of patients who survived, indicating that a predilection toward an anti-inflammatory phenotype may be heritable.

The clinical significance of immunoparalysis

Trauma

Trauma surgeons were among the first clinicians to study the innate immune response in the setting of critical illness. In 1986, Polk and colleagues [16] undertook a systematic evaluation of 20 adults who had severe trauma. The results of their analyses indicated that persistently impaired monocyte antigen-presenting capacity was associated with development of nosocomial sepsis. All of the traumatized patients had reduced monocyte HLA-DR expression compared with healthy controls when first evaluated on ICU admission. It was those who exhibited prolonged HLA-DR down-regulation in whom secondary sepsis developed more often. These findings were confirmed by Livingston and colleagues [18] in a separate series of adult trauma patients. It seems that the initial reduction in monocyte HLA-DR expression is indicative of the CARS state and not itself patho-logic. Rather, it is the failure of HLA-DR expression to recover to normal levels over time that places patients at risk for developing nosocomial sepsis.

The ability of HLA-DR expression profile to predict outcome in trauma-tized adults was strengthened by the work of Cheadle and colleagues [60] in 1989 in a study of serial monocyte HLA-DR measurements in 60 trauma victims beginning the first 24 hours after injury. In their cohort, the depth and persistence of HLA-DR expression was predictive of development of secondary infection. The study differed from previous work in that mono-cytes with low HLA-DR expression underwent ex vivo LPS-induced stimu-lation. Patients who developed secondary sepsis but went on to survive had low initial monocyte HLA-DR expression that was reversible by LPS stim-ulation. In contrast, persistently low HLA-DR expression, even after ex vivo LPS stimulation, was characteristic of patients who died.

Ex vivo TNF-α production also is correlated with outcome in clinical trauma studies. Majetschak and colleagues [28] in 1999 performed ex vivo LPS-induced stimulation of whole blood samples from 46 adult blunt trauma victims. They documented a profound reduction in patients' TNF-α production compared with healthy controls. The degree of reduction in the TNF-α response was associated with the severity of injury and this reduction was detectable in samples obtained within 90 minutes after trauma. Patients requiring surgery to treat their injuries experienced a fur-ther impairment in their TNF-α response.

Septic disease

If innate immune dysfunction can follow the inflammatory insult of trauma then it stands to reason that the hyperinflammation associated with severe sepsis and septic shock also should be associated with the development of immunoparalysis. In the mid-1990s Volk and colleagues [61] studied monocyte HLA-DR expression in 247 adult surgical patients who had septic disease. In their cohort, an HLA-DR expression level less than 30% for 5 days or more was associated with a 12% survival rate. This was in contrast to a survival rate of 88% in patients whose reduction in monocyte HLA-DR expression was transient or less severe ($P < .01$; χ^2). Similarly, patients whose monocyte HLA-DR expression was less than 30% were at increased risk for development of nosocomial sepsis associated with postoperative peritonitis. The authors found similar results in children who had MODS, in that those who demonstrated monocyte HLA-DR expression less than 30% for more than 3 days had significantly increased risks for development of nosocomial infection and death [62].

Monneret and colleagues [14] in 2006 followed 93 adult patients (83 with complete data sets) who had a primary diagnosis of septic shock and evaluated HLA-DR expression. Patients who survived demonstrated recovery of HLA-DR expression by day 3 or 4, whereas those who eventually died failed to recover HLA-DR expression (Fig. 3). Multivariate logistic regression analysis showed that a monocyte HLA-DR expression less than 30% on day 3 or 4 was associated with mortality after adjusting for confounders, including initial severity of illness and presence of comorbidities (odds ratio 6.48; 95% CI, 1.62–25.93).

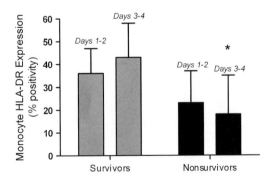

Fig. 3. Prolonged suppression of monocyte HLA-DR expression predicts outcome. In 86 adult patients who had septic shock, monocyte HLA-DR expression was suppressed on days 1–2 in all patients but to a greater degree in nonsurvivors. By days 3–4, survivors had begun to recover HLA-DR expression whereas it remained low in nonsurvivors. *$P < .001$ versus survivors, Mann-Whitney test. Data represent median (25th–75th percentile). (*Data from* Monneret G, Lepape A, Voirin N, et al. Persisting low monocyte human leukocyte antigen-DR expression predicts mortality in septic shock. Intensive Care Med 2006;32(8):1175–83.)

Not all studies of the association between monocyte function and outcome from critical illness are positive. Perry and colleagues [63] in 2003 examined HLA-DR expression in 70 patients on days 1 through 3 after the onset of septic shock. In this study monocyte HLA-DR expression was not found to correlate with mortality. To look for such an association so early in a patient's ICU course may, however, be problematic. A more longitudinal approach to immune monitoring likely is required to identify patients who have prolonged innate immune dysfunction. It is these patients who seem to be at highest risk for development of adverse outcomes.

As in the setting of trauma, impairment of the ex vivo LPS-induced TNF-α response also occurs after septic disease and is associated with adverse outcomes. Ploder and colleagues [64] recently described a series of 19 polytrauma patients who had sepsis in whom the degree of depression of the ex vivo TNF-α response was more predictive of death on the day of sepsis onset than was the level of monocyte HLA-DR expression. The authors' recent cohort of 28 children who had MODS (25 of whom had septic shock) also underwent measurement of their whole blood ex vivo LPS-induced TNF-α responses [52]. These data showed that nonsurvivors demonstrated lower ex vivo LPS-induced TNF-α production over the first 2 weeks of MODS compared with survivors (Fig. 4).

Innate immune dysfunction in other settings

Other types of proinflammatory insults are associated with innate immunodepression. Ho and colleagues [15] showed that suppressed monocyte HLA-DR expression and reduced ex vivo LPS-induced TNF-α production

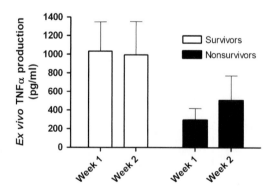

Fig. 4. The ex vivo LPS-induced TNF-α response is lower over time in nonsurvivors of pediatric MODS. Thirty children who had MODS underwent serial measurement of their whole blood ex vivo LPS-induced TNF-α response in the first and second weeks of illness. Nonsurvivors demonstrated a reduced capacity to produce TNF-α when stimulated ex vivo over time compared with survivors ($P = .017$; 2-way ANOVA on log-transformed data). Data represent mean (standard error). (*Data from* Hall MW, Gavrilin MA, Knatz NL, et al. Monocyte mRNA phenotype and adverse outcomes from pediatric multiple organ dysfunction syndrome. Pediatr Res 2007;62(5):597–603.)

on day 10 of acute pancreatitis were predictive of mortality as was the presence of an elevated serum IL-10 level. Monocyte HLA-DR expression on day 10 was better able to predict nosocomial infection and mortality than the Ranson score or Acute Physiology and Chronic Health Evaluation (APACHE) severity of illness score.

Allen and colleagues [65] studied 82 infants and children undergoing CPB for repair of congenital heart defects and documented reduced monocyte HLA-DR expression in all patients post CPB compared with pre-CPB levels. The investigators correlated prolonged reduction of HLA-DR expression with the development of SIRS and sepsis after surgery. A multivariate analysis identified HLA-DR expression as an independent predictor of secondary sepsis after controlling for other variables, including severity of illness, complexity of surgery, and length of CPB. These results were supported by the same group in a 2006 follow-up study [66] in which 36 children undergoing CPB were enrolled. Immune function was monitored serially by ex vivo LPS stimulation assays and IL-10 measurements. Higher levels of plasma IL-10 were associated with the greatest risk for developing more severe innate immune dysfunction. Patients who had more profoundly reduced ex vivo TNF-α responses as early as day 2 after CPB had a greater likelihood of experiencing postoperative complications including nosocomial sepsis.

Reversibility of immunoparalysis

As the natural history of innate immune dysfunction in critical illness becomes clearer, a question arises: Is immunoparalysis simply an epiphenomenon associated with critical illness or does it represent a reversible target for intervention in hopes of improving outcomes? The answer to this question is far from clear, but several lines of evidence suggest that the latter may be true.

Many investigators have described reversal of endotoxin tolerance in vitro with agents, including anti–IL-10 neutralizing antibody [49], IL-12 [67], GM-CSF [37,67,68], and Flt3-ligand [69]. Hershman and colleagues [70] reported in 1989 that monocytes collected from immunoparalyzed adult trauma victims could be made to up-regulate their HLA-DR expression with ex vivo culture with the T_H1 cytokine, IFN-γ. The effects of ex vivo culture with GM-CSF on monocyte function were reported by Flohe and colleagues in 2003 [71]. In this study of 16 adult trauma patients, blood samples were obtained biweekly during the ICU stay. Individual samples were divided into two aliquots, one pretreated with GM-CSF and the other untreated. Monocyte HLA-DR expression and ex vivo LPS-induced TNF-α production then were analyzed for each aliquot and compared. GM-CSF stimulation improved TNF-α production in the treated aliquots and, to a lesser extent, resulted in up-regulation of HLA-DR expression. In patients who went on to recover uneventfully, ex vivo GM-CSF treatment restored monocyte function to the level of normal volunteers.

GM-CSF treatment was unable to improve monocyte function to normal levels in the most severely injured patients, who eventually developed sepsis and MODS. The blood from patients who eventually developed severe MODS with three or more failed organs did not respond to GM-CSF at all. More recently, Lendemans and colleagues [72] showed that ex vivo treatment with IFN-γ or GM-CSF (but not granulocyte colony-stimulating factor [G-CSF]) resulted in improvement in monocyte HLA-DR expression and whole blood LPS-induced cytokine production in blood samples from injured patients.

The administration of immune-stimulating agents directly to patients who had immunoparalysis has been done in a few small case series. In 1997 Kox and colleagues [73] demonstrated restoration of monocyte HLA-DR expression and ex vivo TNF-α response in 9 of 10 adult septic patients who had immunoparalysis and treatment with subcutaneous IFN-γ, 100 μg daily until monocyte HLA-DR expression remained greater than 50% for 3 days. Eight of ten patients showed increased HLA-DR expression within 1 day of treatment. The 28-day mortality in this cohort, with median treatment duration of 6 days, was 40%. This mortality rate represented an improvement over the 58% to 88% mortality previously described by this group in adults who had persistent immunoparalysis [74].

In 2002 Nakos and colleagues [75] conducted a small, randomized, placebo-controlled trial of inhaled interferon in 21 trauma patients who demonstrated reduced HLA-DR expression on alveolar macrophages obtained by bronchoalveolar lavage (BAL). Subjects randomized to the treatment group received 100 μg of inhaled recombinant human (rh) IFN-γ 3 times daily. Although there was no difference in mortality between groups, the IFN-γ–treated subjects showed increased HLA-DR expression on alveolar macrophages, decreased IL-10 levels in subsequent BAL fluid, and a reduced rate of ventilator-associated pneumonia compared with the placebo group.

rhGM-CSF also has been used to systemically treat adult septic patients who have immunoparalysis. In 2003, Nierhaus and colleagues [76] reported a case series in which nine septic adults who had immunoparalysis received rhGM-CSF (5 μg/kg by subcutaneous injection daily for 3 days). All patients experienced increases in monocyte HLA-DR expression and ex vivo LPS-induced TNF-α production within 24 hours of initiation of rhGM-CSF treatment. There was no increase in circulating markers of inflammation (plasma IL-6 and C-reactive protein) associated with rhGM-CSF therapy. Mortality in this series was 33%.

Some trials of immunostimulatory agents in critical illness have not used an a priori measurement of the innate immune response. In 2001 Bilgin and colleagues [77] reported the results of a randomized placebo-controlled trial of rhGM-CSF therapy for neutropenic neonates who had a diagnosis of sepsis. Patients were assigned to experimental groups without a measurement of baseline innate immune function other than absolute neutrophil count. Treated infants received subcutaneous rhGM-CSF (5 μg/kg per day for

7 days). Neonates receiving GM-CSF demonstrated a significant improvement in mortality rate (10%) compared with those in the placebo group (30%; $P < .05$). In another GM-CSF treatment study that did not include measures of innate immune function as inclusion criteria, Rosenbloom and colleagues [78] randomized 40 adult ICU patients who had infection-related SIRS to receive intravenous GM-CSF (125 $\mu g/m^2$) over 72 hours or placebo. Patients treated with GM-CSF demonstrated improved monocyte HLA-DR expression and shorter time to resolution of infection compared with the placebo group. There was no worsening of organ failure or other adverse drug effects in the GM-CSF group.

Not all studies of the use of colony-stimulating factors in ICUs have been positive. For example, a 2003 Cochrane meta-analysis concluded that insufficient evidence existed to recommend for or against the use of GM-CSF or G-CSF for prophylaxis or treatment of critically ill neonates [79]. The studies reviewed for this analysis did not include measurement of parameters, however, such as HLA-DR expression or ex vivo cytokine production in their protocols.

Transplant-related immunosuppression

Patients who have undergone solid organ or hematopoetic stem cell transplantation and remain on exogenous immunosuppression find themselves at high risk for development of secondary infection. Although specific prophylaxis regimens have been recommended for this patient population [80], nosocomial infections often are difficult to prevent. At present, most transplant specialists follow drug levels and monitor end-organ function to titrate immunosuppressive therapy. This approach is most applicable to calcineurin inhibitors, such as cyclosporine or tacrolimus. Although these agents classically are considered T-cell inhibitors, they also exert a polarizing effect, skewing innate and adaptive immune systems toward a T_H2-like phenotype. High plasma IL-10 levels are associated with development of nosocomial infection and death after bone marrow transplantation [81]. Some degree of T_H2 polarization likely is necessary, however, as hepatic graft rejection is associated with low plasma levels of IL-10 [82].

The innate immune-monitoring methods (discussed previously) have been applied to the transplant population with interesting results. In the early 1990s, Settmacher and colleagues [83] described an association between aggressive calcineurin inhibition and reduction in monocyte HLA-DR expression in the setting of induction therapy in adults after liver transplantation. Among 91 patients, those whose monocyte HLA-DR expression dropped below 30% (n = 48) experienced increased rates of bacteremia, viremia, and fungemia compared with those whose HLA-DR levels remained greater than 30% (n = 43). Providing additional evidence for the reversibility of immunoparalysis, Reinke and Volk [84] described a cohort of 45 adult kidney transplant recipients who developed nosocomial sepsis in the setting of immunoparalysis. Patients who underwent rapid tapering of their calcineurin inhibition experienced a 90% survival rate (30/33) with 98% graft survival. In contrast, patients who did not undergo tapering had an 8% survival rate (1/12) with the sole survivor experiencing graft loss.

Pediatric data on this subject are limited, but Hoffman and colleagues [85] described a series of 13 pediatric lung transplant recipients who underwent monocyte HLA-DR monitoring weekly after transplantation. Six of seven patients who developed post-transplant pneumonia demonstrated failure to recover monocyte HLA-DR expression within the first 2 weeks of monitoring. Those who developed pneumonia had lower monocyte HLA-DR expression over the 4-week study period than those who remained infection-free.

Some investigators have used immunostimulatory therapy with IFN-γ or GM-CSF for the treatment of post-transplant septic disease [86,87]; prospective, standardized trials, however, are lacking. Monocyte HLA-DR expression measurement and quantification of the ex vivo LPS-induced TNF-α response seem to have the potential to provide insight into the degree of functional immunosuppression after transplantation and are deserving of future study in this regard.

Other determinants of the immune response in critical illness

Although acquired monocyte dysfunction has been the subject of this review thus far, other factors can influence the immune response of patients in pediatric ICUs. As alluded to previously, the adaptive immune response contributes to the overall immunophenotpe of a given patient. A shift toward a T_H2- or T_{reg}-dominant adaptive immune state also likely results in anti-inflammatory changes in innate immune cells. Cell numbers are similarly important. The cancer literature and HIV literature have taught that patients who have low absolute neutrophil counts or lymphopenia are at high risk for development of secondary infection and death [88–90]. Critical illness itself frequently is associated with unintended immunomodulation. Hyperglycemia [91] and hepatic failure [23] frequently are associated with a proinflammatory state whereas uremia [92,93] and traumatic brain injury [94,95] can be immunosuppressive. Also, many of the therapies that have become mainstays in ICUs have unintended immune effects, including catecholamines (often proinflammatory) [96] and insulin, narcotics, and furosemide (anti-inflammatory) [97–99].

Summary

Historically the battle against hyperinflammation in ICUs has been of primary importance to pediatric intensivists. The notion that many patients are suffering and dying from an occult anti-inflammatory phenotype requires a sea change in clinicians' philosophy. Although some patients will continue to require anti-inflammatory treatments, others may need therapies that augment the immune response. It is likely that the maximum benefit from immunostimulation would be seen in children who have underactive immune responses at the beginning of treatment. To give such agents to children who have normal or high levels of proinflammatory responsiveness would at best be unhelpful and at worst harmful. To that end, the use of immunomodulatory therapies for children in ICUs should be based on development and implementation of prospective, standardized, immune-monitoring regimens. This way, specific children at high risk (eg, those who have immunoparalysis) can be identified as candidates for therapy, avoiding unnecessary or dangerous immunomodulation in low-risk patients. To date, the vast majority of data outlining the natural history of innate immune function in critical illness come from the adult literature. There are only a handful of studies that hint at the developmental aspects of acquired immune dysfunction in neonates, infants, and small children [100–102]. The challenge before the pediatric intensive care community, therefore, is to design and implement multicenter prospective observational and interventional studies to address these important issues and work toward promoting immunologic homeostasis in pediatric ICUs.

References

[1] Prophylactic intravenous administration of standard immune globulin as compared with core-lipopolysaccharide immune globulin in patients at high risk of postsurgical infection. The Intravenous Immunoglobulin Collaborative Study Group. N Engl J Med 1992;327(4):234–40.

[2] Calandra T, Glauser MP, Schellekens J, et al. Treatment of gram-negative septic shock with human IgG antibody to Escherichia coli J5: a prospective, double-blind, randomized trial. J Infect Dis 1988;158(2):312–9.

[3] Bone RC, Balk RA, Fein AM, et al. A second large controlled clinical study of E5, a monoclonal antibody to endotoxin: results of a prospective, multicenter, randomized, controlled trial. The E5 Sepsis Study Group. Crit Care Med 1995;23(6):994–1006.

[4] Greenman RL, Schein RM, Martin MA, et al. A controlled clinical trial of E5 murine monoclonal IgM antibody to endotoxin in the treatment of gram-negative sepsis. The XOMA Sepsis Study Group. JAMA 1991;266(8):1097–102.

[5] McCloskey RV, Straube RC, Sanders C, et al. Treatment of septic shock with human monoclonal antibody HA-1A. A randomized, double-blind, placebo-controlled trial. CHESS Trial Study Group. Ann Intern Med 1994;121(1):1–5.

[6] Fisher CJ Jr, Dhainaut JF, Opal SM, et al. Recombinant human interleukin 1 receptor antagonist in the treatment of patients with sepsis syndrome. Results from a randomized, double-blind, placebo-controlled trial. Phase III rhIL-1ra Sepsis Syndrome Study Group. JAMA 1994;271(23):1836–43.

[7] Opal SM, Fisher CJ Jr, Dhainaut JF, et al. Confirmatory interleukin-1 receptor antagonist trial in severe sepsis: a phase III, randomized, double-blind, placebo-controlled, multicenter trial. The Interleukin-1 Receptor Antagonist Sepsis Investigator Group. Crit Care Med 1997;25(7):1115–24.

[8] Abraham E, Anzueto A, Gutierrez G, et al. Double-blind randomised controlled trial of monoclonal antibody to human tumour necrosis factor in treatment of septic shock. NORASEPT II Study Group. Lancet 1998;351(9107):929–33.

[9] Abraham E, Wunderink R, Silverman H, et al. Efficacy and safety of monoclonal antibody to human tumor necrosis factor alpha in patients with sepsis syndrome. A randomized, controlled, double-blind, multicenter clinical trial. TNF-alpha MAb Sepsis Study Group. JAMA 1995;273(12):934–41.

[10] Cohen J, Carlet J. INTERSEPT: an international, multicenter, placebo-controlled trial of monoclonal antibody to human tumor necrosis factor-alpha in patients with sepsis. International Sepsis Trial Study Group. Crit Care Med 1996;24(9):1431–40.

[11] Panacek EA, Marshall JC, Albertson TE, et al. Efficacy and safety of the monoclonal anti-tumor necrosis factor antibody F(ab')2 fragment afelimomab in patients with severe sepsis and elevated interleukin-6 levels. Crit Care Med 2004;32(11):2173–82.

[12] Fein AM, Bernard GR, Criner GJ, et al. Treatment of severe systemic inflammatory response syndrome and sepsis with a novel bradykinin antagonist, deltibant (CP-0127). Results of a randomized, double-blind, placebo-controlled trial. CP-0127 SIRS and Sepsis Study Group. JAMA 1997;277(6):482–7.

[13] Docke WD, Syrbe U, Meinecke A, et al. Improvement in monocyte function: a new therapeutic approach in sepsis? In: Reinhart K, Eyrich K, Sprung C, editors. Sepsis: current perspectives in pathophysiology and therapy. Berlin: Springer-Verlag; 1994. p. 473–500.

[14] Monneret G, Lepape A, Voirin N, et al. Persisting low monocyte human leukocyte antigen-DR expression predicts mortality in septic shock. Intensive Care Med 2006;32(8):1175–83.

[15] Ho YP, Sheen IS, Chiu CT, et al. A strong association between down-regulation of HLA-DR expression and the late mortality in patients with severe acute pancreatitis. Am J Gastroenterol 2006;101(5):1117–24.

[16] Polk HC Jr, Wellhausen SR, Regan M. A systematic study of host defense processes in badly injured patients. Ann Surg 1986;204(3):282–97.

[17] Hershman MJ, Cheadle WG, Wellhausen SR, et al. Monocyte HLA-DR antigen expression characterizes clinical outcome in the trauma patient. Br J Surg 1990;77(2):204–7.

[18] Livingston DH, Appel SH, Wellhausen SR, et al. Depressed interferon gamma production and monocyte HLA-DR expression after severe injury. Arch Surg 1988;123(11):1309–12.

[19] Chatila TA. Role of regulatory T cells in human diseases. J Allergy Clin Immunol 2005;116(5):949–59 [quiz: 960].

[20] Calandra T, Gerain J, Heumann D, et al. High circulating levels of interleukin-6 in patients with septic shock: evolution during sepsis, prognostic value, and interplay with other cytokines. The Swiss-Dutch J5 Immunoglobulin Study Group. Am J Med 1991;91(1):23–9.

[21] Doughty LA, Kaplan SS, Carcillo JA. Inflammatory cytokine and nitric oxide responses in pediatric sepsis and organ failure. Crit Care Med 1996;24(7):1137–43.

[22] Ghani RA, Zainudin S, Ctkong N, et al. Serum IL-6 and IL-1-ra with sequential organ failure assessment scores in septic patients receiving high-volume haemofiltration and continuous venovenous haemofiltration. Nephrology (Carlton) 2006;11(5):386–93.

[23] Pinsky MR, Vincent JL, Deviere J, et al. Serum cytokine levels in human septic shock. Relation to multiple-system organ failure and mortality. Chest 1993;103(2):565–75.

[24] Steensberg A, Fischer CP, Keller C, et al. IL-6 enhances plasma IL-1ra, IL-10, and cortisol in humans. Am J Physiol Endocrinol Metab 2003;285(2):E433–7.

[25] Diehl S, Rincon M. The two faces of IL-6 on Th1/Th2 differentiation. Mol Immunol 2002;39(9):531–6.

[26] Goldstein B, Giroir B, Randolph A. International pediatric sepsis consensus conference: definitions for sepsis and organ dysfunction in pediatrics. Pediatr Crit Care Med 2005;6(1):2–8.

[27] Docke WD, Hoflich C, Davis KA, et al. Monitoring temporary immunodepression by flow cytometric measurement of monocytic HLA-DR expression: a multicenter standardized study. Clin Chem 2005;51(12):2341–7.

[28] Majetschak M, Flach R, Kreuzfelder E, et al. The extent of traumatic damage determines a graded depression of the endotoxin responsiveness of peripheral blood mononuclear cells from patients with blunt injuries. Crit Care Med 1999;27(2):313–8.

[29] Majetschak M, Krehmeier U, Bardenheuer M, et al. Extracellular ubiquitin inhibits the TNF-alpha response to endotoxin in peripheral blood mononuclear cells and regulates endotoxin hyporesponsiveness in critical illness. Blood 2003;101(5):1882–90.

[30] Hall MW, Carcillo JA. Immune paralysis and the state of immunologic dissonance in pediatric multiple organ dysfunction syndrome. Crit Care Med 2001;29(12):A20.

[31] Docke WD, Randow F, Syrbe U, et al. Monocyte deactivation in septic patients: restoration by IFN-gamma treatment. Nat Med 1997;3(6):678–81.

[32] Flach R, Majetschak M, Heukamp T, et al. Relation of ex vivo stimulated blood cytokine synthesis to post-traumatic sepsis. Cytokine 1999;11(2):173–8.

[33] Heagy W, Nieman K, Hansen C, et al. Lower levels of whole blood LPS-stimulated cytokine release are associated with poorer clinical outcomes in surgical ICU patients. Surg Infect (Larchmt) 2003;4(2):171–80.

[34] Wolk K, Docke W, von Baehr V, et al. Comparison of monocyte functions after LPS- or IL-10-induced reorientation: importance in clinical immunoparalysis. Pathobiology 1999; 67(5–6):253–6.

[35] Wolk K, Docke WD, von Baehr V, et al. Impaired antigen presentation by human monocytes during endotoxin tolerance. Blood 2000;96(1):218–23.

[36] Randow F, Syrbe U, Meisel C, et al. Mechanism of endotoxin desensitization: involvement of interleukin 10 and transforming growth factor beta. J Exp Med 1995;181(5):1887–92.

[37] Bundschuh DS, Barsig J, Hartung T, et al. Granulocyte-macrophage colony-stimulating factor and IFN-gamma restore the systemic TNF-alpha response to endotoxin in lipopolysaccharide-desensitized mice. J Immunol 1997;158(6):2862–71.

[38] Flohe S, Dominguez Fernandez E, Ackermann M, et al. Endotoxin tolerance in rats: expression of TNF-alpha, IL-6, IL-10, VCAM-1 AND HSP 70 in lung and liver during endotoxin shock. Cytokine 1999;11(10):796–804.

[39] Madonna GS, Peterson JE, Ribi EE, et al. Early-phase endotoxin tolerance: induction by a detoxified lipid A derivative, monophosphoryl lipid A. Infect Immun 1986;52:6–11.

[40] Bohuslav J, Kravchenko VV, Parry GC, et al. Regulation of an essential innate immune response by the p50 subunit of NF-kappaB. J Clin Invest 1998;102(9):1645–52.

[41] Kastenbauer S, Ziegler-Heitbrock HW. NF-kappaB1 (p50) is upregulated in lipopolysaccharide tolerance and can block tumor necrosis factor gene expression. Infect Immun 1999;67(4):1553–9.

[42] Wahlstrom K, Bellingham J, Rodriguez JL, et al. Inhibitory kappaBalpha control of nuclear factor-kappaB is dysregulated in endotoxin tolerant macrophages. Shock 1999; 11(4):242–7.

[43] Nakayama K, Okugawa S, Yanagimoto S, et al. Involvement of IRAK-M in peptidoglycan-induced tolerance in macrophages. J Biol Chem 2004;279(8):6629–34.

[44] Escoll P, del Fresno C, Garcia L, et al. Rapid up-regulation of IRAK-M expression following a second endotoxin challenge in human monocytes and in monocytes isolated from septic patients. Biochem Biophys Res Commun 2003;311(2):465–72.

[45] del Fresno C, Otero K, Gomez-Garcia L, et al. Tumor cells deactivate human monocytes by up-regulating IL-1 receptor associated kinase-M expression via CD44 and TLR4. J Immunol 2005;174(5):3032–40.

[46] Dobrovolskaia MA, Vogel SN. Toll receptors, CD14, and macrophage activation and deactivation by LPS. Microbes Infect 2002;4(9):903–14.

[47] Alves-Rosa F, Vulcano M, Beigier-Bompadre M, et al. Interleukin-1beta induces in vivo tolerance to lipopolysaccharide in mice. Clin Exp Immunol 2002;128(2):221–8.

[48] Medvedev AE, Lentschat A, Wahl LM, et al. Dysregulation of LPS-induced Toll-like receptor 4-MyD88 complex formation and IL-1 receptor-associated kinase 1 activation in endotoxin-tolerant cells. J Immunol 2002;169(9):5209–16.

[49] Fumeaux T, Pugin J. Role of interleukin-10 in the intracellular sequestration of human leukocyte antigen-DR in monocytes during septic shock. Am J Respir Crit Care Med 2002;166(11):1475–82.

[50] Pangault C, Le Tulzo Y, Tattevin P, et al. Down-modulation of granulocyte macrophage-colony stimulating factor receptor on monocytes during human septic shock. Crit Care Med 2006;34(4):1193–201.

[51] Pachot A, Lepape A, Vey S, et al. Systemic transcriptional analysis in survivor and non-survivor septic shock patients: a preliminary study. Immunol Lett 2006;106(1):63–71.

[52] Hall MW, Gavrilin MA, Knatz NL, et al. Monocyte mRNA phenotype and adverse outcomes from pediatric multiple organ dysfunction syndrome. Pediatr Res 2007;62(5): 597–603.

[53] Le Tulzo Y, Pangault C, Amiot L, et al. Monocyte human leukocyte antigen-DR transcriptional downregulation by cortisol during septic shock. Am J Respir Crit Care Med 2004; 169(10):1144–51.

[54] Volk T, Schmutzler M, Engelhardt L, et al. Influence of aminosteroid and glucocorticoid treatment on inflammation and immune function during cardiopulmonary bypass. Crit Care Med 2001;29(11):2137–42.

[55] Monneret G, Debard AL, Venet F, et al. Marked elevation of human circulating CD4+CD25+ regulatory T cells in sepsis-induced immunoparalysis. Crit Care Med 2003;31(7):2068–71.

[56] Venet F, Pachot A, Debard AL, et al. Increased percentage of CD4+CD25+ regulatory T cells during septic shock is due to the decrease of CD4+CD25- lymphocytes. Crit Care Med 2004;32(11):2329–31.

[57] Hotchkiss RS, Tinsley KW, Swanson PE, et al. Sepsis-induced apoptosis causes progressive profound depletion of B and CD4+ T lymphocytes in humans. J Immunol 2001;166(11): 6952–63.

[58] Felmet KA, Hall MW, Clark RS, et al. Prolonged lymphopenia, lymphoid depletion, and hypoprolactinemia in children with nosocomial sepsis and multiple organ failure. J Immunol 2005;174(6):3765–72.

[59] Westendorp RG, Langermans JA, Huizinga TW, et al. Genetic influence on cytokine production and fatal meningococcal disease. Lancet 1997;349(9046):170–3.

[60] Cheadle WG, Wilson M, Hershman MJ, et al. Comparison of trauma assessment scores and their use in prediction of infection and death. Ann Surg 1989;209(5):541–5 [discussion: 545–6].

[61] Volk HD, Reinke P, Krausch D, et al. Monocyte deactivation–rationale for a new therapeutic strategy in sepsis. Intensive Care Med 1996;22(Suppl 4):S474–81.

[62] Hall MW, Volk HD, Carcillo JA. Immune paralysis in pediatric multiple organ dysfunction syndrome. Pediatr Res 2000;47(4):57A.

[63] Perry SE, Mostafa SM, Wenstone R, et al. Is low monocyte HLA-DR expression helpful to predict outcome in severe sepsis? Intensive Care Med 2003;29(8):1245–52.

[64] Ploder M, Pelinka L, Schmuckenschlager C, et al. Lipopolysaccharide-induced tumor necrosis factor alpha production and not monocyte human leukocyte antigen-DR expression is correlated with survival in septic trauma patients. Shock 2006;25(2):129–34.

[65] Allen ML, Peters MJ, Goldman A, et al. Early postoperative monocyte deactivation predicts systemic inflammation and prolonged stay in pediatric cardiac intensive care. Crit Care Med 2002;30(5):1140–5.

[66] Allen ML, Hoschtitzky JA, Peters MJ, et al. Interleukin-10 and its role in clinical immunoparalysis following pediatric cardiac surgery. Crit Care Med 2006;34(10):2658–65.

[67] Randow F, Docke WD, Bundschuh DS, et al. In vitro prevention and reversal of lipopolysaccharide desensitization by IFN-gamma, IL-12, and granulocyte-macrophage colony-stimulating factor. J Immunol 1997;158(6):2911–8.

[68] Borgermann J, Friedrich I, Scheubel R, et al. Granulocyte-macrophage colony-stimulating factor (GM-CSF) restores decreased monocyte HLA-DR expression after cardiopulmonary bypass. Thorac Cardiovasc Surg. 2007;55(1):24–31.

[69] Wysocka M, Montaner LJ, Karp CL. Flt3 ligand treatment reverses endotoxin tolerance-related immunoparalysis. J Immunol 2005;174(11):7398–402.

[70] Hershman MJ, Appel SH, Wellhausen SR, et al. Interferon-gamma treatment increases HLA-DR expression on monocytes in severely injured patients. Clin Exp Immunol 1989; 77(1):67–70.

[71] Flohe S, Borgermann J, Dominguez FE, et al. Influence of granulocyte-macrophage colony-stimulating factor (GM-CSF) on whole blood endotoxin responsiveness following trauma, cardiopulmonary bypass, and severe sepsis. Shock 1999;12(1):17–24.

[72] Lendemans S, Kreuzfelder E, Waydhas C, et al. Differential immunostimulating effect of granulocyte-macrophage colony-stimulating factor (GM-CSF), granulocyte colony-stimulating factor (G-CSF) and interferon gamma (IFNgamma) after severe trauma. Inflamm Res 2007;56(1):38–44.

[73] Kox WJ, Bone RC, Krausch D, et al. Interferon gamma-1b in the treatment of compensatory anti-inflammatory response syndrome. A new approach: proof of principle. Arch Intern Med 1997;157(4):389–93.

[74] Docke W, Syrbe U, Meinecke A, et al. Improvement in monocyte function: a new therapeutic approach? In: Reinhart K, Eyrich K, Sprung C, editors. Sepsis: current perspectives in pathophysiology and therapy. New York: Springer-Verlag; 1994. p. 473–500.

[75] Nakos G, Malamou-Mitsi VD, Lachana A, et al. Immunoparalysis in patients with severe trauma and the effect of inhaled interferon-gamma. Crit Care Med 2002;30(7):1488–94.

[76] Nierhaus A, Montag B, Timmler N, et al. Reversal of immunoparalysis by recombinant human granulocyte-macrophage colony-stimulating factor in patients with severe sepsis. Intensive Care Med 2003;29(4):646–51.

[77] Bilgin K, Yaramis A, Haspolat K, et al. A randomized trial of granulocyte-macrophage colony-stimulating factor in neonates with sepsis and neutropenia. Pediatrics 2001; 107(1):36–41.

[78] Rosenbloom AJ, Linden PK, Dorrance A, et al. Effect of granulocyte-monocyte colony-stimulating factor therapy on leukocyte function and clearance of serious infection in nonneutropenic patients. Chest 2005;127(6):2139–50.

[79] Carr R, Modi N, Dore C. G-CSF and GM-CSF for treating or preventing neonatal infections. Cochrane Database Syst Rev 2003;(3):CD003066.

[80] Centers for Disease Control and Prevention; Infectious Disease Society of America; American Society of Blood and Marrow Transplantation. Guidelines for preventing opportunistic infections among hematopoietic stem cell transplant recipients. MMWR Recomm Rep 2000;49(RR-10):1–125.

[81] Hempel L, Korholz D, Nussbaum P, et al. High interleukin-10 serum levels are associated with fatal outcome in patients after bone marrow transplantation. Bone Marrow Transplant 1997;20(5):365–8.

[82] Gras J, Wieers G, Vaerman JL, et al. Early immunological monitoring after pediatric liver transplantation: cytokine immune deviation and graft acceptance in 40 recipients. Liver Transpl 2007;13(3):426–33.

[83] Settmacher U, Docke WD, Manger T, et al. Management of induction phase of immunosuppression in liver graft recipients: prevention of oversuppression by immune monitoring. Transplant Proc 1993;25(4):2703–4.

[84] Reinke P, Volk HD. Diagnostic and predictive value of an immune monitoring program for complications after kidney transplantation. Urol Int 1992;49(2):69–75.

[85] Hoffman JA, Weinberg KI, Azen CG, et al. Human leukocyte antigen-DR expression on peripheral blood monocytes and the risk of pneumonia in pediatric lung transplant recipients. Transpl Infect Dis 2004;6(4):147–55.

[86] Denzel C, Riese J, Hohenberger W, et al. Monitoring of immunotherapy by measuring monocyte HLA-DR expression and stimulated TNFalpha production during sepsis after liver transplantation. Intensive Care Med 1998;24(12):1343–4.

[87] Trindade E, Maton P, Reding R, et al. Use of granulocyte macrophage colony stimulating factor in children after orthotopic liver transplantation. J Hepatol 1998;28(6): 1054–7.

[88] Pizzo PA, Rubin M, Freifeld A, et al. The child with cancer and infection. I. Empiric therapy for fever and neutropenia, and preventive strategies. J Pediatr 1991;119(5):679–94.

[89] Kaplan JE, Masur H, Holmes KK. Guidelines for preventing opportunistic infections among HIV-infected persons–2002. Recommendations of the U.S. Public Health Service and the Infectious Diseases Society of America. MMWR Recomm Rep 2002;51(RR-8): 1–52.

[90] Benson CA, Kaplan JE, Masur H, et al. Treating opportunistic infections among HIV-exposed and infected children: recommendations from CDC, the National Institutes of Health, and the Infectious Diseases Society of America. MMWR Recomm Rep 2004; 53(RR-15):1–112.

[91] Marik PE, Raghavan M. Stress-hyperglycemia, insulin and immunomodulation in sepsis. Intensive Care Med. 2004;30(5):748–56.

[92] Jaber BL, Cendoroglo M, Balakrishnan VS, et al. Apoptosis of leukocytes: basic concepts and implications in uremia. Kidney Int Suppl 2001;78:S197–205.

[93] Massry S, Smogorzewski M. Dysfunction of polymorphonuclear leukocytes in uremia: role of parathyroid hormone. Kidney Int Suppl 2001;78:S195–6.

[94] Woiciechowsky C, Schoning B, Lanksch WR, et al. Mechanisms of brain-mediated systemic anti-inflammatory syndrome causing immunodepression. J Mol Med 1999;77(11): 769–80.

[95] Woiciechowsky C, Volk HD. Increased intracranial pressure induces a rapid systemic interleukin-10 release through activation of the sympathetic nervous system. Acta Neurochir Suppl 2005;95:373–6.

[96] Bergmann M, Sautner T. Immunomodulatory effects of vasoactive catecholamines. Wien Klin Wochenschr 2002;114(17–18):752–61.

[97] Dandona P, Aljada A, Mohanty P, et al. Insulin inhibits intranuclear nuclear factor kappaB and stimulates IkappaB in mononuclear cells in obese subjects: evidence for an anti-inflammatory effect? J Clin Endocrinol Metab 2001;86(7):3257–65.

[98] Singhal PC, Kapasi AA, Franki N, et al. Morphine-induced macrophage apoptosis: the role of transforming growth factor-beta. Immunology 2000;100(1):57–62.

[99] Yuengsrigul A, Chin TW, Nussbaum E. Immunosuppressive and cytotoxic effects of furosemide on human peripheral blood mononuclear cells. Ann Allergy Asthma Immunol. 1999;83(6 Pt 1):559–66.

[100] Kanakoudi-Tsakalidou F, Debonera F, Drossou-Agakidou V, et al. Flow cytometric measurement of HLA-DR expression on circulating monocytes in healthy and sick neonates using monocyte negative selection. Clin Exp Immunol 2001;123(3):402–7.

[101] Yerkovich ST, Wikstrom ME, Suriyaarachchi D, et al. Postnatal Development of Monocyte Cytokine Responses to Bacterial Lipopolysaccharide. Pediatr Res 2007;62(5): 547–52.

[102] El-Mohandes AA, Rivas RA, Kiang E, et al. Membrane antigen and ligand receptor expression on neonatal monocytes. Biol Neonate 1995;68(5):308–17.

ELSEVIER
SAUNDERS

PEDIATRIC CLINICS
OF NORTH AMERICA

Pediatr Clin N Am 55 (2008) 669–686

The Poisoned Child in the Pediatric Intensive Care Unit

Usama A. Hanhan, MD[a,b,*]

[a]Division of Pediatrics, Department of Critical Care Medicine,
University Community Hospital, 3100 East Flecher Ave., Tampa, FL 33613, USA
[b]Department of Pediatrics, Nova Southeastern University, 3200 South University Drive,
Fort Lauderdale, FL 33328, USA

Acutely poisoned children remain a common problem facing pediatricians who work in acute care medicine in the United States and worldwide. The management of such children continues to be challenging, and their care has evolved throughout the years. The concept of gastric decontamination in acute poisoning has changed significantly over the past 10 years, and many of the previously used techniques have been abandoned or fallen out of favor for lack of evidence of their benefit or unacceptable serious risks and side effects. Supportive care continues to be the cornerstone in managing most poisoned children. Only a few patients benefit from antidotes or specific interventions [1–3].

The availability of poison control centers across the nation has significantly improved the outcome of these patients and continues to be an invaluable source of help to parents and medical personnel. Product information leaflets and older textbooks are often out of date and are not a reliable source of information in managing poisoned children. The availability of poison control centers can provide 24-hour on-call staff that are supported by clinical toxicologists. The presence of such centers has significantly decreased the need for most patients to go to the emergency room and directs only patients with significant or potentially life-threatening poisoning to be triaged and cared for in hospital emergency departments and pediatric intensive care units (PICU). The media, and the primary care providers, should play an important role in educating the public about the availability and resources of the poison control centers in their communities.

* University Community Hospital, Pediatric Intensive Care Unit, 3100 East Flecher Ave.,
Tampa, FL 33613.
 E-mail address: uhanhan@uch.mail.org

0031-3955/08/$ - see front matter © 2008 Elsevier Inc. All rights reserved.
doi:10.1016/j.pcl.2008.02.010   *pediatric.theclinics.com*

(The telephone number for the Poison Control Center in the United States is 1-800-222-1222).

Pediatric toxic exposures are a common encounter for pediatric emergency physicians and pediatric intensivists. The American Association of Poison Control Centers (AAPCC) reported more than 1.5 million toxic exposures in children and adolescents in 2005 (Box 1) [4]. This number is probably an underestimate because many cases are not reported and the actual incidence is likely to be even higher. Although toxic exposures in children are common occurrences, most are clinically insignificant and the morbidity and mortality associated with them are uncommon [2,4]. Data from the 2005 AAPCC Toxic Exposure Surveillance System show that toxic exposures caused a major effect in only 0.19% of children and only 114 pediatric deaths were reported [4]. The most common route of toxic exposure was ingestion, and death was most likely associated with ingestion [4].

Gastrointestinal decontamination techniques

The concept of gastrointestinal decontamination has always intrigued physicians who care for poisoned children, and for many years all poisoned patients were treated in a similar way—with aggressive decontamination procedures, including gastric emptying, administration of adsorbent agents, and catharsis. Recent evidence, however, shows that these techniques are unlikely to benefit most poisoned children and may pose a significant risk for these patients [5–9]. Lack of large, controlled studies at this time makes it even more difficult in deciding which patients, if any, would benefit from such techniques, and their application continues to be controversial.

Box 1. Top ten pediatric exposures in children younger than 6 years

1. Cosmetics/personal care products
2. Cleaning substances
3. Analgesics
4. Foreign bodies/miscellaneous
5. Topical preparations
6. Cold and cough preparations
7. Plants
8. Pesticides
9. Vitamins
10. Antihistamines

Data from Lai MW, Klein-Schwartz W, Rodgers GC, et al. 2005 annual report of the American Association of Poison Control Centers' national poisoning and exposure database. Clin Toxicol 2006;44:803–932.

During the past 10 years, however, much has been learned regarding potential risks and benefits, leading to a recent, dramatic change in medical recommendations [2].

Syrup of ipecac, a well-known substance that is used to induce vomiting, was once advocated by the American Academy of Pediatrics. They recommended that parents keep a 1-oz bottle at home to use in the event of accidental poisoning, the assumption being that if it were given within minutes of ingestion, it would recover significant amounts of the substances ingested and consequently mitigate their toxic effects. Unfortunately, even after early administration of ipecac, there has been no clinical evidence that it improves patient outcomes [10,11]. Its unpredictable onset of action and duration of emesis, along with its limitations and contraindications, has led the American Academy of Clinical Toxicology to issue a position statement regarding syrup of ipecac. This statement indicates that syrup of ipecac should not be administered routinely to poisoned patients, and its routine use in the emergency department should be abandoned [6]. This position has led the American Academy of Pediatrics to revise its previous recommendations, currently indicating that ipecac should no longer be used routinely as a home treatment strategy. The Academy has advised parents to safely dispose of (by flushing down the toilet) and remove any existing ipecac in the home [12].

Gastric lavage is another popular method that was routinely used in the emergency department with the hope of removing ingested substances from the stomach and preventing their toxic effects. The procedure involves passing a large-bore orogastric tube (28 Fr in toddlers to 36 Fr in adolescents) and lavaging the stomach with normal saline aliquots. The amount of toxin removed decreases with time—the most benefit occurs when it is completed within 1 hour of ingestion [13,14]. Potential complications include aspiration, vagal stimulation, hypoxia, cardiac arrhythmias, and gastrointestinal perforation. The procedure is contraindicated in situations that involve inappropriately protected airways and corrosive substance ingestions. It is also difficult to properly monitor the acutely ill patient during the procedure.

Similar to syrup of ipecac, there is no evidence that gastric lavage improves patient outcomes, and studies regarding its use have been contradictory [10]. A position statement by the American Academy of Clinical Toxicology implied that gastric lavage should not be used routinely in the management of poisoned patients and that it should only be considered in patients who present within 1 hour of ingesting potentially life-threatening substances [8]. Even then its benefit has been questioned.

Because of its large surface area and adsorptive capacity, activated charcoal has been used by many clinicians as a decontamination strategy for most ingestions. Several studies also have shown no additional benefit for gastric lavage or syrup of ipecac compared with using activated charcoal alone [11,15], which supports its use as the only intervention to be performed in most ingestions when decontamination is deemed necessary or needed. Similar to other modalities of gastrointestinal decontamination, its potential benefit depends on how quickly it is administered, with the greatest benefit being within 1 hour of ingestion. Data that support the use of activated charcoal are extrapolated largely from volunteer studies and a few clinical studies [5,16], with some studies showing evidence of its clinical benefits. There is no direct evidence that the administration of activated charcoal improves clinical outcome, however [5]. The position statement of the American Academy of Clinical Toxicology recommends that activated charcoal not be administered routinely in the management of poisoned patients [5]. A dose of 1 g/kg up to 50 g should be considered in patients who have ingested a potentially toxic or life-threatening overdose within the previous hour, with no contraindications to its use. Activated charcoal is ineffective at adsorbing a small number of substances, including heavy metals, alcohols, and hydrocarbons.

Although there are insufficient data to support or refute its effectiveness in reducing gastrointestinal adsorption of toxins if given beyond 1 hour after ingestion, it can be considered in cases of large overdoses of toxic drugs in which delayed absorption is possible, as in the case of sustained-release preparations. Because of the risk for vomiting and charcoal aspiration, activated charcoal should be used only in patients with adequately protected airways.

The administration of catharsis alone has no role in routine gastrointestinal decontamination of acutely poisoned patients, and the American Academy of Clinical Toxicology recommends against using cathartics with or without activated charcoal [17]. The benefit of using multiple doses of activated charcoal also has been questioned. Berg and colleagues [18] studied the effect of multiple oral doses of activated charcoal on the clearance of intravenously administered phenobarbital to six healthy volunteer men. They showed that activated charcoal enhanced the nonrenal clearance of phenobarbital. Although theoretically using multiple doses of activated charcoal may interrupt the enterohepatic and enteroenteric recirculation of certain drugs such as theophylline, carbamazepine, and phenobarbital, its clinical benefit has never been proven [19]. Multiple doses of activated charcoal can lead to increased risk for charcoal aspiration and bowel obstruction, and its use is contraindicated in the presence of decreased peristalsis.

The concept of whole bowel irrigation to try to push ingested toxins through the gastrointestinal tract and out of the body has gained more interest in recent years. The procedure entails the administration of a polyethylene glycol solution orally or through a nasogastric tube until the resulting rectal effluent is clear. Large volumes are usually recommended, with a goal of approximately 2 L/h in adults and 500 mL/h in preschool children. Polyethylene glycol is an osmotically balanced solution that is not absorbed and does not produce fluid or electrolyte imbalance [9]. Data regarding its potential benefit have been largely obtained from case reports and volunteer studies [9]. The procedure may be considered in large ingestions of heavy metals or enteric-coated tablets and illegal drug packets. The American Academy of Clinical Toxicology's position statement indicates that there is no conclusive evidence that whole bowel irrigation improves clinical outcome in acutely poisoned patients [20]. Contraindications to whole bowel irrigation include unprotected airways, ileus or intestinal obstruction, and gastrointestinal hemorrhage or perforation.

History and physical examination

After the initial stabilization of the patient, a detailed history and a thorough examination should be performed. Small children often present after unknown or unsuspected ingestions. Such children typically become intoxicated with drugs or substances that are attractive and available. Adolescent poisonings are most often the result of substance abuse or intentional overdose in the act of a suicidal attempt, and obtaining a reliable history may be crucial to subsequent management. Any child who presents with unexplained altered mental status, respiratory or hemodynamic compromise, seizures, or metabolic derangement should be considered for a toxic ingestion. A thorough examination should include special attention to vital signs, mental and neurologic status, pupillary size and reactivity, skin color and hydration, respiratory effort, pulses, and perfusion.

Vital sign abnormalities are often seen with certain ingestions. For example, hypothermia may be seen with opiates, sedatives, and alcohol ingestions. Hyperthermia is common after salicylate, anticholinergic, and amphetamine ingestions. Tachycardia is associated with anticholinergics, antihistamines, sympathomimetics, and tricyclic antidepressants. Bradycardia is seen with beta-blocker, calcium channel blocker, and clonidine ingestions. Tachypnea may result from direct pulmonary insult or noncardiogenic pulmonary edema or as a compensatory mechanism in the setting of metabolic acidosis. Respiratory depression, including apnea, is more common in young children after clonidine, opiate, or sedative-hypnotic ingestion.

Profound hypotension may result from tricyclic antidepressants, beta-blockers, and calcium channel blocker overdose, whereas cocaine, sympathomimetics, and anticholinergics frequently cause hypertension in children.

Focused laboratory investigations should be directed by the information obtained from the detailed history and physical examination findings. Initial studies should include measurement of serum glucose, electrolytes, acid–base status, and chemistry panel. Measurement of serum osmolality and anion gap is valuable in cases of alcohol poisoning. Urinalysis may reveal crystals or myoglobinurea. Co-oximetry measurements detect carbon monoxide poisoning and methemoglobinemia. An EKG may detect occult cardiac conduction problems, including dysrhythmias, and early signs of cardiotoxic drugs, such as prolonged QRS and QT intervals.

Urine drug screens are generally not helpful in managing acutely poisoned patients and rarely influence acute intervention decisions [2,21]. They are generally nonspecific and do not provide reliable information regarding time of drug exposure. By design, urine drug screens detect the parent drug or its metabolite up to several days after use. False-positive and -negative results are not uncommon, and the interpretation of results should be done within the context of clinical findings and with the understanding of the test limitations. Similarly, with few exceptions, measurement of serum drug concentrations is generally not routinely helpful in treating poisoned children. Exceptions include acetaminophen level, which should be ordered on nearly all poisoned patients to ensure that this common and potentially serious ingestion is not overlooked, particularly because acetaminophen ingestions initially produce few to no symptoms. Other drug levels that should be considered are salicylates, ethanol, serum iron, and lithium levels—especially in the presence of impaired renal function. Other specific laboratory investigations not mentioned herein may be necessary in certain toxic exposures.

General management

The main challenge for physicians who care for poisoned children is identifying, as early as possible, patients who are at risk for developing serious and life-threatening toxicities and deciding whether any decontamination techniques would be of benefit or if any specific antidotes or special interventions are required. Although most accidental pediatric poisoning cause minor or no effects, a few substances—even when ingested in small amounts—can lead to severe toxicities or even death [4,22]. Identifying those high-risk patients allows clinicians to provide therapeutic and life-saving measures, and with the appropriate toxicologic and supportive care, such patients have the potential for a lifetime of well-being. Patients who present with serious signs and symptoms or have potentially life-threatening toxic exposures should be admitted to the PICU for close monitoring and management.

The initial stabilization of an acutely poisoned child starts with providing standard resuscitation procedures and initiating life-saving measures, including maintaining airway and checking protective reflexes, ensuring adequate ventilation and oxygenation, monitoring heart rate and blood pressure, obtaining intravenous access, assessing level of consciousness and mental status, and providing the necessary interventions to support vital organs. Treatment of cardiorespiratory arrest and circulatory collapse in a poisoned child generally follows the Pediatric Advance Life Support/Advanced Cardiac Life Support (PALS/ACLS) guidelines [23]. There are situations in which different early interventions are also required. For example, using sodium bicarbonate in tricyclic antidepressant overdose, atropine and oximes for organophosphate insecticides and nerve gas exposure, naloxone for opiate toxicity, digoxin immune Fab for digitalis poisoning, and other specific antidotes in certain known life-threatening exposures is required for early intervention [23].

Inadequate ventilation or reduced respiratory effort may require intubation and mechanical ventilation. Hypotension should be treated initially with intravenous fluids and volume expansion. An initial bolus of 20 mL/kg of normal saline should be given and titrated to effect. The use of specific antidotes also should be considered in treating hypotension that results from certain intoxications such as beta-blockers, calcium channel antagonists, and digoxin. Hypotension resistant to intravenous fluids and appropriate antidotes should be treated with vasopressors and close monitoring for any arrhythmias, because the use of inotropic agents may cause further cardiovascular toxicity. Although dopamine traditionally has been used to support circulation and blood pressure, often it is ineffective in poisoned children. Norepinephrine should be considered in poisonings that produce peripheral vasodilation. Epinephrine and dobutamine are more likely to be effective when there is direct toxin-induced myocardial depression.

Arrhythmias are often the result of metabolic derangements, such as acidosis, hypokalemia, hypoxia, and hypomagnesemia. Treatment of these metabolic derangements is crucial in poisoned children. Most antiarrhythmic agents have negative inotropic effects and may potentially be proarrhythmic. Their use in poisoned patients should be avoided and only cautiously considered after correcting and treating any possible precipitating factors or metabolic derangements [24]. It is preferable to use specific measures to alleviate the toxic effects of certain poisons, such as the use of sodium bicarbonate in tricyclic antidepressant-related arrhythmias, digoxin-specific antibodies for digoxin toxicity, and glucagon or, more recently, glucose and insulin in cases of calcium channel antagonists and beta-blocker toxicities. Correction of any precipitating factors, including electrolyte abnormalities and acid base status disturbances, with the appropriate use of antidotal agents when indicated might negate the need for antiarrhythmic drugs in most cases.

Hypoglycemia is another metabolic derangement that may be encountered in poisoned children, and correcting it is crucial and important to the success of treatment. Significant hypoglycemia is often seen with insulin overdose or sulfonylurea toxicities. Symptomatic hypoglycemia requires an intravenous administration of a dextrose bolus (D25, 2–4 mL/kg in young children and D50, 1–2 mL/kg in older children and adolescents). Hypoglycemia often may be prolonged and require continuous infusion of high glucose concentration with careful monitoring of blood glucose levels and correcting any electrolyte abnormalities, particularly hypokalemia. Refractory hypoglycemia may be encountered in significant sulfonylurea ingestions. In such patients, adjunct treatment with Octreotide, a somatostatin analog, should be considered [25]. Octreotide is capable of directly inhibiting insulin secretion and minimizes the risk of glucose-stimulating insulin release in these patients. The dose is 4 to 5 μg/kg/d subcutaneously in divided doses every 6 hours, up to a maximum dose of 50 μg every 6 hours [26]. Glucagon is another agent that has been used for many years in the treatment of drug-induced hypoglycemia [22]. It increases serum glucose levels by stimulating hepatic glycogenolysis and gluconeogenesis. It can be administered intravenously, subcutaneously, or intramuscularly at a dose of 0.025 to 0.1 mg/kg, with a maximum dose of 1 mg repeated every 20 minutes as needed [22,27]. Glucagon, however, does not inhibit sulfonylurea-induced insulin release. It carries the risk of vomiting and aspiration, and its use should be considered as a temporary measure in the emergency management of hypoglycemia associated with sulfonylurea toxicity.

Agitation and irritability are often encountered in poisoned patients and may require the administration of sedatives. The drug of choice in most patients is intravenous benzodiazepines such as diazepam and lorazepam [24]. The dose administered should be given in increments every 3 to 5 minutes to achieve the desired sedative effect while avoiding excessive central nervous system and respiratory depression. Phenothiazines and butyrophenones are best avoided because they can potentially increase the toxicity of cardiotoxic drugs and may reduce the seizure threshold in these patients [28].

Seizures should be treated with benzodiazepines as first-line antiepileptic drugs [29]. Diazepam, 0.3 mg/kg up to 10 mg intravenously, and lorazepam, 0.1 mg/kg up to 4 mg, are appropriate initial drugs and would adequately stop seizures in most patients. Phenytoin should be avoided in treating seizures, especially with tricyclic antidepressant overdose, because of its sodium channel-blocking properties, which can theoretically exacerbate the cardiotoxicity of some drugs such as cocaine and tricyclics [30]. Refractory seizures and patients in status epilepticus are best managed with continuous intravenous midazolam drip or pentobarbital coma [29]. This group of patients usually requires intubation and mechanical ventilation with continuous EEG monitoring and supportive care in the PICU. Although the detailed management of the various toxic exposures in children is beyond the scope of this article, the following discussion is a review of a few of the potentially serious and life-threatening ingestions in children.

Acetaminophen intoxication

Acetaminophen is widely available in hundreds of over-the-counter and prescription medications. It is an effective analgesic/antipyretic drug that, although safe when used in recommended doses, can cause significant hepatic toxicity with an acute ingestion of more than 7.5 g in adults or 150 mg/kg in children [31,32]. Its widespread availability and the underestimation of its toxicity have resulted in large numbers of accidental and suicidal intoxications. Acetaminophen accounts for more overdoses and more overdose deaths each year in the United States than any other pharmaceutical agent [33]. In a retrospective review of 322 cases of acetaminophen overdose in children, 43% were intentional, 53% were unintentional, and 3% were dosing errors [34]. Hepatocellular toxicity occurred in 27 patients (8%), 25 of whom ingested it intentionally.

Acetaminophen is rapidly absorbed after a therapeutic oral dose with peak levels achieved within 1 to 2 hours. In the event of an overdose, however, peak serum levels are reached within 4 hours after overdose of an immediate release preparation and may be delayed even later with extended-release forms [35].

The main site of metabolism is the liver, and under the usual therapeutic circumstances, more than 90% of the drug is conjugated with sulfate and glucuronate to form inactive, nontoxic compounds that are excreted by the kidney. Only approximately 4% is conjugated with glutathione by the cytochrome P-450 enzyme system to form mercapturic acid and cysteine conjugates, which are then excreted by the kidney. It is along this pathway to the mercapturic acid conjugates that excess amounts of a toxic intermediate metabolite N-acetyl-p-benzoquinoneimine are accumulated after a toxic overdose when glutathione stores become depleted and the detoxification capacity of the liver is exceeded. N-acetyl-p-benzoquinoneimine accumulates and binds to intracellular hepatic macromolecules and produces cell necrosis and damage [36–38]. Because of its protective role, exogenous glutathione would be the ideal therapeutic agent in acetaminophen toxicity, but glutathione does not readily enter the hepatocytes [39]. N-acetylcysteine (NAC), a glutathione precursor, is currently regarded as the antidote of choice for the treatment of acetaminophen poisoning. Although the precise mode of action of NAC is unclear after being taken up by the liver cells, it is metabolized to cysteine, a precursor of glutathione that binds the toxic intermediate metabolites of acetaminophen and prevents their hepatotoxic effects [40].

Several risk factors can influence the propensity of acetaminophen to cause hepatotoxicity, including patient age, nutritional status, pattern of ingestion, and coingestions [41,42]. Children younger than 5 years seem to be less susceptible to hepatotoxicity than older children and adults after an acute overdose [43,44]. In children and adults, repeated excessive dosing is associated with greater morbidity and mortality than a single acute overdose [45]. Fasting or malnutrition depletes hepatic stores of glucuronide and glutathione, which predisposes to hepatic injury. Concomitant ingestions or use of agents that induce the cytochome P-450 enzymes also may worsen the outcome and increase the risk of hepatotoxicity when an intentional overdose of acetaminophen has occurred [46]. Examples of such agents include anticonvulsants and antituberculosis drugs.

The clinical course of acute single-dose ingestions can be divided into four stages. The first 12 to 24 hours are remarkable for mild or no symptoms. The initial manifestations are nonspecific and include nausea, vomiting, and anorexia. Other patients remain asymptomatic, and the initial manifestations do not predict subsequent hepatotoxicity [47]. It is crucial, however, that clinicians promptly recognize acetaminophen poisoning, because NAC, the antidote for acetaminophen, is most effective if administered within 8 to 10 hours of ingestion [48–50].

The second stage is marked by resolution of the early gastrointestinal symptoms. This resolution of symptoms, however, is of no prognostic importance because most patients become asymptomatic for a period even if severe liver dysfunction subsequently appears. Biochemical evidence of hepatic injury with elevation of transaminases, bilirubin, and prothrombin time usually appears approximately 36 hours after ingestion and reaches its peak during the third stage, on the third and fourth day, with recurrence of symptoms such as nausea, vomiting, anorexia, and symptoms of hepatitis. Although extraordinarily high transminase levels in excess of 10,000 IU/mL may occur, fulminant liver failure with jaundice, encephalopathy, and bleeding is an infrequent occurrence. Stage four is the recovery stage and lasts approximately 7 to 8 days.

Management

The risk of toxicity is best predicted by measuring serum acetaminophen concentration in relation to the time of ingestion. Liver damage is uncommon with ingestions of less than 125 mg/kg, but severe damage occurs in approximately 50% of adults with intoxications of 250 mg/kg and in almost all patients who ingest 350 mg/kg [31]. Although the dose history helps guide treatment decisions, it is not sufficient evidence on which to base treatment after an acute overdose. Studies by Rumack and colleagues [40,44,51] resulted in the formulation of the Rumack-Matthew nomogram, which defines—with good correlation—the risk of hepatic damage in terms of serum levels and lapse time since ingestion. The serum acetaminophen level should be measured between 4 and 24 hours after an acute overdose of an immediate-release preparation and then plotted in the nomogram to determine the need for NAC therapy. Additional laboratory tests that should be monitored include electrolytes, aspartate aminotransferase, alanin transaminase, blood urea nitrogen and creatinine, prothrombin time, and international normalized ratio. Acetaminophen levels obtained more than 24 hours after ingestion are difficult to interpret. Patients with an unknown time of ingestion and a serum acetaminophen concentration more than 10 μg/mL or elevation of aminotransaminases are usually treated with NAC.

NAC is the antidote of choice for the treatment of acetaminophen poisoning. It can be administered orally or intravenously in patients with intractable vomiting or whose medical condition precludes enteral use. The standard oral NAC treatment regimen in the United States, which was approved by the US Food and Drug Administration, consists of a 72-hour oral course given as a 140-mg/kg loading dose followed by 17 doses of 70 mg/kg every 4 hours (Table 1). Although most effective when given within 8 to 10 hours after ingestion, several studies have shown that when administered less than 16 hours—and even up to 24 hours—after ingestion, NAC therapy has a profound effect of lowering morbidity and mortality [40,49,50,52].

Table 1
N-acetylcysteine therapy

Oral (NAC) (72-h regimen)	Loading dose: 140 mg/kg Subsequent doses: 70 mg/kg (every 4 hours for a total of 17 doses)
IV (NAC) continuous infusion (21-h regimen)	Loading dose: 150 mg/kg IV over 60 min 50 mg/kg IV over 4 hours 100 mg/kg IV over 16 hours
IV (NAC) (48-h regimen)	Loading dose: 140 mg/kg Subsequent doses: 70 mg/kg every 4 hours for a total of 12 doses (each dose infused over 60 min)

Intravenous regimens for NAC have been used for more than 20 years in Europe and Canada. The Food and Drug Administration in the United States approved an intravenous formulation of NAC (Acetadote) in early 2004, using a continuous 20-hour infusion protocol. In February 2006, the package insert was revised and extended the loading dose infusion time from 15 to 60 minutes, making it a 21-hour infusion [53]. The recommended dosing is a loading dose of 150 mg/kg infused over 60 minutes, followed by 50 mg/kg for 4 hours and 100 mg/kg for 16 hours, with a cumulative total dose of 300 mg/kg [53].

Another effective and shorter alternative to the 72-hour oral regimen was demonstrated using a pyrogen-free form of intravenous NAC for 48 hours [48]. The regimen included a 140-mg/kg loading dose followed by 12 maintenance doses of 70 mg/kg every 4 hours. All doses were infused intravenously over 1 hour. The incidence of hepatotoxicity in the 48-hour intravenous protocol was comparable to the standard 72-hour oral protocol and the 20-hour intravenous protocol.

In an open-label clinical trial, Perry and Shannon [54] studied intravenous versus oral NAC in a pediatric population. The intravenous NAC regimen was 140 mg/kg loading dose over 1 hour, followed by 12 maintenance doses of 70 mg/kg every 4 hours. The control group included patients treated with the standard accepted oral NAC protocol, with the same eligibility requirements as the intravenous NAC groups. No patients in the intravenous group had hepatic toxicity if treated within 10 hours, and 9.8% of patients had toxicity if treated within 10 to 24 hours. Intravenous NAC was also found to be as effective as oral NAC in reducing hepatic toxicity.

The use of NAC in children with delayed ($>$24 hours) presentation of acetaminophen intoxication has not been studied. In a prospective controlled trial among 50 adults with acetaminophen-induced fulminant hepatic failure, the use of intravenous NAC greatly reduced mortality rates (20% versus 48%) [55]. Although no controlled studies have evaluated the use of NAC in patients with delayed presentation and hepatoxicity without signs of hepatic failure, many toxicologists would recommend the use of NAC in these patients. Children with delayed presentation and hepatic toxicity should be managed in consultation with a medical toxicologist and the poison control center.

Calcium channel blockers

Calcium channel antagonists are used in the treatment of various disorders, including hypertension, cardiac arrhythmias, and coronary artery disease. The widespread availability of these drugs increases the likelihood for accidental ingestions in children. More than 9500 cases of calcium channel blocker intoxications were reported to United States poison control centers during 2005 [4]. Although calcium channel antagonists represent only 16% of all cardiovascular drug exposures, this group of medications accounted for 38% of deaths [56]. Calcium channel blockers are available in immediate-release and extended-release preparations. Children can develop substantial toxicity with exposure to as few as one or two tablets [57–62].

Calcium channel antagonists block the entry of calcium through the L-type calcium channels in the myocardium and the vascular smooth muscles. Toxic exposures in children may result in hypotension, depressed contractility, conduction abnormalities, and dysrhythmias [63]. The onset of symptoms may be delayed for up to 24 hours with extended-release preparations. Other symptoms in children include unsteady gait, dizziness, altered mental status, and seizures caused by cerebral hypotension [59,60,62]. Inhibition of insulin release may lead to hyperglycemia, lactic acidosis may result from tissue hypoperfusion, and bowel hypoperfusion may lead to ischemia [58–60]. Nausea, vomiting, and ileus also have been described.

All children suspected of having calcium channel antagonist exposure should be admitted to the PICU for close monitoring and management. Diagnostic evaluation should include serum electrolytes, BUN, creatinine, calcium, and glucose. Hyperglycemia may be seen; however, it is rarely of clinical significance. An electrocardiogram also should be obtained to help in identifying any conduction abnormalities or dysrhythmias. A chest radiograph should be obtained for patients with any signs of respiratory distress or hypoxia to evaluate for pulmonary edema.

Treatment

The main focus in the treatment of calcium channel blocker toxicity is the support of circulation. Intravenous fluids are the initial therapy for hypotension. Additional vasopressor therapy may be required. Choices include drugs such as dopamine, epinephrine, and norepinephrine. Norepinephrine seems to be the vasopressor of choice for hypotension in the presence of failure of vascular resistance. Atropine should be administered to any patient with symptomatic bradycardia; however, often it is ineffective. More recently, hyperinsulinemia euglycemic treatment, which has been shown to have positive inotropic effects, has gained acceptance as an early intervention in toxin-induced shock [64]. Although the mechanism of action is not clear, high-dose insulin seems to overcome the state of carbohydrate dependence and insulin resistance within the myocardium that is created by calcium channel blocker toxicity [65]. Although the ideal dose has not been well established, a continuous infusion of 0.5 to 1 U/kg/h has been used to reverse the cardiovascular collapse associated with calcium channel blocker overdose [65,66]. Patients should be given supplemental glucose—a bolus of D25 and a dextrose infusion at 0.5 g/kg/h titrated to maintain normal serum glucose concentrations (Table 2). Glucose and potassium levels should be monitored (at least hourly at the initiation of therapy) with correction of any electrolyte abnormalities.

Intravenous calcium chloride, although theoretically antidotal, is frequently ineffective in maintaining perfusion; however, high-dose continuous infusion has been used successfully in anecdotal reports [67,68]. Some believe that an infusion rate of 0.5 mEq/kg/h of calcium is reasonable; however, close monitoring of ionized and serum calcium levels and an electrocardiogram are necessary in such patients (Table 2). Calcium gluconate may be administered through a peripheral vein; however, calcium chloride should be administered via a central venous line.

Glucagon has been shown to increase heart rate in calcium channel blocker overdose; however, it has minimal effects on the mean arterial pressure. Glucagon increases intracellular levels of cyclic AMP and has been effective in treating human cases of calcium channel blocker toxicities [69–71]. A systematic review of use of glucagon in animal models of beta-blocker and calcium channel blocker toxicity indicates that glucagon does not improve survival [72].

Table 2
Medication guidelines in the management of calcium channel blockers toxicity

Intravenous fluids	Normal saline 20 mL/kg bolus	May repeat as needed/titrate to effect
Norepinephrine	Initial dose 0.05–0.1 µg/kg/min Titrate up to 1–2 µg/kg/min	Higher doses may be required in calcium channel blocker toxicity
Atropine	0.02 mg/kg IV Minimum dose 0.1 mg Maximum dose 1 mg	May repeat after 10 minutes
Calcium chloride	Initial bolus 20 mg/kg IV Continuous infusion 20–50 mg/kg/h or 0.5 mEq/kg/h	Consider infusion if good response with initial bolus dose Monitor serum Ca levels and EKG
Glucagon	Initial bolus 0.025–0.1 mg/kg IV Adolescents 1–5 mg IV Maximum infusion rate 10 mg/h	Consider continuous infusion if good response with initial boluses
Insulin/glucose	Insulin: bolus 0.1 U/kg Insulin infusion 0.2–1 U/kg/h D25 2–4 mL/kg bolus Continuous dextrose infusion 0.5 g/kg/h	Titrate dextrose infusion to maintain euglycemia Monitor serum glucose and electrolytes

Animal studies of calcium channel blocker toxicity have shown improved survival associated with hyperinsulinemia/euglycemia therapy compared with other treatment modalities, including calcium and glucagon [73,74]. Clinical experience with this novel therapy, however, is still limited, and ideal dosing has not been established. Although toxicologists and clinicians feel that hyperinsulinemia/euglycemia therapy should be recommended as first-line treatment in calcium channel blocker poisonings, further research is greatly needed in this area. Other treatment modalities include the insertion of a transvenous pacemaker to assist with electrical conduction; however, it does not counteract the negative inotropic effects of these medications and may not correct the patient's low blood pressure [75]. Calcium channel blockers are highly protein bound, and their removal by hemodialysis is ineffective.

Clonidine

Clonidine, originally developed as a nasal decongestant, has been approved by the Food and Drug Administration in the United States for the treatment of hypertension. It is a commonly prescribed, centrally acting antihypertensive agent that has gained expanded therapeutic use in the treatment of attention deficit hyperactivity disorder, Tourette syndrome, and ethanol or opioid withdrawal. With its widespread use in all age populations, clonidine toxic exposures in children have increased, with more than 1700 exposures in children younger than 6 years reported to the AAPCC in 2005 [4].

Clonidine is a central alpha-adrenoreceptor agonist, and because of a functional overlap in the mu receptors targeted by opioids and the alpha-2-receptors targeted by clonidine, the clinical manifestations that have been described with clonidine poisoning largely resemble an opioid toxidrome [76,77]. Symptoms include meiosis, respiratory depression, mental status depression, bradycardia, and hypotension. Most children become symptomatic within 30 to 90 minutes after ingestion [76]. Toxicity can occur with just one or two tablets of clonidine. Toddlers may present in a deeply comatose state with apnea and bradycardia; when stimulated, they may respond with increased pulse and respiration and improved level of consciousness. When not stimulated, however, the child may quickly return to the previous state or even go into cardiopulmonary arrest [76].

Treatment of clonidine overdose is mainly supportive. Activated charcoal should be administered if the patient presents early—within 1 hour of the ingestion. Adequate patent airway should be maintained, and continuous cardiorespiratory monitoring and an EKG should be done. Bradycardia usually responds to atropine, and hypotension usually responds to fluids but may require direct-acting vasopressors, such as dopamine or norepinephrine. Naloxone has been used with variable success and has been shown to reverse cardiovascular and respiratory depression in up to 50% of case reports [76,78–82]. This is probably caused by opioid receptor overlap, as described previously. Its use is generally considered in treating severe clonidine overdose that results in significant respiratory depression. The suggested naloxone dose is 0.1 mg up to a maximum of 10 mg [76,80,82]. All patients who present with altered mental status, cardiac abnormalities, or respiratory depression should be admitted and managed in the PICU.

References

[1] Tenenbein M. Recent advancements in pediatric toxicology. Pediatr Clin North Am 1999;46: 1179–88.

[2] Barry JD. Diagnosis and management of the poisoned child. Pediatr Ann 2005;34(12): 937–46.

[3] Bryant S, Singer J. Management of toxic exposure in children. Emerg Med Clin North Am 2003;21:101–19.

[4] Lai MW, Klein-Schwartz W, Rodgers GC, et al. 2005 annual report of the American Association of Poison Control Centers' national poisoning and exposure database. Clin Toxicol 2006;44:803–932.

[5] American Academy of Clinical Toxicology and European Association of Poisons Control Centers and Clinical Toxicologists. Position statement: single-dose activated charcoal. J Toxicol Clin Toxicol 1997;35:721–41.

[6] American Academy of Clinical Toxicology and European Association of Poisons Control Centers and Clinical Toxicologists. Position statement: ipecac syrup. J Toxicol Clin Toxicol 1997;35:699–709.

[7] American Academy of Clinical Toxicology and European Association of Poisons Control Centers and Clinical Toxicologists. Position statement and practice guidelines on the use of multi-dose activated charcoal in the treatment of acute poisoning. J Toxicol Clin Toxicol 1999;37:731–51.

[8] American Academy of Clinical Toxicology and European Association of Poisons Control Centers and Clinical Toxicologists. Position statement: gastric lavage. J Toxicol Clin Toxicol 1997;35:711–9.

[9] American Academy of Clinical Toxicology and European Association of Poisons Control Centers and Clinical Toxicologists. Position statement: whole bowel irrigation. J Toxicol Clin Toxicol 1997;35:753–62.

[10] Pond SM, Lewis-Driver DJ, William GM, et al. Gastric emptying in acute overdose: a prospective randomized controlled trial. Med J Aust 1995;163(7):345–9.

[11] Merigian KS, Woodard M, Hedges JR, et al. Prospective evaluation of gastric emptying in the self-poisoned patient. Am J Emerg Med 1990;8(6):479–83.

[12] Poison treatment in the home. American Academy of Pediatrics committee on injury, violence, and poison prevention. Pediatrics 2003;112(5):1182–5.

[13] Comstock EG, Faulkner TP, Boisaubin EV, et al. Studies on the efficacy of gastric lavage as practiced in a large metropolitan hospital. Clin Toxicol 1981;18(5):581–97.

[14] Knlig K, Bar-Or D, Cantrill SV, et al. Management of acutely poisoned patients without gastric emptying. Ann Emerg Med 1985;14(6):562–7.

[15] Kornberg AE, Dolgin J. Pediatric ingestions: charcoal alone versus ipecac and charcoal. Ann Emerg Med 1991;20(6):648–51.

[16] Smilkstein MJ. Techniques used to prevent gastrointestinal absorption of toxic compounds. In: Goldfrank LR, Flomenbaum NE, Lewin NA, et al, editors. Goldfrank's toxicologic emergencies. 7th edition. New York: McGraw-Hill; 2002. p. 44–57.

[17] Position paper: cathartics. J Toxicol Clin Toxicol 2004;42(3):243–53.

[18] Berg MJ, Berlinger WG, Goldberg MJ, et al. Acceleration of the body clearance of phenobarbital by oral activated charcoal. N Engl J Med 1982;307(11):642–4.

[19] Bradberry SM, Vale JA. Multiple-dose activated charcoal: a review of relevant clinical studies. J Toxicol Clin Toxicol 1995;33(5):407–16.

[20] Position paper: whole bowel irrigation. J Toxicol Clin Toxicol 2004;42(6):843–54.

[21] Dawson AH, Whyte IM. Evidence in clinical toxicology: the role of therapeutic drug monitoring. Ther Drug Monit 2002;24:159–62.

[22] Henry K, Harris CR. Deadly ingestions. Pediatr Clin North Am 2006;53:293–315.

[23] Albertson TE, Dawson A, de Latorre F, et al. American Heart Association; international liaison committee on resuscitation. TOX-ACLS: toxicologic-oriented advanced cardiac life support. Ann Emerg Med 2001;37:578–90.

[24] Greene SL, Dargan PI, Jones AL. Acute poisoning: understanding 90% of cases in a nutshell. Postgrad Med J 2005;81:204–16.

[25] McLaughlin SA, Crandall CS, McKinney PE. Octreotide: an antidote for sulfonylurea-induced hypoglycemia. Ann Emerg Med 2000;36(2):133–8.

[26] Little G, Boniface K. Are one or two dangerous? Sulfonylurea exposure in toddlers. J Emerg Med 2005;28(3):305–10.

[27] Pollack CV. Utility of glucagon in the emergency department. J Emerg Med 1993;11: 195–205.

[28] Markowitz JC, Brown RP. Seizures with neuroleptics and antidepressants. Gen Hosp Psychiatry 1987;9:135–41.

[29] Hanhan UA, Fiallos MR, Orlowski JP. Status epilepticus. Pediatr Clin North Am 2001; 48(3):683–94.

[30] Callaham M, Schumaker H, Pentel P. Phenytoin prophylaxis of cardiotoxicity in experimental amitriptyline poisoning. J Pharmacol Exp Ther 1988;245:216–20.

[31] Linden CH, Rumack BH. Acetaminophen overdose. Emerg Med Clin North Am 1984; 2:103–19.

[32] Lewis RK, Paloucek FP. Assessment and treatment of acetaminophen overdose. Clin Pharm 1991;10:765–74.

[33] Benson GD. Hepatotoxicity following the therapeutic use of antipyretic analgesics. Am J Med 1983;75:85–93.

[34] Alander SW, Dowd MD, Bratton SL, et al. Pediatric acetaminophen overdose: risk factors associated with hepatocellular injury. Arch Pediatr Adolesc Med 2000;154:346–50.

[35] Forrest JA, Clements JA, Prescott LF. Clinical pharmacokinetics of paracetamol. Clin Pharmacokinet 1982;7:93–107.

[36] Mitchell JR, Thorgeirson SS, Potter WZ, et al. Acetaminophen-induced hepatic injury; protective role of glutathione in man and rationale for therapy. Clin Pharmacol Ther 1974; 16:676–84.

[37] Miner DJ, Kissinger PT. Evidence for the involvement of N-acetyl-p-quinonimine in acetaminophen metabolism. Biochem Pharmacol 1979;28:3285–90.

[38] Prescott LF, Critchley J. The treatment of acetaminophen poisoning. Annu Rev Pharmacol Toxicol 1983;23:87–101.

[39] Prescott LF, Newton RW, Swainson CP, et al. Successful treatment of severe paracetamol overdose with cysteamine. Lancet 1974;1:588–92.

[40] Rumack BN, Peterson RG, Koch CG, et al. Acetaminophen overdose: 662 cases with evaluation of oral acetylcysteine treatment. Arch Intern Med 1981;141:380–5.

[41] Sztajnkrycer MJ, Bond GR. Chronic acetaminophen overdosing in children: risk assessment and management. Curr Opin Pediatr 2001;13:177–82.

[42] Lee WM. Drug-induced hypatotoxicity. N Engl J Med 2003;349:474–85.

[43] Rumore MM, Blaiklock RG. Influence of age-dependent pharmacokinetics and metabolism on acetaminophen hepatotoxicity. J Pharm Sci 1992;81:203–7.

[44] Rumack BH. Acetaminophen overdose in young children: treatment and effects of alcohol and other additional ingestants in 417 cases. Am J Dis Child 1984;138:428–33.

[45] Rivera-Penera T, Gugig R, Davis J, et al. Outcome of acetaminophen overdose in pediatric patients and factors contributing to hepatotoxicity. J Pediatr 1997;130:300–4.

[46] Bray GP, Harrison PM, O'Grady JG, et al. Long-term anticonvulsant therapy worsens outcome in paracetamol-induced fulminant hepatic failure. Hum Exp Toxicol 1992;11:265–70.

[47] Smilkstein MJ. Acetaminophen. In: Goldfrank LR, Flomenbaum NE, Lewin NA, editors. Goldfrank's toxicologic emergencies. Stamford (CT): Appleton and Lange; 1998. p. 541–64.

[48] Smilkstein MJ, Bronstein AC, Linden C, et al. Acetaminophen overdose: a 48-hour intravenous N-acetylcysteine protocol. Ann Emerg Med 1991;20(10):1058–63.

[49] Prescott LF, Illingworth RN, Critchley JA, et al. Intravenous N-acetylcysteine: the treatment of choice for paracetamol poisoning. Br Med J 1979;2:1097–100.

[50] Smilkstein MJ, Knapp GL, Kulig KW, et al. Efficacy of oral N-acetylcysteine in the treatment of acetaminophen overdose: analysis of the national multicenter study (1976–1985). N Engl J Med 1988;319:1557–62.

[51] Rumack BH, Matthew H. Acetaminophen poisoning and toxicity. Pediatrics 1975;55:871–6.

[52] Rumack BH, Peterson RG. Acetaminophen overdose: incidence, diagnosis and management in 46 patients. Pediatrics 1978;62:898–903.

[53] Acetadote (acetylcysteine) injection [package insert]. Nashville (TN): Cumberland Pharmaceuticals Inc; 2006.

[54] Perry HE, Shannon MW. Efficacy of oral versus intravenous N-acetylcysteine in acetaminophen overdose: results of an open-label clinical trial. J Pediatr 1998;132(1):149–52.

[55] Keays R, Harrison PM, Wendon JA, et al. Intravenous acetylcysteine in paracetamol induced fulminant hepatic failure: a prospective controlled trial. BMJ 1991;303:1026–9.

[56] Watson WA, Litovitz TL, Rodgers GC Jr, et al. 2002 Annual report of the American Association of Poison Control Centers toxic exposure surveillance system. Am J Emerg Med 2003;21:353–421.

[57] Michael J, Sztajnkrycer M. Deadly pediatric poisons: nine common agents that kill at low doses. Emerg Med Clin North Am 2004;22:1019–50.

[58] Bar-Oz B, Levichek Z, Koren G. Medications that can be fatal for a toddler with one tablet or teaspoonful: a 2004 update. Paediatr Drugs 2004;6(2):123–6.

[59] Anderson AC. Calcium channel blockers overdose. Clin Pediatr Emerg Med 2005;6:109–15.

[60] Ramoska EA, Spiller HA, Myers A. Calcium channel blocker toxicity. Ann Emerg Med 1990;19(6):649–53.

[61] Bryer AF, Wax P. Accidental ingestion of sustained release calcium channel blockers in children. Vet Hum Toxicol 1998;40(2):104–6.

[62] Lee DC, Green T, Dougherty T, et al. Fatal nifedipine ingestions in children. J Emerg Med 2000;19(4):359–61.

[63] Katz AM. Cardiac ion channels. N Engl J Med 1993;328:1244–51.

[64] Boyer EW, Shannon M. Treatment of calcium channel blocker intoxication with insulin infusion. N Engl J Med 2001;344(22):1721–2.

[65] Kline JA, Raymond RM, Schroeder JD, et al. The diabetogenic effects of acute verapamil poisoning. Toxicol Appl Pharmacol 1997;145:357–62.

[66] Yuan TH, Kerns WP II, Toamszewski CA, et al. Insulin-glucose an adjunctive therapy for severe calcium channel antagonist poisoning. J Toxicol Clin Toxicol 1999;37(4):463–74.

[67] Isbister GK. Delayed asystolic cardiac arrest after diltiazem overdose: resuscitation with high dose intravenous calcium. Emerg Med J 2002;19:355–7.

[68] Lam YM, Tse HF, Lau CP. Continuous calcium chloride infusion for massive nifedipine overdose. Chest 2001;119:1280–2.

[69] Mahr NC, Valdes A, Lamas G. Use of glucagon for acute intravenous diltiazam toxicity. Am J Cardiol 1997;79:1570–1.

[70] Walter FG, Frye G, Mullen JT, et al. Amelioration of nifedipine poisoning associated with glucagon therapy. Ann Emerg Med 1993;22:1234–7.

[71] Doyon S, Roberts JR. The use of glucagon in a case of calcium channel blocker overdose. Ann Emerg Med 1993;22:1229–33.

[72] Bailey B. Glucagon in beta-blocker and calcium channel blocker overdose: a systematic review. J Toxicol Clin Toxicol 2003;41:595–602.

[73] Kline JA, Leonova E, Raymond RM. Beneficial myocardial metabolic effects of insulin during verapamil toxicity in the anesthetized canine. Crit Care Med 1995;23:1251–63.

[74] Kline JA, Tomaszowski CA, Schroeder JD, et al. Insulin is a superior antidote for cardiovascular toxicity induced by verapamil in the anesthetized canine. J Pharmacol Exp Ther 1993; 267:744–50.

[75] Salhanick SA, Shannon MW. Management of calcium channel antagonist overdose. Drug Saf 2003;26:65–79.

[76] Henretig FM. Clonidine and central-acting antihypertensives. In: Ford MD, Delaney KA, Ling LJ, et al, editors. Clinical toxicology. Philadelphia: WB Saunders; 2001. p. 391–6.

[77] Kuhar MJ. Receptors for clonidine in brain: insights into therapeutic actions. J Clin Psychiatry 1982;43:17–9.

[78] Bizovi K. Antihypertensives, beta-blockers, and calcium antagonists. In: Erickson TB, Aherns WR, Aks SE, et al, editors. Pediatric toxicology: diagnosis and management of the poisoned child. New York: McGraw-Hill; 2005. p. 245–52.

[79] Klein-Schwartz W. Trends and toxic effects from pediatric clonidine exposure. Arch Pediatr Adolesc Med 2002;156:392–6.

[80] Tenenbein M. Naloxone in clonidine toxicity. Am J Dis Child 1984;138:1084–5.

[81] Abbruzzi G, Storks C. Pediatric toxicologic concerns. Emerg Med Clin North Am 2002; 20(1):223–46.

[82] Wiley JF, Wiley CC, Torrey SB, et al. Clonidine poisoning in young children. J Pediatr 1990; 116(4):654–8.

ELSEVIER
SAUNDERS

PEDIATRIC CLINICS
OF NORTH AMERICA

Pediatr Clin N Am 55 (2008) 687–708

Pediatric Intensivist Extenders in the Pediatric ICU

Cheryl L. Cramer, RN, MSN, ARNP[a],
James P. Orlowski, MD, FAAP, FCCP, FCCM[b],*,
Lucian K. DeNicola, MD, FAAP, FCCM[c]

[a]*Pediatric Intensive Care Unit, University Community Hospital, 3100 East Fletcher Avenue, Tampa, FL 33613, USA*
[b]*University Community Hospital, 3100 East Fletcher Avenue, Tampa, FL 33613, USA*
[c]*4976 Maybank Way, Jacksonville, FL 32225-1054, USA*

Without change there is no innovation, creativity, or incentive for improvement. Those who initiate change will have a better opportunity to manage the change that is inevitable.   —Thomas Pollard

The use of physician extenders, primarily advanced registered nurse practitioners (NPs) and physician assistants (PAs), has existed for many years but has recently escalated, especially in pediatric critical care, with the imposition by the Accreditation Council on Graduate Medical Education (ACGME) of limits on the long hours traditionally worked by house officers. On July 1, 2003 the ACGME mandated that residents were to work no more than 24 hours of continuous patient care (with an added 6-hour transition and education period), 1 day in 7 free of patient care responsibilities, and a minimum of 10 rest hours between duty periods [1]. These rules were based on a considerable body of scientific literature demonstrating that sleep deprivation affects cognitive performance and possibly patient care [1]. To the largest extent, these limits on resident duty hours were the result of a single case, the Libby Zion case, which occurred at New York Hospital–Cornell Medical Center in 1984 [2]. This landmark case has forced hospitals and other medical institutions to use manpower in more resourceful ways.

The Libby Zion case

Libby Zion was the 18-year-old daughter of a former federal prosecutor and columnist for the *New York Times*. In January of 1984 Libby Zion commenced psychiatric treatment for stress, which over the next few months

---

* Corresponding author.
E-mail address: jameso@mail.uch.org (J.P. Orlowski).

included prescriptions for phenelzine, imipramine, flurazepam, and diazepam. In late February she underwent a dental extraction and her dentist prescribed aspirin–oxycodone hydrochloride for pain. A few days later she
began complaining of fever and otalgia, and subsequently developed chills,
myalgias, and arthralgias. On March 4 her temperature reached 41°C and
her father contacted his doctor, an attending physician at the New York
Hospital–Cornell Medical Center, who advised that Libby be brought to
the emergency department (ED) [2–4].

   She arrived at the ED around 2330 and was seen by a junior medical resident. Libby did not disclose her previous prescriptions for imipramine, flurazepam, or diazepam, but stated that she had not taken her phenelzine that
day because she felt too ill. She admitted to frequent use of marijuana but
reported no use of cocaine or any other illicit drugs. She was noted to be
writhing during her physical examination, which the resident believed to
be volitional. She was febrile with a temperature of 39.7°C and mild orthostatic blood pressure changes. Her right tympanic membrane was hyper-
emic; she had a soft systolic murmur, a clear chest, and petechiae on her
right thigh. Her leukocyte count was 18,000 per cubic millimeter, and a chest
radiograph was normal. She was given intravenous fluids and a set of blood
cultures was obtained. After discussing the case with the referring physician,
the resident admitted the patient to the medical service around 0200 and
gave her acetaminophen. On admission she was examined by both an intern
and a junior resident, who obtained separate histories that did not disclose
any use of illicit drugs. They both noted shivering and agitation, and made
tentative diagnoses of a viral syndrome. They ordered blood, urine, and stool
cultures, and recommended that antibiotics be withheld and that the phenelzine be discontinued. The resident ordered 25 mg of meperidine be given for
agitation and shivering, despite knowledge that the patient had been on
a monoamine oxidase inhibitor (MAOI) (phenelzine). Both the resident
and intern had been working for more than 18 hours without a break [2–4].

   The house officers left the floor to care for other patients, and around
0330 Libby Zion was given the meperidine intramuscularly for agitation
and shivering. Between 0400 and 0430 the patient became more restless, confused, and began thrashing about in bed. The intern was called twice by the
nurses during this period of time, and first ordered the use of physical
restraints, and later ordered 1 mg of haloperidol for continued agitation
and confusion. Between 0430 and 0600 the patient was noted to be resting
comfortably, and the restraints were removed. She was able to take acetaminophen by mouth. Shortly after 0600 she again became agitated and
was found to have an axillary temperature of 42°C. The intern was called
and ordered cold compresses and a cooling blanket. At 0630 Libby Zion
went into cardiorespiratory arrest and could not be resuscitated.

   The medical examiner's preliminary report on March 6, 1984, listed the
cause of death as bilateral bronchopneumonia and stated that the patient
had hyperpyrexia and sudden collapse shortly after injection of meperidine

and haloperidol while in restraints for toxic agitation. Toxicology specimens detected cocaine in her nostrils and serum samples obtained before death were positive for cocaine.

Because of his political connections, Libby's father was able to persuade the New York County District Attorney to convene a grand jury investigation into her death. The grand jury returned no criminal indictments against the New York Hospital–Cornell Medical Center nor its physicians and house officers, but cited five circumstances that they believed contributed to Libby Zion's death: inadequate resident supervision in the emergency department, inadequate resident supervision on the hospital wards, sleep deprivation among the treating residents, lack of regulation of the use of physical restraints, and the absence of a computerized system to prevent adverse drug interactions. The grand jury report was issued at a time when media coverage of the Libby Zion case was prompting questions about the quality of care in teaching hospitals and focusing on the long hours that house officers work and their lack of adequate supervision by attending physicians. At the same time, a politically motivated New York City council president published a health department study suggesting that mistakes were to blame for many deaths in New York City hospitals. In response to these reports, the commissioner of the New York State Department of Health appointed Dr. Bertrand Bell to chair an ad hoc Advisory Committee on Emergency Services, composed of nine distinguished New York physicians. The Bell Commission ultimately endorsed the grand jury report and suggested limits on working hours, such that house staff and attending physicians in emergency departments should only work 12-hour shifts, and that physicians caring for patients on hospital wards should only work 16-hour shifts, with at least 8 hours off between shifts. The Bell Commission subsequently heard testimony from many organizations, including the ACGME, the American College of Physicians, the American College of Surgeons, the American Medical Association, the Association of American Medical Colleges, the Committee of Interns and Residents, and the Greater New York Hospital Association. Testimony included potential problems with implementation of the Bell Commission recommendations, including effects on graduate medical education, hospital staffing, malpractice litigation, and health care financing. The Greater New York Hospital Association estimated that the proposed changes would require an additional 2045 full-time attending physicians, 974 full-time ancillary personnel, and an annual cost of more than $200 million for the 50 New York City hospitals. In response to these testimonies, the Bell commission upheld its recommendations of a 12-hour limit on emergency department coverage by attending physicians and residents and 24-hour supervision of acute care inpatient units by experienced physicians, but altered its work hour limits for house offices outside the emergency department to 80 hours per week averaged over 4 weeks, with no more than 24 consecutive hours per shift and one 24-hour period of nonworking time per week.

This situation may be one in which a bad case resulted in a good law. The *Physicians' Desk Reference* for phenelzine states in two sentences buried in a full column of contraindications that it "should not be used in combination with dextromethorphan or with CNS depressants such as alcohol and certain narcotics. Excitation, seizures, delirium, hyperpyrexia, circulatory collapse, coma and death have been reported in patients receiving MAOI therapy who have been given a single dose of meperidine" [5]. Libby Zion's excitation, delirium, and hyperpyrexia all preceded her dose of meperidine, and are just as likely as her death to have been caused by cocaine toxicity. Other possible diagnoses include the serotonin syndrome attributable to the combination of phenelzine and meperidine, the neuroleptic malignant syndrome attributable to haloperidol alone or in combination with phenelzine, malignant hyperthermia attributable to the phenelzine, or cocaine-induced hyperpyrexia [6–9].

The father subsequently sued the hospital for $2 million in a wrongful death suit, on the grounds that his daughter had received inadequate care in the hands of overworked and undersupervised medical house officers. The trial finally occurred in late 1994 and early 1995. The jury absolved New York Hospital–Cornell Medical Center in the death of Libby Zion, stating that its system of training and supervision for young doctors was not to blame. They found three of the four physicians were culpable for having given her the wrong drug, but found that Libby Zion was herself partly at fault for not telling the doctors that she had taken cocaine and a host of other prescription drugs. The jury awarded Mr. Zion $375,000, but he was not happy with the verdict because it included reference to cocaine, and he had been seeking to clear her name of the taint of cocaine. Three months later, the judge of the New York State Supreme Court in Manhattan got both parties to agree to the settlement of $375,000, but threw out the jury's finding that Libby Zion's use of cocaine had made her 50% responsible for her own death [10,11].

Changes in manpower

As early as 1995 adult and pediatric critical care fellowship funding was being reduced because of a 1994 report from the Council on Graduate Medical Education. They predicted a 22% physician surplus by the year 2000 because of an excess of specialists and a deficiency of generalists [12]. A 1996 survey of 59 pediatric ICU (PICU) directors or division chiefs showed that 75% believed that the number of PICU fellowships were "just right" or "too many," 80% believed that there would be "too many" pediatric intensivists within 10 years, and although 71% believed that it would lead to increased quality of care, 75% believed that it would hurt intensivist compensation and 86% believed that it would lead to reduced job security [13].

In contrast, a rigorous, prospective data-based study by the Committee on Manpower of the Pulmonary and Critical Care Societies in 2000 indicated that demand would outstrip supply of adult intensivists by the year 2007 and there would be a 35% manpower deficiency by 2035 [14]. Similarly Stromberg [15] found that of the 81 pediatric cardiac intensivists required by 2008 there would only be 18 to 24 trained by then in the United States and Canada.

In 2007 John Birkmeyer, writing for the Leapfrog Group, identified ICU physician staffing (IPS) as the leading safety standard to judge the quality of care in hospitals. Hospitals fulfilling the IPS standard operate adult and pediatric ICUs that are managed or comanaged by intensivists who:

Are present during daytime hours and provide clinical care exclusively in the ICU and,

When not present on site or by way of telemedicine, return pages at least 95% of the time within 5 minutes and arrange for a Fundamentals of Critical Care Support–certified physician or physician extender to reach ICU patients within 5 minutes [16].

Furthermore, they found that only 26% of responding hospitals met the Leapfrog IPS standard because some non-intensivist physicians are unwilling to relinquish care, or hospitals are unable to hire intensivists because of manpower shortages. These shortages are attributable to decreased numbers of critical care fellowships based on decreased training funds and many board-certified intensivists choosing not to work in ICUs related to reimbursement issues. Meeting these standards is estimated to save 53,000 lives and $5.4 billion annually [17].

Pediatric ICU demographics

From 1995 to 2001 the number of PICUs in the United States increased from 306 to 349 (+13.7%) and the number of PICU beds increased by 34.4%, with the largest growth in units with more than 15 beds. In 1993, 73% of PICUs had an intensivist on staff. By 2001, 94% of PICUs had an intensivist on staff with 30% in-house at night. The number of PICU beds is growing more rapidly than the rate of the pediatric population [18]. Between 1993 and 2005 the median number of beds per unit did not increase and stands at 12, but the number of admissions per unit increased from 528 to 696 (31.8%) per year (Table 1) [19].

As of September 2007, there were 141 PICU positions listed in the jobs database of the Pediatric Section of the Society of Critical Care Medicine [20] and 59 pediatric critical care fellowships (up from 40 fellowships in 1992) that graduate approximately 110 board-eligible pediatric intensivists per year. The attrition rate is unknown. Hospitals are increasingly demanding continuous physician staffing in the ICUs. A recent survey described the penetrance of 24-hour staffing in 98 Canadian ICUs. Sixty percent of 88 responding units reported dedicated, continuous coverage. In 15% of these, staff intensivists with a median level of 3 postgraduate years of experience

Table 1
Pediatric intensive care unit use over 10-year period

	1993 (1995)	2001 (2005)	% Increase
PICUs	306	349	13.7
PICU Beds	2901	3899	34.4
Admits/PICU	528	696	31.8

provided coverage. Those units with in-house physicians had more ICU beds and fewer ICU staff physicians. Eighty three percent worked shifts that were more than 20 hours long [21].

Many hospitals are using pediatric intensive care extenders to supplement the board-certified intensivists and pediatric residents. These extenders are advanced practice nurses (APNs), certified PAs, and hospital-based acute care pediatricians (hospitalists). The Academy of Pediatrics has endorsed extenders in the care of hospitalized children [22].

Hospitalist

For many years community hospitals have employed "house physicians" to care for patients without primary or specialist physicians. Teaching hospitals traditionally used residents for the same purpose. In the 1990s, with the reduction in residents' hours, increasing demands of the uninsured and aging population, and growth of managed care, many hospitals increased their employment of house physicians. Efforts to improve the efficiency and quality of hospital inpatient care have led to the movement to replace the primary care physician with the hospitalist as the inpatient physician of record. A hospitalist serves as the physician of record after accepting referrals of hospitalized patients from primary care physicians or the ED. One of the forces promoting the hospitalist movement is the assumption that inpatient care provided by a small number of physicians is less costly, of higher quality, and less variable than the care provided by primary care physicians, who see patients only briefly once a day. Hospitalists are accessible throughout their shifts and can better respond to changing patient needs [23]. In 1999, a survey by the National Association of Inpatient Physicians found that most were young and most were men, and only 48% had practiced hospital-based medicine for more than 2 years. Eighty-nine percent of respondents were internists; of these, 51% were generalists and 38% were subspecialists. Most hospitalists limited their practices to the inpatient setting, but 37% practiced outpatient general internal medicine or subspecialty medicine in a limited capacity. In addition to providing care for inpatients, 90% of hospitalists were engaged in consultative medicine. Quality assurance and practice guideline development were the most frequently reported nonclinical activities (53% and 46%, respectively). Small group practices (31%) and staff-model health maintenance organizations

(25%) were the most common practice settings, and 78% of participants were reimbursed through salary. Financial incentives were common (43%) but modest [24].

Studies did demonstrate that hospitalists decreased length of stay and produced cost savings to hospitals and third party payers. Halasyamani and colleagues [25] compared risk-adjusted length of stay, variable costs, 30-day readmission rate, and mortality of 10,595 patients admitted to a tertiary community hospital by community physicians, private hospitalists, and academic hospitalists. There was a 20% reduction in length of stay on the academic hospitalist service and 8% on the private hospitalist service, compared with community physicians. Similarly, total costs were 10% less on the academic hospitalist and 6% less on the private hospitalist services compared with community physicians. The length of stay of academic hospitalists was 13% shorter than that of private hospitalists. Differences in costs, 30-day mortality, and 30-day readmission rate between hospitalist groups were not statistically significant [25]. Similar results were found on pediatric services. Bellet and Whitaker [26] studied 1440 hospitalizations at the Cincinnati Children's Hospital. Average length of stay was reduced by 11% and hospital charges were reduced by 10% for patients admitted to hospitalists versus those admitted to the traditional ward service [26]. Dwight and colleagues [27] compared staff-only hospitalist services to staff/resident services at an academic teaching hospital adjusted for age, gender, and comorbidity. Patients cared for by staff physicians only had a mean length of stay reduced by 14% without a difference in mortality, subspecialty consultation, or readmission rates [27]. Several studies looked at community physicians' attitudes toward the development of hospitalist services [28–30]. In general, community physicians believed that the care of inpatients was inefficient use of their own time. Hospitalists improved patient satisfaction and improved quality of care but diminished the community physician's career satisfaction, diminished their ability to keep up-to-date with medical knowledge, and adversely affected the doctor–patient relationship.

The use of hospitalists in the PICU began with the new century and may be linked with the expansion of telemedicine and the desire of smaller and more rural hospitals, under pressure from managed care, to provide lower-level critical care services at the local community hospital. Many of these hospitals had already incorporated hospitalists to care for the general ward patients. Intensivist groups could provide consultation to these "step down" units on rounds or by telemedicine and continue to provide tertiary services at their primary institution. Similarly, hospitalists could "cross cover" PICUs at night, thus reducing the pressure to enlarge intensivist groups while still providing continuous care. Although this model is being expanded there are few reports attesting to the usefulness or outcomes. Tenner and colleagues [31] compared the severity-adjusted survival and length of stay of patients in a teaching hospital PICU, in which residents provided after-hours in-house coverage, with survival in the same unit, with hospitalists providing this coverage. The same group of academic pediatric intensivists managed the patients in this study of 1211 children over an 18-month period in two PICUs in San Antonio. Although overall mortality was the same during both eras, severity-adjusted mortality was more than twice as high in the resident era as in the hospitalist era. Similarly, both actual and severity-adjusted length of stay were longer in the resident era [31].

Physician assistants

The first PA program was created at Duke University in 1965. There are now 136 training programs accredited by The American Medical Association's Committee on Allied Health Education and Accreditation. One hundred and eight of these programs offer a master's degree curriculum [32]. A PA is registered by the state after 2 or more years of undergraduate education followed by 9 to 12 months of preclinical didactic studies and 9 to 15 months of physician-supervised clinical education. The formal training is divided into didactic and clinical portions of equal length. The didactic phase consists of courses in anatomy, physiology, microbiology, and clinical laboratory studies, and a wide variety of medical specialty and patient examination courses. The clinical phase is divided into 4- to 6-week rotations that cover family practice, pediatrics, surgery, emergency medicine, internal medicine, and other specialties. Some educational programs for PAs graduate child health associates, who receive specialized training in pediatrics. By law, PAs may perform medical services, but only when supervised by a physician and only when such acts and duties are within the scope of practice of the supervising physician. The National Commission on Certification of Physician Assistants certifies PAs. To sit for the examination, a PA must be a graduate of an accredited PA program. PAs are re-registered every 2 years based on 100 hours of continuing medical education and are recertified every 6 years by examination [32]. Currently, there are 75,800 PAs working in all 50 states and the District of Columbia [33].

Advanced practice nurse

APN is a title used to signify the registered nurse who has acquired additional nursing education beyond that required for licensure. This APN title can signify the clinical nurse specialist (CNS), certified registered nurse anesthetist (CRNA), certified nurse midwives (CNM), and the nurse practitioner (NP). The CNM and CRNA do not fall under the scope of PICU extenders and are excluded from discussion.

NP training programs exist in every state (Table 2) [34]. The variability among states on NP scope of practice is of interest to note and is generally governed by the Nurse Practice Act of the state. NP programs currently require a master's degree for admission or one is granted at the program's completion. In the near future, the practicing NP may be required to hold a doctorate degree. The NP title is further divided into subspecialties including pediatric nurse practitioner (PNP), pediatric critical care nurse practitioner (PCCNP), family nurse practitioner, neonatal nurse practitioner (NNP), and acute care nurse practitioner (ACNP).

The role of the NP was developed in 1965 as a joint effort of a pediatric physician and a nursing professor at the University of Colorado. This program was created as a solution to assist the physician in the care of children because of lack of physician availability [35]. This NP program was begun at Denver Children's Hospital and graduated NPs in pediatric primary care (PNPs). Further NP role development prompted the NNP programs in the 1970s, which focused on the acute care of the neonate.

The education of these early NNPs varied widely because the education was institutionally based with the primary responsibility assumed by the neonatologists. Titles, certification, and scope of practice were variable and based on the state's nursing practice act. There was no reciprocity between states and not all states recognized APNs. It was not until 1994 that The National Association of Neonatal Nurses issued its Guidelines for Neonatal Nurse Practitioners Education Program, which included the general curriculum and entry-level competency standards, eventually leading to the development of graduate NNP programs. The history of other ACNP roles is less clear because they originated sporadically to fill the needs of expanding pediatric services during cutbacks in pediatric residency programs. In 1995, The American Association of Critical Care Nurses and the American Nursing Association published *Standards of Clinical Practice and Scope of Practice for the Acute Care Nurse Practitioner*, which became the basis for the development of the ACNP role [36].

Another APN is the master's-prepared CNS, who exists in some inpatient acute care facilities. They function as clinicians, educators, and researchers in pediatric areas, such as pediatric critical care, pediatric oncology, pediatric infectious disease, pediatric gastroenterology, pediatric neurology, pediatric orthopedics, pediatric cardiology, pediatric cardiac surgery, and pediatric general surgery. The pediatric CNS role probably exists in every subspecialty area of pediatrics. The main difference between the CNS and NP is the amount of time spent in direct patient care. One study by Williams and Valdivieso [37], in 1994, found that the CNS spent only 33% of work time in direct patient-care activities, whereas the NP spent 63% of work time in direct patient care. Apparently, the CNS role is predominantly one of education. Because the Centers for Medicare and Medicaid Services funds only 40% to 50% of residency programs, and resident duty hours are severely restricted now, many hospital administrators are employing acute care or critical care NPs as cost-effective alternatives to resident-managed care in the acute care setting. The days of the CNS role may be limited because health care systems cannot continue to support indirect advanced nursing practice roles not involved in providing direct patient care and generating revenue.

Table 2
Nurse practitioner state practice requirements

State	National certification	Physician required chart review	Type of mandated physician involvement	Independent practice	Prescriptive authority
Alabama	Yes	Yes	Collaborative/protocols	No	No controlled medications
Alaska	Yes	No	None	Yes	Yes
Arizona	Yes	No	None	Yes	Yes
Arkansas	Yes	Yes	Collaborative/protocols	No	Yes
California	No	No	Collaborative/supervise/protocols	No	Yes
Colorado	Yes	No	Collaborative	No	Yes
Connecticut	Yes	No	Collaborative/direct/protocols	No	No
Delaware	Case by case	No	Collaborative	No	Yes with Board of Medicine approval
District of Columbia	Yes	No	Collaborative/protocols	Yes	Yes
Florida	Yes	No	Supervise/protocols	No	No
Georgia	Yes	Yes	Protocols	No	Yes
Hawaii	No	No	Collegial relationship	Yes	Yes
Idaho	Yes	No	Collaborative/supervise/protocols	Yes	Yes
Illinois	Yes	Yes	Collaborative	No	No schedule I or II
Indiana	No	No	Collaborative	No	Yes
Iowa	No	No	Collaborative	Yes	Yes
Kansas	No	No	Protocols	No	Yes
Kentucky	Yes	No	Collaborative	Yes	Yes
Louisiana	Yes	No	Collaborative/protocols	No	Yes
Maine	Yes	No	Collaborative/supervise[a]/protocols none after 24 mo	Yes after 2 yrs of practice	Yes
Maryland	Yes	Yes	Collaborative/direct	No	Yes
Massachusetts	Yes	Yes	Collaborative/protocols	No	Yes
Michigan	Yes	No	Collaborative	Yes	No schedule I or II
Minnesota	Yes	No	Collaborative/delegation	No	Yes
Mississippi	Yes	Yes	Collaborative/protocols	No	Yes

Missouri	Yes	Yes	Collaborative/protocols	No
Montana	Yes	No	Referral process	Yes
Nebraska	Yes	No	Supervise/collaborative	Yes
Nevada	Yes	Yes	Collaborative/protocols	Yes
New Hampshire	Yes	No	None	Yes
New Jersey	Yes	No	Collaborative/protocols	Yes
New Mexico	Yes	No	None	Yes
New York	No	Yes	Collaborative/protocols	Yes
North Carolina	Yes	Yes	Supervise/protocols	Yes
North Dakota	No	No	Collaborative	Yes
Ohio	Yes	Yes	Standard care agreement	Yes
Oklahoma	Yes	No	Supervise/direct	No schedule I or II
Oregon	No	No	None	Yes
Pennsylvania	Yes	Yes	Direct/protocols/collaborative	Yes
Rhode Island	Yes	No	Collaborative for prescription only	Yes
South Carolina	Yes	No	Protocols/collaborative	No schedule I or II
South Dakota	Yes	Yes	Collaborative	Yes
Tennessee	Yes	No	Supervise/collaborative	Yes
Texas	Yes	Yes	Collaborative/supervise/protocols	Yes
Utah	Yes	No	Consultation/referral plan	Yes
Vermont	Yes	Yes	Collaborative/protocols	Yes
Virginia	Yes	Yes	Collaborative/direct/protocols	Yes
Washington	Yes	No	None	Yes
West Virginia	Yes	No	Collaborative/protocols	No schedule I or II
Wisconsin	Yes	No	Collaborative	Yes
Wyoming	Yes	No	Collaborative	Yes

[a] None after 24 months.

The NPs and PAs who are used in ICU positions necessitate additional precepted education beyond that required for certification. The additional precepted education should be the responsibility of the pediatric unit director and should include orientation to hospital and departmental policies, protocols, and direct teaching of clinical skills needed for the specific unit. The NPs and PAs should work under the direct supervision of an attending physician, who is readily available to answer questions and provide backup to the NP or PA. Decisions regarding the need for admission, management plans, and appropriateness for discharge must be made with the involvement of the attending physician [38].

ACNPs are different from PAs. PAs are educated to assist physicians; their role allows for no independent or autonomous functions. They may perform diagnostic and therapeutic interventions without the physical presence of a supervising physician, who is available by telephone. Legally, PAs must work under the supervision of physicians. The ACNP collaborates with a physician and provides advanced nursing care with a holistic versus a disease-oriented approach [36]. An ACNP is independently licensed and may operate without the supervision of a licensed physician. Both provide continuity of patient care and often act as liaisons between the intensivist, other specialists, house staff, and nursing staff to provide interdisciplinary practice [22,36]. Despite these differences in philosophy, studies of the roles of PAs and ACNPs in ICUs show few differences [39].

Studies of pediatric critical care nurse practitioners and physician assistants

Undoubtedly, the first uses of critical care physician extenders were NPs staffing the neonatal ICU (NICU) in the early 1970s [40,41]. Comparisons to traditional physician staffing were not published until 1994, when Schultz and colleagues [42] compared NNPs to pediatric house officers in a transitional care unit. This nonrandomized, nonconcurrent study evaluated the effectiveness of NNPs at a level III NICU through a retrospective review of medical records. Two groups of infants cared for in a transitional care unit were evaluated, with one group cared for by pediatric residents and the other group by two Master's prepared NNPs in collaboration with a neonatologist. The NNPs cared for infants who were significantly smaller, with younger gestational ages, than those cared for by the pediatric residents. The care provided by the NNPs resulted in a mean 2.4-day reduction in length of stay, and a mean reduction in hospital charges of $3,491 per patient [42].

An excellent study by Mitchell-DiCenso and colleagues [43] randomized patients over a 1-year study period (821 infants), to either an NP/CNS team during the daytime hours and residents at night (414 infants) or exclusive care by pediatric residents and neonatology fellows (407 neonates). Outcome measures included mortality, number of complications, length of stay, quality of care, and cost. There were 19 deaths (4.6%) in the NP/CNS group and 24 (5.9%) in the resident group (relative risk [RR], 0.78%; CI, 0.43–1.40). In the NP/CNS group, 230 (55.6%) neonates had complications, in comparison with 220 (54.1%) in the resident group (RR, 1.03; CI, 0.91–1.16). Complications were defined by a list of 28 events compiled through consensus by a group of neonatologists, and included medical outcomes, such as pneumothorax; self-extubation; procedure-related problems, such as malpositioned catheters and skin breakdown; fluid and electrolyte problems; blood transfusions; and readmission to the NICU. Mean lengths of stay were 12.5 days in the NP/CNS group and 11.7 days in the resident group (difference in means, 0.8 days; CI, 1.1–2.7 days). The performance on the quality indicators was comparable in the two groups except for two instances, jaundice and charting, both of which favored the NP/CNS group. Mean scores on the Neonatal Index of Parent Satisfaction were 140 in the NP/CNS group and 139 in the resident group (difference in means, 1.0; CI, 3.6 to 5.6). In the NP/CNS group, 6 infants (2.6%) performed 30% or more below their age level in the Minnesota Infant Development Inventory, in comparison with 2 infants (0.9%) in the resident group (RR, 2.87; CI, 0.59–14.06). The cost per infant in the NP/CNS group was $14, 245 and in the resident group, $13, 267 (difference in means, $978; CI, $1313.18–$3259.05). The authors concluded that NP/CNS and resident teams were similar with respect to all tested measures of performance [43]. These results support the use of NPs as an alternative to pediatric residents in delivering care to critically ill neonates. Similar results were found in subsequent studies [43–46]. A more recent study found that advanced NNPs performing preterm neonatal resuscitation intubated at the same rate but more quickly than did residents, administered surfactant sooner, and caused less hypothermia [47].

Another study in neonatology, called the Ashington experiment, was not randomized and used historical controls [48]. The Ashington experiment involved an innovative neonatal service run entirely by advanced NNPs. They found that mortality, defined as intrapartum deaths and deaths during the first 28 days of life, for singletons born to mothers booked for delivery in Ashington, declined from 5.12/1000 singletons in 1991 to 1995, before the introduction of the NNP service, to 3.11/1000 in 1996 to 2000 after the NNPs came into post. On six of seven dimensions of quality, Ashington performed better than the average of five comparator hospitals and overall ranked second. Quality of resuscitation was assessed, and there was no evidence of substandard care. Quality of care as measured by detection rates of congenital heart disease, congenital dislocation of the hip, and parental satisfaction were high, and costs were marginally lower, than comparable units. The authors concluded that the Ashington experiment showed that NNPs could provide a high standard of neonatal care without a doctor on site [48].

Numerous NNP studies are reported but there was little mention of NPs in the adult ICU until the mid 1980s, when there were discussions about the role of the APN in the ICU [49]. A training program was developed for adult critical care NPs at the University of Pittsburgh in 1993 [50]. Presently, several similar programs are available [51]. A comparison of activities and outcomes between ACNPs, PAs, and medical residents in a Pittsburgh ICU showed that residents cared for more patients, older and sicker patients, worked more hours, and took a more active role on rounds. NPs and PAs were more likely to discuss patients with the bedside nurses and patients' families and spent more time in research and administrative activities. Compared with residents, the extenders performed fewer invasive procedures. Outcomes between the extenders and residents were no different [52].

Although a letter to the editor in *Chest* (January, 1992) mentioned that PAs had been used in the postoperative cardiothoracic ICU at Emory University Hospital since 1980 [53], the first evaluation of PAs in intensive care was published in 1991. Dubaybo and colleagues [54] evaluated the operation of the medical ICU at Allen Park, Michigan Veterans Administration Hospital during a 2-year period when residents staffed the unit as compared to a 2-year period when specially trained PAs staffed the unit. They found that there was a decrease in admissions but an increase in length of stay and laboratory evaluations without any change in severity, mortality, or complications during the period when PAs were acting as house staff [54].

More recently, Thourani and Miller [55] discussed a 30-year experience using PAs in the adult cardiothoracic ICU at Emory. During those 30 years the number of PAs employed increased from 2 to 23, with no further increase in resident coverage, while cases increased from 400 to 4000. Retention was 50%. The PAs took histories, did physicals, performed conduit harvesting, inserted invasive catheters and chest tubes, acted as surgical first assistants, and closed chests. Salaries ranged from $50,000 to $100,000. They concluded that the addition of PAs resolved problems in work assignments and enabled the expansion of the service without increasing the number of resident trainees [55].

Martin [56] conducted a retrospective chart review study that evaluated the medical records of 25 children, cared for by two PCCNPs, to the same number of children managed by pediatric residents. Parents and staff nurses described a high level of satisfaction with NP practice, and discharge planning documentation appeared earlier in the NP patient records [56].

Manpower shortages led to the development of a program using PNPs in the department of surgery at a children's hospital [57]. A questionnaire was used to survey attending surgeons, house staff, and parents about their satisfaction with the PNPs. All of the attending physicians were pleased with the PNPs caring for their patients and believed that the program reduced the residents' workload. Junior and senior residents believed the PNPs reduced their workload and they considered the PNPs as valuable resources. None of the residents believed that the PNPs interfered with their training. In fact, 73% of the junior residents and 55% of the senior residents believed that the PNPs contributed to their learning. Ninety-six percent of parents surveyed were satisfied with the involvement of the PNPs in their child's care, with the remaining 4% undecided. Ninety-two percent of the parents believed that the PNPs kept them well informed of their child's progress [57].

A recent study compared, by way of work sampling analysis, the time spent doing essential tasks in an adult ICU of an ACNP and physicians-in-training. Hoffman and colleagues [58] found that ACNPs and ICU fellows spent similar amounts of time performing daily tasks. They noted the NPs spent more time communicating with patients, families, and other team members and were more involved in activities that led to better coordination of care, whereas the residents spent more time performing non-unit activities.

Nurse practitioners and physician assistants as pediatric ICU extenders

Because of a contraction in the pediatric residency in Jacksonville, Florida, and a previous good experience staffing the NICU [59], physician extenders were incorporated into staffing the PICU in 1984. In 1988, the Pediatric Section of the Society of Critical Care Medicine undertook a national manpower study and in 1990 to 1991 surveyed 148 hospitals, which represented 50% of hospitals listed as having a PICU [33]. At that time, 69 of the responding hospitals employed physician extenders and 12 employed them in the PICU. Of these, 75% were NPs and 25% were PAs. The only distinguishing characteristic of hospitals employing extenders in the PICU was availability of child-care physicians. Hospital size, affiliation, location, size of catchment area, number of pediatric beds, and number of admissions did not influence the employment of extenders. Fifty percent of hospitals employing extenders were university teaching hospitals. These NPs and PAs acted the same as pediatric house staff, which included the performance of invasive procedures of intubation, ventilation, and lumbar puncture. Extenders in the PICU were twice as likely as extenders in the NICU to insert central catheters, arterial catheters, and chest tubes. They were also twice as likely to initiate muscle relaxants and cardiotonic drugs. Attitudes toward the employment of extenders differed between attending and administrative staff of hospitals that had or did not have child care residents. Those that had residents believed that the extenders compared most favorably with second-year pediatric residents, whereas the staff of hospitals that did not have residents believed that the extenders performed equal to third-year residents (Fig. 1). Acceptance of extenders was strongest by attendings and residents, moderate by nurses and administrators, and weakest by medical students. At that time, 45% of responding institutions planned to employ or increase their employment of pediatric critical care extenders [33].

Recently Mathur and colleagues [60] reported a 5-year experience with PAs in the PICU at Downstate Medical College. They described the background and training of these PAs and the problems encountered when the PAs, who are familiar and consistent members of the PICU team, encounter

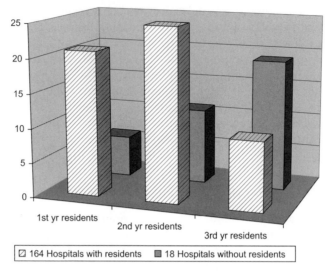

Fig. 1. Pediatric physician extenders compare most favorably to second- or third-year residents based on type of hospital.

the rotating resident who has only a 1- to 2-month rotation on-service, but has the higher responsibility. This dynamic undermines a collegial relationship and has resulted in retention difficulties [60].

The American College of Critical Care Medicine of the Society of Critical Care Medicine and the American Academy of Pediatrics published in 2004 "Guidelines and levels of care for pediatric intensive care units" [61], which included the statement that:

> Studies suggest that having a full-time pediatric intensivist in the PICU improves patient care and efficiency. At certain times of the day, the attending physician in the PICU may delegate the care of patients to a physician of at least the postgraduate year 2 level, or to an advanced practice nurse or physician assistant with specialized training in pediatric critical care [61].

Likewise, the Committee on Hospital Care of the American Academy of Pediatrics published a statement in 1999 entitled "The role of the nurse practitioner and physician assistant in the care of hospitalized children" [22], which supported the role of NPs and PAs in pediatric inpatient units, with the caveat that:

> The NPs and PAs who are used in such positions require additional precepted education, beyond that required for certification. The additional precepted education should be the responsibility of the pediatric unit director and should include orientation to hospital and departmental policies and protocols and direct teaching of clinical skills needed for the specific unit [22].

The American Nurses Association standards of practice state that the role of the ACNP is:

To assess, think critically, provide advanced therapeutic interventions, and perform diagnostic reasoning and case management in the care of acutely ill patients [62].

By 1997, the University of Maryland had developed an educational program and curriculum for the PCCNP. They were able to demonstrate that the PCCNP was successfully managing children in the PICU, with an average pediatric risk for mortality score of 28 [63]. Several authors have discussed the role of the PCCNP in the PICU [56,62–64]. They have been well accepted, work well with bedside nurses and physician staff, and seem to document and discharge plan better than residents.

Verger and colleagues [65] conducted a national survey soliciting descriptive information and the skills and responsibilities of the PCCNP. This extensive review surveyed 74 NPs in 29 hospitals, who subscribed to one of two list servers for APNs, and graduates of pediatric masters programs and attendees at national nursing conferences who identified themselves as PCCNPs. All respondents were master's prepared, with 54% of the NPs receiving master's or post–master's degrees from a pediatric acute or critical care graduate program. The terminal degrees of other respondents were obtained from pediatric primary care programs (39%), family NP programs (5%), or adult acute care NP programs. Seventy-two percent of NPs had been awarded their degrees within the previous 5 years. Sixty-seven percent were employed by university hospitals, with 73% working in children's hospitals. Ninety-five percent worked with trained pediatric intensivist physicians, with the remaining 5% working with cardiac surgeons. Sixty percent worked with pediatric critical care fellows, 68% with pediatric residents, and 54% with CNSs. Eighty-one percent possessed national certification as an NP. Ninety-one percent of those certified were certified as an NP in pediatric primary care by the Pediatric Nursing Certification Board of the American Nurses Credentialing Center. They had a mean of 13 years of nursing experience and all had critical care experience, with a mean of 10.6 years, and a mean of 5.7 years as a staff nurse in the pediatric critical care unit. Forty percent possessed 1 year or less of experience in their NP role, with a mean of 2.9 years [65].

Few studies have documented the clinical responsibilities and technical skills of NPs in PICUs. Verger and colleagues [65] report 49% of NPs were supervised by a combined nurse and physician leadership team, 18% by nursing alone, and 32% by a physician only. Sixty-four percent of NPs were paid from a nursing budget, 29% from the physicians practice plan or physician line hospital budget, and 7% by a combination. All NPs participated in direct patient care, accounting for 71.5% of their time. They worked an average of 50 hours per week, and 48% provided in-house patient coverage during weekends or nights. Fifty percent were on call with residents, 53% with fellows, and 72% with attending physicians.

Salaries in 2004 ranged from $45,000 to $95,000 with 44% earning between $65,000 and $75,000 for an average of 50 hours per week. These PCCNPs filled identical roles as pediatric residents with more than 85% performing endotracheal intubation, initiating ventilation and vasoactive/cardiotonic drips, placing central vein and arterial catheters, performing lumbar punctures, and inserting chest tubes. More experienced and more senior NPs took on leadership roles in education and training nurses and resident physicians, along with nursing management [65].

All the NPs surveyed performed history and physical examinations, documented progress and procedure notes, initiated and adjusted nutrition and hydration, ordered and interpreted laboratory/diagnostic tests, interpreted EKGs, ordered medications, and interpreted radiographs (Table 3). Other skills performed by more than 90% of respondents included initiating and adjusting intravenous therapy (100%), adjusting oxygen delivery (98%), initiating and adjusting mechanical ventilation (97%), ordering blood therapy (97%), and initiating and titrating vasoactive drips (91%) (see Table 3). More than 80% of NPs performed venipuncture (99%), intravenous line insertion (99%), lumbar puncture (94%), feeding tube placement (93%), suture removal (93%), endotracheal intubation (85%), arterial line insertion (83%), chest tube removal (81%), and central line placement (81%). Percutaneously inserted central lines (PICC) were performed by 55% of respondents (Table 4) [65].

The only information about hospitalists in the PICU is the study by Tenner [31], which was previously mentioned.

The future

The position of extenders in the medical center is well established. NPs and PAs have performed at least as well (if not better) as residents in clinics,

Table 3
Nurse practitioner patient management skills

Skill	% Participation	Self skill rating scale: (1) novice, (3) proficient, (5) expert	Respondent numbers
Initiate/adjust IV fluids	100	4.50	74
Initiate/adjust vasoactive drugs	91	3.79	67
Adjust oxygen therapy	98	4.40	72
Initiate/adjust mechanical ventilation	97	3.51	72
Needle thoracentesis	78	3.00	58
Initiate/adjust nutritional support	100	4.45	74
Order/interpret lab and diagnostic tests	100	4.45	74
Interpret radiologic tests	100	3.54	74
Order blood therapy	97	4.33	72
Interpret EKGs	97	3.41	72
Order medications	100	4.09	74

Table 4
Nurse practitioner technical skills

Skill	% participation	Self skill rating scale: (1) novice, (3) proficient, (5) expert	Number of respondents
Peripheral IV insertion	99	4.26	71
Venipuncture	99	4.38	71
Lumbar puncture	94	4.00	68
Feeding tube insertion	93	4.5	67
Suturing	37	3.21	27
Intubate	85	3.34	61
Insert arterial lines	83	3.17	60
Insert central lines	81	2.84	58
Insert PICC lines	55	3.53	58
Insert umbilical lines	17	2.75	12
Chest tube removal	81	No data	58
Chest tube insertion	78	3.00	58
Remove intracardiac lines	36	3.24	26

on the wards, in emergency departments, and in adult, neonatal, specialty, and pediatric ICUs. With the increase in demand for hospital services, aging population, and restriction in resident hours, there seems to be an increasing need for hospital-based medical professionals. Although there may be some friction between trainees (medical students and residents) and extenders who may be competing for procedures and hierarchy, these issues usually resolve with time and familiarity. Some subspecialists strongly object to referring to, or having their patients covered by, non-physician extenders in units closed to admission by non-intensivists. There continue to be issues as to the status of the extender, partially based on remuneration and partially based on funding source. Should extenders be thought of as substitute physicians with open-ended hours, academic requirements, ultimate responsibility and liability, and even job security and academic rank paid directly (or indirectly) by patient payment, or as shift workers with regular hours, minimal continuity, limited liability, and no access to tenure (or some other form of job security) paid from corporate entities [60]? Emergency physicians have traditionally worked as shift workers. The demand for 24-hour in-house coverage in ICUs has made the intensivist a shift worker and the hospitalist movement is certainly shift oriented. It is unclear how these changes will affect the academic medical center.

Will the hospitalist displace the non-physician extenders? Will office-based physicians have less resistance in referring to specialty board eligible/certified hospitalists than they have to non-physician extenders? Will hospitals prefer a practice plan–paid hospitalist physician with liability insurance for provision of off-hour coverage to extenders that are paid and insured by the hospital? Will government, HMOs, and corporate entities (Leapfrog) have a voice in determining the medical provider [66–69]?

The future is uncertain, but what we know for fact is the availability and quality of the NP and PA are nearly equal to that of the resident physician. Given time and appropriate training these PICU extenders can be a gift, to be used by the facility with enough stamina to embrace change. For the time being it seems that all players are necessary, but the system is dynamic so change is inevitable.

References

[1] Weinstein DF. Duty hours for resident physicians—tough choices for teaching hospitals. N Engl J Med 2002;347:1275–8.
[2] Asch DA, Parker RM. The Libby Zion case: one step forward or two steps backward? N Engl J Med 1988;318:771–5.
[3] Brensilver JM, Smith L, Lyttle CS. Impact of the Libby Zion case on graduate medical education in internal medicine. Mt Sinai J Med 1998;65:296–300.
[4] Friedman WA. Resident duty hours in American neurosurgery. Neurosurgery 2004;54: 925–33.
[5] Parke-Davis Company. In: Nardil. Physicians desk reference. Montvale (NJ): Medical Economics Publishing; 1985. p. 1793–5.
[6] Lannas PA, Pachar JV. A fatal case of neuroleptic malignant syndrome. Med Sci Law 1993; 33:86–8.
[7] Staufenberg EF, Tantam D. Malignant hyperpyrexia syndrome in combined treatment. Br J Psychol 1989;154:577–8.
[8] Crandall CG, Vongpatanasin W, Victor RG. Mechanism of cocaine-induced hyperthermia in humans. Ann Intern Med 2002;136:785–91.
[9] Rosenberg J, Pentel P, Pond S, et al. Hyperthermia associated with drug intoxication. Crit Care Med 1986;14:964–9.
[10] Hoffman J. Jurors find shared blame in '84 death. New York Times, February 7, 1995.
[11] Robins N. The girl who died twice; every patient's nightmare: the Libby Zion case and the hidden hazards of hospitals. New York: Delacorte Press; 1995.
[12] Council on Graduate Medical Education. Recommendations to improve access to health care through physician workforce reform. Washington, DC: US Dept of Health and Human Services; 1994.
[13] Workforce survey results. Available at: http://pedsccm.org/org-meet/aap/aap_sept96.htm. Accessed February 13, 2007.
[14] Angus DC, Kelly MA, Schmitz RJ, et al. Committee on manpower for pulmonary and critical care societies: current and projected workforce requirements for care of the critically ill and patients with pulmonary disease; can we meet the requirements of an aging population? JAMA 2000;284:2762–70.
[15] Stromberg D. Pediatric cardiac intensivists: are enough being trained? Pediatr Crit Care Med 2004;5:414–5.
[16] Pronovost P, Rainey TG, Birkmeyer JD. ICU physician staffing (IPS). The leapfrog group fact sheet. Available at: www.leapfroggroup.org. Accessed February 21, 2007.
[17] Pronovost PJ, Waters H, Dorman T. Impact of critical care physician workforce for intensive care unit physician staffing. Curr Opin Crit Care 2001;7:456–9.
[18] Randolph AG, Gonzales CA, Cortellini L, et al. Growth of pediatric intensive care units in the United States from 1995 to 2001. J Pediatr 2004;144:792–8.
[19] Odetola FO, Clark SJ, Freed GL, et al. A national survey of pediatric critical care resources in the United States. Pediatrics 2005;115:e382–6.
[20] The Pediatric Critical Care Medicine website. Available at: http://pedsccm.org/jobs. Accessed February 13, 2007.

[21] Parshuram CS, Kirpalani H, Mehta S, et al. In-house, overnight physician staffing: a cross-sectional survey of Canadian adult and pediatric intensive care units. Crit Care Med 2006;34: 1674–5.

[22] American Academy of Pediatrics Committee on Hospital Care 1997–1998. The role of the nurse practitioner and physician assistant in the care of hospitalized children. Pediatrics 1999;103:1050–2.

[23] Anderson S. The hospitalists. Radiol Manage 2000;22:57–60.

[24] Lindenauer PK, Pantilat SZ, Katz PP, et al. Hospitalists and the practice of inpatient medicine: results of a survey of the national association of inpatient physicians. Ann Intern Med 1999;130:343–9.

[25] Halasyamani LK, Valenstein PN, Friedlander MP, et al. A comparison of two hospitalist models with traditional care in a community teaching hospital. Am J Med 2005;118:536–43.

[26] Bellet PS, Whitaker RC. Evaluation of Pediatric Hospitalist Service: impact on length of stay and hospital charges. Pediatrics 2000;105:478–84.

[27] Dwight P, MacArthur C, Friedman JN, et al. Evaluation of staff only hospitalist system in a tertiary care children's hospital. Pediatrics 2004;114:1545–9.

[28] Auerbach AD, Aronson MD, Davis RB, et al. How physicians perceive hospitalist services after implementation: anticipation vs. reality. Arch Intern Med 2003;163:2330–6.

[29] Exline JL, Topping S, Baxter C. CEO's perceptions of hospitalists: diffusion of the strategy. Hosp Top 2004;82:18–24.

[30] Srivastava R, Norlin C, James BC, et al. Community and hospital-based physician's attitudes regarding pediatric hospitalist systems. Pediatrics 2005;115:34–8.

[31] Tenner PA, Dibrell H, Taylor RP. Improved survival with hospitalists in a pediatric intensive care unit. Crit Care Med 2003;31:847–52.

[32] Jones PE. Physician assistant education in the United States. Acad Med 2007;82:882–7.

[33] DeNicola L, Kleid D, Brink L, et al. Use of physician extenders in pediatric and neonatal intensive care units. Crit Care Med 1994;22:1856–64.

[34] The American journal of nurse practitioners: state by state listings for 2007. Available at: http://www.webnp.net/ajnp.html. Accessed February 13, 2007.

[35] Buppert C. What is a nurse practitioner? In: Nurse practitioner's business practice and legal guide. 2nd edition. Boston: Jones & Bartlett; 2004. p. 6–7.

[36] Lott JW, Polak JD, Kenyon TB, et al. Acute care nurse practitioner. In: Hamric AB, Spross JA, Hanson CM, editors. Advanced nursing practice. Philadelphia: WB Saunders; 1996. p. 351–73.

[37] Williams CA, Valdivieso GC. Advanced practice models: a comparison of clinical nurse specialist and nurse practitioner activities. Clin Nurse Spec 1994;8:311–8.

[38] SK&A Healthcare Information Solutions. Available at: http://www.SKAinfo.com. Accessed February 13, 2007.

[39] Available at: http://www.sccm.org/specialties/physician_assistants/index.asp. Accessed February 13, 2007.

[40] Slovis TL, Comerci GD. The neonatal nurse practitioner. Am J Dis Child 1974;128:310–4.

[41] Barnett SI, Sellers P. Neonatal critical care nurse practitioners: a new role in neonatology. MCN Am J Matern Child Nurs 1979;4:279–86.

[42] Shultz JM, Liptak GS, Fioravanti J. Nurse practitioners' effectiveness in NICU. Nurs Manag 1994;10:50–3.

[43] Mitchell-DiCenso A, Guyatt G, Marrin M, et al. A controlled trial of nurse practitioners in neonatal intensive care. Pediatrics 1996;98:1143–8.

[44] Schulman M, Lucchese KR, Sullivan AC. Transition from housestaff to nonphysicians as neonatal intensive care providers: cost, impact on revenue and quality of care. Am J Perinatol 1995;12:442–6.

[45] Karlowicz MG, McMurray JL. Comparison of neonatal nurse practitioners and pediatric residents' care of extremely low-birth-weight infants. Arch Pediatr Adolesc Med 2000;154: 1123–6.

[46] Bissinger RL, Allred CA, Arford PH, et al. A cost effectiveness analysis of neonatal nurse practitioners. Nurs Econ 1997;15:92–9.
[47] Aubrey WR, Yoxall CW. Evaluation of the role of the neonatal nurse practitioner in resuscitation of preterm infants at birth. Arch Dis Child Fetal Neonatal Ed 2001;85:F96–9.
[48] Hall D, Wilkinson AR. Quality of care by neonatal nurse practitioners: a review of the Ashington experiment. Arch Dis Child Fetal Neonatal Ed 2005;90:F195–200.
[49] Keane A, Richmond T, Kaiser L. Critical care nurse practitioners: evolution of the advanced practice-nursing role. Am J Crit Care 1994;3:232–7.
[50] Watts RJ. The critical-care nurse practitioners curriculum at the University of Pennsylvania: update and revision. AACN Clin Issues 1997;8:116–22.
[51] Available at: http://www.allnursingschools.com/featured/acute-care-nurse-practitioner/. Accessed February 13, 2007.
[52] Rudy EB, Davidson LJ, Clochesy JM, et al. Care activities and outcomes of patients cared for by acute care nurse practitioners, physician assistants, and resident physicians: a comparison. Am J Crit Care 1998;7:267–81.
[53] Grabenkort WR, Ramsay JG. Role of physician assistants in critical care units. Chest 1992; 101:293 [letter].
[54] Dubaybo BA, Samson MK, Carlson RW. The role of physician-assistants in critical care units. Chest 1991;99:89–91.
[55] Thourani VH, Miller JI. Physician assistants in cardiothoracic surgery: a 30 year experience in a university center. Ann Thorac Surg 2006;81:195–9.
[56] Martin SA. The pediatric critical care nurse practitioner: evolution and impact. Pediatr Nurs 1999;25:505–10.
[57] Nemes J, Barnaby K, Shamberger RC. Experience with a nurse practitioner program in the surgical department of a children's hospital. J Pediatr Surg 1992;27:1038–42.
[58] Hoffman L, Tasota F, Scharfenberg C, et al. Management of patients in the intensive care unit: comparison via work sampling analysis of an acute care nurse practitioner and physicians training. Am J Crit Care 2003;12:436–43.
[59] Carzoli RP, Martines-Cruz M, Cuevas LL, et al. Comparison of neonatal nurse practitioners, physician assistants, and residents in the neonatal intensive care unit. Arch Pediatr Adolesc Med 1994;148:1271–6.
[60] Mathur M, Rampersad A, Goldman GM. Physician assistants as physician extenders in the pediatric intensive care unit setting—a 5-year experience. Pediatr Crit Care Med 2005;6: 14–9.
[61] Rosenberg DI, Moss MM, ACCM of SCCM. Guidelines and levels of care for pediatric intensive care units. Crit Care Med 2004;32:2117–27.
[62] Molitor-Kirsch S, Thompson L, Milonovich L. The changing face of critical care medicine: nurse practitioners in the pediatric intensive care unit. AACN Clin Issues 2005;16:172–7.
[63] Derengowski SL, Irving SY, Koogle PV, et al. Defining the role of the pediatric critical care nurse practitioner in a tertiary care center. Crit Care Med 2000;28:2626–30.
[64] Delametter GL. Advanced practice nursing and the role of the pediatric critical care nurse practitioner. Crit Care Nurs Q 1999;21:16–21.
[65] Verger JT, Marcoux KK, Madden MA, et al. Nurse practitioners in pediatric critical care: results of a national survey. AACN Clin Issues 2005;16:396–408.
[66] Roberts KB. A hospitalist movement? Where to? Pediatrics 1999;103:497.
[67] Sox HC. The hospitalist model: perspective of the patient, the internist and internal medicine. Ann Intern Med 1999;130:368–72.
[68] Colle RC. Hospitalists redefine the future of inpatient medicine. Cost Qual 2000;6:8–11.
[69] Williams MV. The future of hospital medicine: evolution or revolution? Am J Med 2004;117: 446–50.

PEDIATRIC CLINICS

OF NORTH AMERICA

ELSEVIER
SAUNDERS

Pediatr Clin N Am 55 (2008) 709–733

Ventilation Strategies and Adjunctive Therapy in Severe Lung Disease

Niranjan Kissoon, MD[a],*,
Peter C. Rimensberger, MD[b], Desmond Bohn, MD[c]

[a]Department of Pediatrics, University of British Columbia, Children's Hospital,
Room K4-105, 4480 Oak Street, Vancouver, BC V6H 3V4, Canada
[b]Department of Pediatrics, University Hospital of Geneva, Rue Willy–Donze 6,
Geneve 14, CH 1211 Switzerland
[c]Critical Care Medicine, Hospital for Sick Children, 555 University Avenue,
Toronto, ON M5G 1X8, Canada

Respiratory failure caused by severe lung disease is a common reason for admission to the pediatric and neonatal intensive care units (ICUs). Efforts to decrease morbidity and mortality have fueled investigations into innovative methods of ventilation, kinder gentler ventilation techniques, pharmacotherapeutic adjuncts, and extracorporeal life support modalities. This article discusses the rationale for and experience with some of these techniques.

Noninvasive ventilation

Technique

Noninvasive ventilation in the management of children has been recognized as feasible in several clinical situations [1,2]. Noninvasive positive pressure ventilation (NPPV) is defined by the interface between the patient and the ventilator. It usually refers to continuous positive airway pressure (CPAP) or bilevel positive airway pressure (BiPAP).

CPAP is delivered to the lower airways through nasal prongs, facemasks, or head boxes. In its simplest form, the positive pressure is created by putting the expiratory limb of the circuit on a column of water (bubble system) [3]. However, mechanical ventilators or other noninvasive CPAP devices are also used. CPAP improves oxygenation and reduces the work of breathing as it unloads the inspiratory muscles and also limits alveolar collapse.

---

* Corresponding author.
E-mail address: nkissoon@cw.bc.ca (N. Kissoon).

0031-3955/08/$ - see front matter © 2008 Elsevier Inc. All rights reserved.
doi:10.1016/j.pcl.2008.02.012   *pediatric.theclinics.com*

BiPAP provides an inspiratory positive pressure or CPAP and an end expiratory pressure or EPAP. BiPAP works best when there is a relatively fixed small leak and high variable gas flow to generate an assisted breath. In expiration, gas flow again must also be relatively high to ensure carbon dioxide (CO_2) clearance. Most devices "leak" at 20 L to 40 L per minute, and can generate 40 L to 80 L per minute gas flow in inspiration. Most also have a mandatory minimal EPAP of 4 centimeters of water to ensure CO_2 removal. High gas flow, while necessary, is responsible for many of the complications in using bilevel ventilation, including discomfort, drying of eyes, difficulty in humidification, and difficulty in providing supplementary oxygen. An integral component of a bilevel ventilator is a triggering system to enable spontaneous assisted ventilation.

BiPAP devices can be used in several modes. Although originally marketed as a "ventilatory assist device" capable of only CPAP or spontaneous bilevel ventilation, most devices have additional modes, such as spontaneous/timed (S/T), timed, and more recently pressure control (PC). The S/T mode provides intermittent asynchronous mandatory breaths on a background of spontaneous triggered assisted breaths. The T mode provides asynchronous mandatory breaths without the option of spontaneous triggered assisted breaths. The PC mode allows simulation of the time-cycled, pressure-limited mode of neonatal ventilators with an important difference: the "extra" breaths can be triggered and are synchronous. In the assisted spontaneous mode (pressure support), the patient triggers the required breath. All three modes can be used to "take-over" ventilation, however S/T and T are limited to a maximum of 30 breaths per minute. The maximum setting for the PC mode is currently 30 breaths per minute; however, because it is an "assist control" mode of ventilation, the patient might be capable of generating a higher respiratory rate.

Clinical experience

In a retrospective study cohort over a 5-year period, 83 of a 114 subjects (77%) were treated successfully with NPPV. Success rate was highest in patients with acute chest syndrome (100%), followed by immuno-compromised patients (92%) and those with community acquired pneumonia (87%). The success rate of NPPV was lowest in patients with acute respiratory distress syndrome (ARDS) (22%), with treatment for respiratory failure after extubation having an intermediate outcome (67%) [4].

CPAP has been used for decades for neonates with respiratory distress syndrome caused by hyaline membrane disease. It is well known to maintain functional residual capacity, decrease upper airway resistance, inflate collapsed alveoli, and promote progressive alveoli recruitment and decrease intra-pulmonary shunting. The application of CPAP via noninvasive means is relatively inexpensive and results in significant short-term survival and trend toward long-term survival in infants in a resource limited environment in South Africa [5]. A retrospective case controlled series has shown significantly less need for supplemental oxygen and a decreased incidence of bronchopulmonary dysplasia with the introduction of synchronized nasal intermittent positive pressure ventilation [6].

Noninvasive ventilation has also been used in asthma and bronchiolitis with favorable outcomes [7]. Beers and colleagues [8], in a retrospective review of 73 patients with status asthmaticus treated with BiPAP, reported that 77% of these patients showed an improvement in their respiratory rate and 88% showed an improvement in oxygen saturation and were less likely to need pediatric intensive care unit (PICU) admission. Their experience is similar to others [9]. The use of noninvasive ventilation in acute respiratory distress syndrome in children is very limited. In the study by Essouri and colleagues [4], only nine subjects with a diagnosis of ARDS were afforded noninvasive ventilation, with a success rate of only 22%. It would seem therefore that until further experience is gained, noninvasive ventilation cannot be recommended routinely in the management of ARDS in children. However, studies in adults have suggested that it may be a better option to support patients who are immuno-suppressed, as avoiding endotracheal intubation reduces the risk of ventilator associate pneumonia [10]. Noninvasive ventilation is also an effective method for reducing left ventricular afterload in patients with dilated cardiomyopathy [11].

Pressure-limited (permissive hypercapnia) ventilation

Clinical experience

The traditional approach to mechanical ventilation has always been one targeted on the objective of a normal PaO_2 and $PaCO_2$, and the accepted practice was to use tidal volumes of 10 mL/kg to 15 mL/kg to achieve this. With the increasing recognition that these volumes can injure the already damaged lung, has come the realization that ventilation with reduced tidal volume with a pressure-limited target rather than $PaCO_2$ may be a safer option. The origin of this revolutionary approach can be traced back to a landmark article by Darioli and Perret [12]. In this article, they described a series of adult patients ventilated using the volume control mode, but with tidal volumes of 8 mL/kg to 12 mL/kg, a low inspiratory flow rate, and a rate of 6 to 10 cycles per minute. They set the maximum peak inspiratory pressure (PIP) at 50 cm H_2O. If this was exceeded with the initial settings, the tidal volume was reduced further and the $PaCO_2$ allowed to rise. All patients survived. The duration of ventilation was short (less than 3 days), and this in an era where 10% to 20% mortality was the norm for ventilated patients with status asthmaticus. What was even more important was that the investigators enunciated the principle that normocarbia should not be the objective in this situation, as the measures required to achieve it are potentially harmful, if not lethal. They defined the objective to be correction of hypoxemia, while ignoring hypercarbia up to the level of 90 mm Hg.

Hickling and colleagues [13], in a series of studies, adopted a similar approach in adult patients with ARDS. In many instances this resulted in significant degrees of hypercarbia, but no attempt was made to correct this. This resulted in a substantial reduction in hospital mortality. Both of these studies have used the volume control mode with limitation of tidal volume as a method of reducing the PIP. The alternative option as a method of preventing volume distention of the injured lung is to use the pressure control mode with limitation of the PIP. It has been suggested that this may be preferable for, as well as allowing for a decelerating gas flow pattern, it guarantees that the preset PIP will not be exceeded.

Based on the accumulated experimental data from animals and human experience, a pressure limited permissive hypercapnia strategy would seem to make eminent sense. While few would argue that modest elevations of $PaCO_2$ in the range of 50 mm Hg are of little concern, levels of greater than 100 mm Hg cause great anxiety to a generation of critical care physicians trained to strict adherence to the physiologic norm. Acute elevations in CO_2 result in the rapid development of an intracellular acidosis. A rising hydrogen ion concentration produces an increase in pulmonary vascular resistance and in cerebral blood flow, which may be harmful in cerebral injury or pulmonary hypertension. Apart from this, there is little evidence that pH levels as low as 7.2 have any adverse effect on myocardial performance or tissue oxygen delivery, while hypocapnia has the opposite effects [14,15]. Indeed, experimental evidence would suggest the contrary. In animal models of ischemia, reperfusion of the lung and sepsis hypocapnia has been shown to worsen, while hypercarbia and acidosis has been shown to attenuate the injury [16–18]. In the clinical situation, as long as the kidneys are working, patients can compensate for pH levels that drop as low as 7.1 with effective renal retention of bicarbonate. There is also anecdotal evidence in the literature that in children a very high (greater than 200 mm Hg) level of $PaCO_2$ is not associated with adverse consequences, such as myocardial performance, as long as oxygenation is maintained [19].

Amato and colleagues [20], in a randomized, controlled clinical trial in adult patients with ARDS, compared a standard volume control mode with a ventilation strategy that used a low tidal volume combined with a positive end-expiratory pressure (PEEP) level set above the inflection point, with the goal of reducing the fraction of inspired oxygen (FiO_2) to less than 0.5. They were able to demonstrate an improved survival to ICU discharge in the lung protective group. However, one has to be cautious in interpreting this as the definitive study, given the fact that the tidal volumes (10 mL/kg–15 mL/kg) used in the conventional arm of this study resulted in $PaCO_2$ levels of 35 mm Hg to 38 mm Hg, which were not in keeping with current conventional practice. Three more randomized, controlled trials also failed to demonstrate a beneficial effect using tidal volume reduction in ARDS patients, but none used the aggressive lung recruitment strategies advocated by Amato [21–23].

The single most influential study in heightening awareness of the issue of ventilation-induced lung injury in ARDS was the ARDSNet randomized trial of 6 mL/kg versus 12 mL/kg tidal volume [24]. Eight hundred subjects were randomized and the results showed a relative risk reduction in mortality of 22% in the low tidal volume group. Although this is a landmark study in ARDS, it cannot be assumed that 6mL/kg tidal volume should be adopted as the standard ventilator setting for patients. In the first instance, a large number of subjects were screened for study entry but not included, and a significant number of subjects in the 12 mL/kg arm of the study actually had their tidal volumes increased following randomization, which begs the question as to whether at least part of the outcome difference was because of injurious ventilation in that group rather than a protective effect of 6 mL/kg [25]. Clearly, it would be unwise to assume that this low tidal volume represents a standard that should be adopted for all patients with ARDS [26]. Rather, the study should be interpreted as showing that high tidal volume ventilation contributes to mortality in ARDS, and that tidal volume reduction with hypercarbia is safe and may improve outcome. A second ARDSNet study, as well as two others comparing a high lung volume recruitment strategy with PEEP compared with a more conventional pressure-limited approach, have not shown a survival benefit [23,27,28]. However, it is generally accepted in pediatric practice that the ventilation strategy in patients with acute hypoxic respiratory failure (AHRF) should be to keep the PIP less than 35 cm H_2O by reducing the tidal volume, allowing the $PaCO_2$ to rise when the situation demands, and to use a sufficient level of PEEP to prevent lung collapse (Fig. 1).

High-frequency ventilation

Techniques

High-frequency ventilation is defined by a frequency that greatly exceeds the normal respiratory rate and low tidal volume (V_T), approximating anatomic deadspace. There are three major types of high-frequency ventilation:

High-frequency positive-pressure ventilation (HPPV) (rate 60–150 per minute);
High-frequency jet ventilation (HFJV) (rate 100–600 per minute); and
High-frequency oscillatory ventilation (HFOV) (rate 180–1,500 per minute or 3 Hz–25 Hz).

HPPV and HFJV promote gas exchange in a conventional way, with tidal volume greater than deadspace volume. Expiration is passive. In contrast, HFOV uses tidal volumes that are less than dead space and expiration is active.

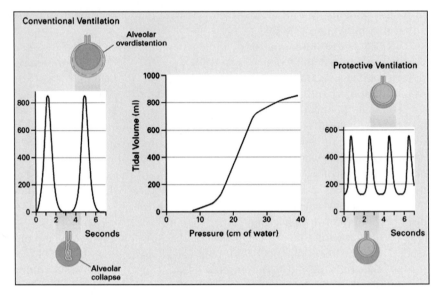

Fig. 1. Tidal volumes and pressure volume curve representing traditional and lung protective ventilation strategies in a 70-kg adult. The upper and lower inflection points on the pressure volume curve are 14 cm H_2O and 26 cm H_2O (*center graph*). The use of a traditional tidal volume of 12 mL/kg and no PEEP (*left graph*) results in alveolar over-distention when pressure exceeds the upper inflection point, and alveolar collapse at end expiration as end-expiratory lung volume falls below the lower inflection point. The pressure-limited ventilation strategy using 6 mL/kg (*right graph*) prevents over distention at the open inflection point, and PEEP 2 cm H_2O above the lower inflection point prevents alveolar collapse at end volume. (*From* Tobin MJ. Advances in mechanical ventilation. N Engl J Med 2001;344:1986–96; with permission. Copyright © 2001, Massachusetts Medical Society.)

HFJV is used mainly during (adult) laryngeal surgery; few randomized, controlled trials exist in neonates, with conflicting results [29,30]. Concerns have been raised about prolonged HFJV—not only in neonates but in adults—regarding airway damage, ranging from focal necrosis to complete airway obstruction with mucus and severe necrotizing tracheobronchitis [31,32]. Increased risk of adverse cerebral outcome [33] has been reported. Studies, however, have not used consistent criteria for assessment, and HFJV systems have varied widely. HFOV is the most commonly used method, and has become so with the good and long-lasting experience in the neonatal and PICU [34–38].

Specific characteristics of high-frequency oscillatory ventilation

HFOV can be described by the following four characteristics: (1) ventilation at a high rate of 3 Hz to 25 Hz, (2) the use of a continuous distending pressure to maintain lung volume with (3) superimposed ventilation with extremely small tidal volumes that are less than the anatomic dead space, and (4) active expiration. In other types of high-frequency ventilation (eg, high-frequency jet ventilation, high-frequency percussive ventilation, high-frequency flow interruption), expiration is mainly passive, and therefore dependent on chest wall and lung recoil, with the exception, to a certain extent, of systems that use a method to generate negative pressure swings in the system to enhance lung emptying. HFOV employs a piston or a diaphragm to oscillate a bias flow of gas (between 10 L to 40 L per minute according to patient size and demands) to produce positive and negative pressure swings (oscillation amplitude) in the circuit system in which continuous distending pressure is maintained by a low pass-filter that acts as a resistor. Operator selected parameters include mean airway pressures (ie, continuous distending pressure), frequency, inspiratory time, pressure amplitude, and oxygen concentration of inspired gas. The presence of a bias flow allows the premature infant, especially, to maintain spontaneous respiration during HFOV. In children and adults, the inspiratory flow demands from the patient cannot be matched by the bias flow system, and therefore deep sedation and sometimes muscle paralysis are required.

Basic mechanisms of gas exchange during high-frequency oscillatory ventilation

One attraction of HFOV in neonatal and pediatric use has been the way in which HFOV uncouples the regulation of oxygenation and CO_2 elimination into two separate control systems, unlike the situation with conventional ventilators where it is often difficult to adjust one (ie, CO_2 level) without also affecting the other.

Oxygenation

The strategy of improving oxygenation during HFOV and controlled mechanical ventilation (CMV) is similar. In both circumstances, it is important to maximize ventilation-perfusion matching while avoiding impairment of cardiac output (optimize oxygen delivery). During CMV, inflation breaths (ie, plateau pressure) recruit lung volume and, by using PEEP, avoid recollapse or atelectasis [39]. During HFOV, a high mean airway pressure is used to recruit alveoli and maintain lung volume relatively constant above functional residual capacity. Practically, oxygenation is regulated by first increasing airway pressures (stepping up the inflation limb of the pressure-volume curve of the respiratory system) for reversing atelectasis, and then by reducing airway pressures (sliding down the deflation limb of the pressure-volume curve) for finding the mean distending pressure that maintains alveolar expansion.

Removal of carbon dioxide

During CMV, CO_2 removal is accomplished by bulk convection and is directly related to minute ventilation, the product of tidal volume and frequency. HFOV achieves gas transport with stroke volumes that are below anatomic deadspace; therefore, gas cannot be "washed out" from the alveolar space by bulk movements. Because alveolar ventilation during HFOV is defined as $F \times V_T^2$ (where F equals frequency), changes in volume delivery (as a function of pressure-amplitude, frequency, or % inspiratory time) have the most significant affect on CO_2 elimination. Because of technical characteristics of the device, the delivered tidal volume is inversely related to frequency, with frequency controlling the time allowed (distance) for the piston to move (the lower the frequency, the greater the volume displaced, and the higher the frequency, the smaller the volume displaced). In short, HFOV is much more dependent on amplitude than on rate. Accordingly, and in the interest to use the smallest tidal volume possible, it can be recommended for neonatal, pediatric, and even adult patients to use the maximum pressure-amplitude coupled with the highest tolerated frequency [40].

Pathophysiologic rationale

Recruitment of nonaerated tissue, prevention of lung unit recollapse, and the avoidance of overdistention have become the three cornerstones of these concepts of lung protection [41,42]. This can be best achieved by a minimal stress open lung strategy, such as small tidal volumes and high PEEP levels, that should be high enough to prevent recollapse of recruited lung units [39,42]. However, small tidal volume ventilation may cause complications resulting from the effects of acute respiratory acidosis on hemodynamics, gas exchange, and oxygen transport or consumption [43] that require an increased use of sedatives and often muscle relaxants, and may lead to alveolar instability and lung collapse [44]. Within the context of ventilator-induced lung injury and lung protective strategies, high frequency ventilation could be considered to be the optimal protective ventilator mode, providing by design small tidal volume ventilation (even extremely small) and allowing for lung recruitment and the maintenance of optimal lung volume without concomitant lung overdistention. Side effects, such as the acute respiratory acidosis during conventional ventilation, are not associated with its use.

Clinical experience

Although data suggest significant benefits in pulmonary outcomes when HFOV is applied with a recruitment strategy in preterm infants with respiratory distress syndrome, when compared with classical conventional ventilation, it is still not clear whether HFOV is really superior in terms of overall outcome in this population [45], as careful conventional ventilation may allow investigators to achieve similar outcome data. Two large multicenter trials [37,38] that emphasized alveolar recruitment as part of the strategy for high frequency ventilation—one, a United States trial [38] also using a strategy in the conventional ventilation arm that targeted a tidal volume of 5 mL/kg to 6 mL/kg of body weight—were recently published in an effort to clarify the role of high-frequency ventilation for lung protection in the management of respiratory distress syndrome in preterm infants. The latter study [38] showed a clear but statistically nonsignificant reduction in days on the ventilator (13 days in the HFOV group versus 21 days in the CMV group) and a significant decrease in the need for supplemental oxygen at 36 weeks of gestational age for the HFOV arm. The other trial, the UK Oscillation Study [37], not as vigorously controlling ventilator protocols, could show no difference in outcome between the two study arms.

Use of HFOV in the pediatric population with diffuse alveolar disease or ARDS has been shown to be safe in improving physiologic short-term endpoints, but has not been associated with significant improvements in clinically important outcome measures [35,36].

Indications and timing

HFOV is most beneficial when initiated early, before major lung injury has developed [34,46]. When transitioning the patient to HFOV from CMV, the airway pressure (P_{aw}) is typically set 4 cm H_2O to 5 cm H_2O above the P_{aw} last used on the conventional ventilator to match previous oxygenation; amplitude is set by adjusting the pressure swings amplitude to observe visible chest wall vibrations. The adequacy of the chosen pressure amplitude has to be controlled rapidly by a Pco_2 measurement (eventually by transcutaneous measurements), especially in the preterm infant, to avoid as much as possible hypocarbia that is undesirable because of increasing the risk of cerebral adverse outcome [40]. In actual clinical application, frequencies are mainly adjusted according to the age of the patient (Fig. 2), although this might not be the best approach, at least on theoretic grounds—the best choice being to use the maximum amplitude coupled with the highest frequency affordable to achieve acceptable CO_2 values [47,48].

In applying an open lung strategy, P_{aw} is gradually increased by steps of 1 cm H_2O to 2 cm H_2O, with the goal of reducing the FiO_2 to less than or equal to 0.6 while achieving adequate oxygen saturation (SaO_2) values (greater than or equal to 90%, and greater than or equal to 85% in the premature infant). During this phase, hemodynamics should be carefully monitored, and at the occurrence of a minimal decrease of blood pressures (ie, more than 2 mm Hg in the preterm infant), airway pressures have to be reduced and the oxygen response conserved before eventually further increasing airway pressures again. Once appropriate saturation is achieved and FiO_2 could be lowered to less than or equal to 0.6, airway pressure should be reduced stepwise in increments of 1 cm H_2O to 2 cm H_2O (moving downward on the deflation limb of the pressure/volume curve that exhibits hysteresis) [39,49] as long as SaO_2 can be maintained, the ultimate goal being to find the lowest pressure allowable to maintain "good" saturation. Chest radiography is recommended after finding the optimal P_{aw} to ensure adequacy of lung

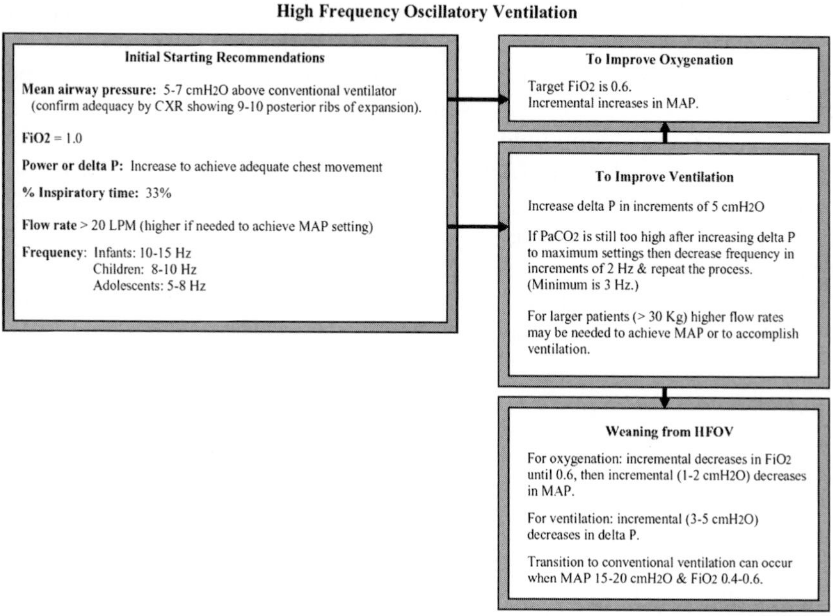

High Frequency Oscillatory Ventilation

Initial Starting Recommendations

Mean airway pressure: 5-7 cmH2O above conventional ventilator (confirm adequacy by CXR showing 9-10 posterior ribs of expansion).

FiO2 = 1.0

Power or delta P: Increase to achieve adequate chest movement

% Inspiratory time: 33%

Flow rate > 20 LPM (higher if needed to achieve MAP setting)

Frequency: Infants: 10-15 Hz
            Children: 8-10 Hz
            Adolescents: 5-8 Hz

To Improve Oxygenation

Target FiO2 is 0.6.
Incremental increases in MAP.

To Improve Ventilation

Increase delta P in increments of 5 cmH2O

If PaCO2 is still too high after increasing delta P to maximum settings then decrease frequency in increments of 2 Hz & repeat the process. (Minimum is 3 Hz.)

For larger patients (> 30 Kg) higher flow rates may be needed to achieve MAP or to accomplish ventilation.

Weaning from HFOV

For oxygenation: incremental decreases in FiO2 until 0.6, then incremental (1-2 cmH2O) decreases in MAP.

For ventilation: incremental (3-5 cmH2O) decreases in delta P.

Transition to conventional ventilation can occur when MAP 15-20 cmH2O & FiO2 0.4-0.6.

Fig. 2. Recommendations for instituting high-frequency oscillation and transition to conventional ventilation. (*Courtesy of* Martha Curley, RN, PhD, Boston, MA.)

recruitment and to exclude signs of overinflation. Both hemidiaphragms should be displaced to the level of the eighth to ninth rib, although this lacks any scientific evidence. If signs of overinflation are present, airway pressures have to be reduced further.

Classical indications for HFOV in the neonatal population are respiratory distress syndrome, congenital diaphragmatic hernia usually associated with alveolar and pulmonary vascular hypoplasia [50], air leak syndrome such as pneumothoraces or interstitial emphysema, and persistent pulmonary hypertension of the newborn. Classical indications for HFOV in the pediatric population include diffuse alveolar disease (eg, primary or secondary ARDS) [51], with growing experiences of lower airway disease, at least when conventional ventilation fails (bronchiolitis, status asthmaticus, and acute chest syndrome) [52–54]. High-frequency ventilation has become a valuable alternative to conventional ventilation in acute lung injury and largely proven to be safe in neonates, children, and adult patients. Within the context of ventilator-induced lung injury and lung protective strategies, high-frequency ventilation can be considered to be the optimal protective ventilator mode, providing by design small tidal volume ventilation, allowing for lung recruitment and the maintenance of optimal lung volume without concomitant lung overdistention. It should be considered at least as an early rescue ventilatory therapy.

Nitric oxide

Physiologic rationale

The only United States Food and Drug Administration approved indication for inhaled nitric oxide presently is to improve oxygenation in term neonates with hypoxic respiratory failure associated with pulmonary hypertension. Despite this, nitric oxide has been used in other situations. The importance of nitric oxide in the management of acute respiratory failure lies in it being a selective pulmonary vasodilator and in its ability to be delivered directly to the pulmonary circulation without discernable systemic adverse effects. These actions render nitric oxide very attractive for treatment of acute respiratory distress syndrome because ventilation–perfusion mismatch, intrapulmonary right to left shunt, pulmonary hypertension, and hypoxemia are important components of ARDS [55].

Clinical experience

Many reports have been published in pediatric and adult patients treated with inhaled nitric oxide for ARDS [56–59]. In general, about 75% of children and adults with ARDS respond to inhaled nitric oxide, with a 20% improvement in oxygenation and a 10% to 15% reduction in pulmonary artery pressure. However, despite these improvements in oxygenation, randomized, controlled trials in adults and children with ARDS have found no effect on mortality or duration of mechanical ventilation.

Two recent reports in preterm infants offer some hope that the use of inhaled nitric oxide in preterm infants may lead to pulmonary benefit, perhaps through mechanisms independent of pulmonary vasodilatation. Kinsella and colleagues [60] randomly assigned preterm neonates who were less than 48 hours of age and receiving mechanical ventilation to receive inhaled nitric oxide, and found that inhaled nitric oxide reduced mortality and bronchopulmonary dysplasia in infants with a birth weight of 1,000 g to 1,250 g. In contrast, Ballard and colleagues [61] enrolled infants who were ventilator dependent at 7 to 21 days of age, all receiving continuous positive airway pressure to a 24-day course of inhaled nitric oxide at decreasing doses. These investigators found nitric oxide treatment improved survival at 36 weeks gestational age after menstrual age without pulmonary dysplasia in infants who were 7 to 14 days of age at randomization. Studies in newborns with hypoxic respiratory failure, who are extracorporeal membrane oxygenation (ECMO) candidates, have shown positive outcomes with the use of inhaled nitric oxide in several trials [62–65]. In fact, during mechanical ventilation inhaled nitric oxide (up to 50 parts per million) was shown to significantly reduce pulmonary shunt fraction. However, the improvement may be limited by both high and low mean airway pressure [66].

Methods of delivery

Inhaled nitric oxide can be delivered effectively during HFJV [67], during CMV [68], and also during HFOV [69]. However, in all cases the inhaled nitric oxide should be connected with the inspiratory limb of the breathing circuit as proximally as possibly to minimize contact of nitric oxide administered with oxygen and achieve maximal nitric oxide and minimal nitrogen dioxide concentration during inspiration [70]. Another recent development has been the situation that administration of nitric oxide can be more effectively delivered to well-ventilated lung regions using the pulse method [71]. It is important to monitor the concentration of nitric oxide as close as possible to the patient, regardless of the method of delivery or the concentration used.

Nitric oxide has been successfully delivered using HFJV, initially at a concentration of 20 parts per million. During high-frequency ventilation, the nitric oxide source can be connected to the secondary flow circuit immediately after the humidifier. With this method, nitric oxide delivered to the secondary flow mixes in the patient module with the oxygen mixture from the primary flow and the final gas is then delivered to the endotracheal tube. In this system, because the system is open and contains no valves, only a portion of the nitric oxide mixture is entrained into the endotracheal tube, while a significant portion bypasses the patient module through the expiratory limb. The concentration can be measured in the endotracheal tube using a catheter placed in the endotracheal tube and connected to a nitric oxide analyzer [72].

Adverse effects

Once nitric oxide enters the circulation, it quickly combines with hemoglobin and forms methemoglobin, thus making it a selective pulmonary vasodilator with minimal or no systemic side effects. Methemoglobin reductase within erythrocytes converts methemoglobin to hemoglobin. The incidence of methemoglobinemia is low when inhaled nitric oxide is administered within the accepted dose range of less than 40 parts per million. Normal methemoglobin concentration is less than 2% and levels less than 5% do not require treatment. If levels are gradually increasing, a lower but still effective inhaled nitric oxide dose may be used. At higher levels, inhaled nitric oxide should be discontinued and methylene blue should be infused. Milrinone has been used to alleviate rebound pulmonary hypertension on discontinuation of inhaled nitric oxide [73]. In the presence of oxygen, inhaled nitric oxide is rapidly oxygenized to nitrogen dioxide. To minimize this effect, both the concentration of oxygen and nitric oxide should be kept to its lowest amount. Inhaled nitric oxide has also been reported to cause coagulation related abnormalities, which may lead to bleeding if it is used before extracorporeal membrane oxygenation [74]. However, in general inhaled nitric oxide administration is safe.

Assessment of medical personnel exposure
to toxic nitrogen oxide metabolites

The Occupational Health and Safety Administration (OHSA) has established legal permissible exposure limits for nitric oxide (NO) and nitrogen dioxide (NO_2) [75]. The OSHA limit for NO is 25-ppm average throughout an 8-hour work shift. This limit is chosen because it is believed to offer adequate protection against the risk of methemoglobinemia [76]. In addition, because of the acute irritant properties of NO_2, OHSA established a ceiling limit of 5 ppm for NO_2, which should not be exceeded at any time during the work shift. The National Institute of Occupational Safety and Health recommends that the average NO_2 exposure throughout any 15-minute period should not exceed 1 ppm [76].

In a study assessing the potential exposures of medical personnel to nitric oxide during simulated and actual inhaled nitric oxide treatment of neonatal and pediatric patients, detectable exposures to NO and NO_2 were infrequent and well below permissible exposure limits for OHSA and other exposure guidelines [77]. A total of 28 bedside nurses and 18 respiratory therapists were monitored during six different patient treatments. The highest measured concentration of NO and NO_2 in the personal breathing zones were peak readings of 6.7 ppm of NO and 3.1 ppm of NO_2. Exposure averages throughout 15 periods and throughout the work shift were below the limit of detection (0.8-ppm NO and 0.5-ppm NO_2) [77]. It should be noted, however, that this study was conducted with a single inhaled nitric oxide ventilator delivery system operating in the patient rooms. Exposure levels could be affected by changes in the NO treatment protocol, delivery method, and by the characteristics of the treatment room. Providing adequate ventilation in the NO treatment room and ensuring free circulation of the air around release points can control exposures. If necessary, treatment gas vented from the NO delivery system or the ventilator circuit could be scavenged by suction or by passing it through a chemical solvent trap for toxic NO gas. However, in most instances this does not seem to be necessary.

Heliox

Physiologic rationale

Heliox is an inert gas with a very low atomic weight (6 g/mol and density of 0.18g/liter). Its low density allows it to pass through narrowed passages with less turbulence than nitrogen or oxygen, and for many years helium oxygen mixtures (heliox) have been used for patients with severe airway obstruction. Because helium is nontoxic and biologically inert it can be safely mixed with oxygen. In general, helium is available in mixtures of 80% helium and 20% oxygen (80/20 heliox) or 70% helium and 30% oxygen (70/30 heliox). Heliox decreases turbulent gas flow because the rate of turbulent gas flow is proportionate to the density of the gas. Advantages of heliox are improved delivery of aerosolized medications and ease of breathing, and it may facilitate weaning from mechanical ventilation [78].

Administration and delivery systems

Currently available nebulizers are designed to be powered by nitrogen/oxygen mixtures. By using heliox and reducing the density of the gas, heliox may decrease the fraction of the total dose and the respirable mass of the drug, compared with powering the nebulizer with air [79]. In a pediatric model of mechanical ventilation, heliox was noted to provide a better deposition of albuterol from a metered dose inhaler [80], and lung deposition of a significantly higher dose of albuterol when compared with a nitrogen/oxygen mixture [81]. Incorrect adaptations of ventilator equipment to deliver heliox pose a problem because tidal volumes may be unpredictably altered by heliox [79]. Because flow-through valves, regulators and tubing, and flow differences are difficult to predict [82], some of the physiologic changes attributed to heliox may in fact be because of unrecognized changes in ventilator flow and tidal volume delivery [83].

The initiation of heliox therapy does not require any additional equipment beyond the standard equipment in most respiratory departments once the specialty-mix gas cylinders of heliox are available. If a patient requires supplemental oxygen because of hypoxemia, this limits the heliox concentration that can be administered. Standard concentrations are usually 80/20 heliox, though it is also available in 70/30 and 60/40 mixtures. It has been suggested that a patient needing an oxygen concentration greater than 40% achieves limited benefit from heliox, because the limited amount of helium in 60/40 heliox causes more turbulent flow and higher gas density through the airways [84].

In most cases, clinicians have modified circuits to apply the heliox gas mixture because the low density of helium causes inaccurately high readings from flow meters for air or oxygen. However, if regular oxygen flow meters are used based on the density of the helium, a correction factor can be used to determine the liter flow. This is as follows:

- For the 80/20 mixture (1.8 times the liter flow);
- For the 70/30 mixture (1.6 times the liter flow); and
- For the 60/40 mixture (1.4 times the liter flow).

The delivery of the heliox during mechanical ventilation has its challenges. Certain ventilators perform relatively well with heliox and are not substantially affected by it; however, others are. Understanding the effects of heliox on ventilator performance requires vigilance and continuous monitoring because helium can interfere with ventilator function and the accuracy of the pneumotachometer. In addition, understanding the principles of valve design and gas flow of the individual ventilators is useful. Several studies have examined the effects of heliox and ventilator performance [85–89].

Important considerations during the delivery of heliox is to ensure consistency of inspired oxygen delivered as well as tidal volumes. Regardless of the ventilator used, to ensure consistent delivery of FiO_2, supplemental oxygen values must be measured close to the patient by devices that are density independent. To ensure consistent tidal volume delivery, one can use the conversion factor for each ventilator as suggested by Tassaux and colleagues [86], and estimate the delivered tidal volume from the set tidal volume or the eschaled tidal volume. Alternatively, one can measure the tidal volume directly at the endotracheal tube, using a density independent pneumothachometer or one that is calibrated for helium.

For spontaneously breathing patients, heliox is most efficiently delivered with a closed system that eliminates leaks and air entrapment. Administration through a snuggly fitting nonrebreather facemask reduces the chance of room air contamination. Typically, clinical set up for heliox administration to a spontaneously breathing patient can be achieved using a facemask and reservoir bag or a nonrebreather system. A Y-piece attachment can be placed between the mask and the reservoir bag to add a nebulizer for concurrent beta-agonist administration [89]. This type of delivery system needs to be continuously supplying a flow of 12 L to 15 L per minute to maintain reservoir bag inflation, and will require a 2 H to 5 H size cylinder (1,200 L of gas at approximately 2,200 pounds per square inch) per day.

It is well recognized that traditional methods of oxygen delivery to children, including nasal cannula, oxygen hood, oxygen tents, and other mask types may entrain quantities of room air and hence may not be very effective in delivering heliox mixtures. However, there are methods to circumvent room air entrainment. For instance, heliox delivery was greater when a nonrebreathing mask and a simple mask were used, as compared with nasal cannula [89]. In a laboratory bench study of heliox delivered via a hood, concentrations were noted to vary: concentrations were higher at the top of the hood, well above the patients mouth and nares, implying that oxyhood method of delivery may be suboptimal. The bottom line is that heliox should be delivered with a closed system that prevents or at least minimizes the entrapment of room air, ensuring that a fraction of inhaled helium is greater than 50%. There are different methods to achieve this goal. However, the standardization of the equipment is often difficult to accomplish.

Clinical experience

A small retrospective review of 28 pediatric subjects who were mechanically ventilated with heliox for an asthma exacerbation revealed that heliox decreased peak inspiratory pressure and $PaCO_2$ and increased pH (the heliox concentration ranged from 32% to 74% and the patients served as their own control) [90]. In an uncontrolled case series of 10 infants with bronchiolitis (age ranging from 1 to 9 months), who were mechanically ventilated with varying concentrations of heliox and nitrogen-oxygen mixtures, the investigators found that heliox mixtures did not result in a significant or no-ticeable improvement in ventilation and oxygenation [91]. In case reports and case series, heliox has been delivered by various nonconventional tech-niques, including high-frequency oscillatory ventilation [92], high frequency jet ventilation [93], and high frequency percussive ventilation [94] in different pulmonary pathologies. Using high frequency jet ventilation in a series of five children with acute respiratory distress syndrome, heliox administration resulted in a decrease in $PaCO_2$ by 24% within 45 minutes of initiating he-liox [92]. Insufficient experience exists to recommend heliox in patients with severe lung disease.

Extracorporeal membrane oxygenation

The first successful use of a membrane oxygenator to support a patient with acute hypoxic respiratory failure was published in 1972 [95]. Following the publication of further anecdotal reports [96], a National Institutes of Health sponsored randomized trial was set up in 1975 to compare ECMO in ARDS with what was then standard-of-care positive pressure ventilation [97]. The disappointing survival of 10% in both arms of this study led to ECMO being largely abandoned as a treatment for AHRF in adults in North America. Bartlett and colleagues [98] then pioneered the use of ECMO in neonatal respiratory failure and published the first case series of 45 subjects from the University of Michigan in 1982 with a 50% survival. Since then, over 20,000 neonates have been treated with an overall survival of 80% [99]. Beginning in the late 1980s, an increasing number of pediatric patients greater than 28 days with AHRF unresponsive to conventional treatments have had ECMO used as a rescue therapy. The most recent Ex-tracorporeal Life Support Organization (ELSO) Registry reports show data on over 3,000 patients where ECMO was used for respiratory support, with an overall survival of 60% [99].

Indications and contraindications

Indications for the initiation of ECMO support for AHRF in neonates have been defined based on the use of the Oxygenation Index (OI), which incorporates the PaO_2, FiO_2, and a measure of the intensity of ventilation (MAP or mean airway pressure). Thus, $OI = MAP \times FiO_2 \times 100/PaO_2$. Ne-onates whose OI exceeds 40 are predicted to have a greater than 80% mor-tality, and this number has been used to enter patients in a number of prospective trials of alternative therapies in AHRF. The situation is less clear in older children, particularly those with ARDS, which frequently in-volves other organ systems apart from the lungs. However, recent studies have shown that there is a relationship between both OI, as well as the PaO_2/FiO_2 ratio, and outcome in older children with AHRF [100,101]. In a multi-institutional retrospective cohort analysis of over 300 patients with AHRF from 32 centers over a 1-year period, the use of ECMO was associated with reduced mortality in the group of patients with the highest OI, compared with those who received conventional or high frequency ventilation [102]. Despite this, the most common indication to initiate ECMO support in older children is failure to adequately oxygenate following a trial of conventional and alternate therapies, in the absence of clear contraindications. These contraindications include greater than 10 days of positive pressure ventilation, an irreversible underlying disease process, and major central nervous system abnormalities. In the past, immuno-suppressed patients with underlying malignancies were excluded, but this is also being rethought.

Pump flow, ventilator settings, anticoagulation, and fluid management

ECMO pump flows for supporting pediatric patients with AHRF are set to deliver 80 mL/kg to 100 mL/kg per minute depending on patient size, sufficient to keep the venous oxygen saturation at 70% to 75% on veno-arterial bypass or on SaO_2 of 90% on veno-venous. The hematocrit is maintained to 40% to 45%, to maximize oxygen delivery. The sweep gas flow is adjusted to achieve a $PaCO_2$ of 40 mm Hg to 45 mm Hg. The key objective of ECMO is to provide lung rest by removing the ongoing injury from positive pressure and oxygen on the lung. The peak inspiratory pressure on ventilator should be reduced to 25 cm H_2O to 30 cm H_2O and the rate to 5 to 10 breaths per minute. PEEP at a level of 5 cm H_2O to 10 cm H_2O is added in an attempt to prevent further derecruitment. Patients may also be turned into the prone position [103].

Maintaining adequate anticoagulation in patients on ECMO is a fine balance between preventing thrombus developing in the circuit and not causing bleeding, especially in the central nervous system. Heparin is infused at a rate of 20 units/kg to 50 units/kg per hour, with the objective of maintaining the activated clotting time at 180 to 200 seconds. In the event of bleeding, the activated clotting time target can be reduced to 160 to 180 seconds. Platelets are infused to maintain the count above 100,000/mm [97]. Monitoring of fibrinogen and D-dimers are also routinely performed. Both aminocaproic acid and activated factor VIIa have been used to treat hemorrhage in ECMO patients [104,105].

The management of fluid balance has been shown to affect the outcome in ECMO patients. Failure to return the patient to dry weight has been associated with nonsurvival in a large series of ECMO support for pediatric AHRF from the University of Michigan [106]. Therefore, diuresis should be maintained with a furosemide infusion or, if that fails, hemofiltration. At the same time, it is important that patients receive nutritional support to prevent protein breakdown, negative nitrogen balance, and tissue edema. Enteral feeding is the preferred route to prevent bacterial translocation from the gut [107].

Weaning and decannulation

Following the initiation of ECMO, the systemic inflammatory response associated with the exposure of blood to the oxygenator and circuit results in diffuse capillary leak and worsening edema of the injured lung. There is a further reduction in pulmonary compliance and opacification of the chest X-ray. Signs of improvement in lung function indicating that an attempt at weaning from ECMO may be feasible include the onset of diuresis, an increase in lung compliance, and clearing of the chest X-ray. In pediatric AHRF this rarely occurs within the first week of support [106]. Once pulmonary function improves, the weaning process can commence. For patients on veno-arterial support, flows are reduced while positive pressure is increased. The final test is to clamp the cannulas and circulate through the bridge while the patient is on full ventilation. Cannulas must be unclamped and flushed at regular intervals. For patients on veno-venous bypass, the lung can be tested by switching off the sweep gas while fully ventilating the patient. ECMO can be discontinued and the patient decannulated if an SaO_2 greater than 90% can be maintained on an FiO_2 less than or equal to 0.6 and a PEEP less than or equal to 10 cm H_2O.

Complications

With a highly invasive complex technology such as ECMO, complications can be expected. These can be divided into patient and device related (Tables 1 and 2).

Outcome in extracorporeal membrane oxygenation
support for acute hypoxic respiratory failure

The survival of pediatric patients with AHRF placed on ECMO support reported to the ELSO registry as of the end of 2006 is 55% in 3,500 patients. The average duration of support was 10 days, with occasional very

Table 1
Principal technical (device) complications

Complication	Comments
Oxygenator failure	It is unusual for an oxygenator to fail completely, but they do lose efficiency over time
Pump tubing (raceway) rupture	Only occurs in the roller pump system
Cannula malposition	More common with the venous cannula; leads to high negative pressures and inadequate flows
Clots in circuit	May occur in oxygenator, bridge, bladder of hemofilter
Air embolism	Can occur if there are cracks in the tube or through stopcocks
Pump failure	A rare event; pumps have a battery back up system which can also be used for transport
Hemolysis	Formerly a significant problem with the centrifugal pump system

Table 2
Principal patient complications

Complication	Comments
Seizures and other central nervous system complications	May be caused by intracerebral hemorrhage or infarction; commonly manifested by the onset of seizures
Systemic hypertension	May be predisposing factor to above
Renal dysfunction and fluid overload	The development of renal failure or the inability to maintain patient within 10% of dry weight has been negatively correlated with outcome [106]
Culture proven infection	Can be seen in up to 20% of patients [99]
Hepatic failure and hyperbilirubinemia	Hepatic failure developing on ECMO is associated with poor outcome [106]
Failure to separate from ECMO	Failure of lung recovery or major neurologic damage are the most common reasons

prolonged runs of up to 3 months. The underlying disease process has an impact on outcome, with the highest survival in patients with viral pneumonia in the ELSO registry. Within this category, recent series of formerly premature infants with respiratory syncytial virus showed an 80% survival to hospital discharge, but with a 60% neurodisability rate [108]. Good outcomes have been reported in small case series for pulmonary hemorrhage [109,110], burns and smoke inhalation [111,112], and post traumatic lung injury [113]. Two disease categories remain particularly challenging. AHRF secondary to pertussis that presents in the first 3 months of life is associated with a particularly severe form of pulmonary hypertension, which does not resolve. The mortality in these patients, even with ECMO support, is 80% [114,115]. The second group consists of those patients with hematologic malignancies. Data from the ELSO registry on patients placed on ECMO following bone marrow transplantation published up to 2006 showed only one survivor to hospital discharge in 19 patients [116]. For children with immuno-suppression and pneumocystis pneumonia, the outcomes are substantially better with 75% of children surviving in one small case series [117].

Summary

A better understanding of respiratory physiology in severe lung disease have spurred investigations into a various techniques and therapies to decrease morbidity and mortality. No single approach is appropriate for all patients; hence, therapies and techniques used should be tailored depending on the individual patient, resources available, and the experience of the treating team.

References

[1] Millar D, Kirpalani H. Benefits of noninvasive ventilation. Indian Pediatr 2004;41: 1008–17.

[2] Elliott MW, Ambrosino N. Noninvasive ventilation in children. Eur Respir J 2002;20: 1332–42.

[3] Morley CJ, Lau R, De Paoli A, et al. Nasal continuous positive airway pressure: does bubbling improve gas exchange. Arch Dis Child Fetal Neonatal Ed 2005;90:343–4.

[4] Essouri S, Chevret L, Durand P, et al. Noninvasive positive pressure ventilation: five years of experience in a pediatric intensive care unit. Pediatr Crit Care Med 2006;7:329–34.

[5] Pieper CH, Smith J, Maree D, et al. Is CPAP of value in extreme preterms with no access to neonatal intensive care? J Trop Pediatr 2003;49:148–52.

[6] Kulkarni A, Ehrenkranz RA, Bhandari V. Effect of introduction of synchronized nasal intermittent positive pressure ventilation in a neonatal intensive care unit on bronchopulmonary dysplasia and growth in preterm infants. Am J Perinatol 2006;23:233–40.

[7] Larrar S, Essouri S, Durand P, et al. The effects of nasal continuous positive airway pressure ventilation in infants with severe acute bronchiolitis. Arch Pediatr 2006;13: 1397–403.

[8] Beers SL, Abramo TJ, Bracken A, et al. Bi-level positive airway pressure in the treatment of status asthmaticus in pediatrics. Am J Emerg Med 2007;25(1):6–9.

[9] Thill PJ, Macguire JK, Baden HP, et al. Noninvasive positive pressure ventilation in children with low airway obstruction. Pediatr Crit Care Med 2004;5:337–42.

[10] Hilbert G, Gruson D, Vargas F, et al. Noninvasive ventilation in immuno-suppressed patients with pulmonary infiltrates, fever, and acute respiratory failure. N Engl J Med 2001; 344:481–7.

[11] Mehta S, Nava S. Mask ventilation and cardiogenic pulmonary edema: "another brick in the wall". Intensive Care Med 2005;31:757–9.

[12] Darioli R, Perret C. Mechanical controlled hypoventilation in status asthmaticus. Am Rev Respir Dis 1984;129(3):385–7.

[13] Hickling KG, Henderson SJ, Jackson R. Low mortality associated with volume pressure limited ventilation with permissive hypercapnia in severe adult respiratory distress syndrome. Intensive Care Med 1990;16:372–7.

[14] Laffey JG, Kavanagh BP. Carbon dioxide and the critically ill—too little of a good thing? Lancet 1999;354(9186):1283–6.

[15] Laffey JG, Kavanagh BP. Hypocapnia. N Engl J Med 2002;347(1):43–53.

[16] Laffey JG, Engelberts D, Duggan M, et al. Carbon dioxide attenuates pulmonary impairment resulting from hyperventilation. Crit Care Med 2003;31(11):2634–40.

[17] Laffey JG, Engelberts D, Kavanagh BP. Buffering hypercapnic acidosis worsens acute lung injury. Am J Respir Crit Care Med 2000;161(1):141–6.

[18] Laffey JG, Tanaka M, Engelberts D, et al. Therapeutic hypercapnia reduces pulmonary and systemic injury following in vivo lung reperfusion. Am J Respir Crit Care Med 2000; 162(6):2287–94.

[19] Goldstein B, Shannon DC, Todres ID. Supercarbia in children: clinical course and outcome. Crit Care Med 1990;18:166–8.

[20] Amato MBP, Barbas CSV, Medeiros DM, et al. Effect of a protective-ventilation strategy on mortality in the acute respiratory distress syndrome. N Engl J Med 1998;338(6): 347–54.

[21] Brochard L, Roudot-Thoraval F, Roupie E, et al. Tidal volume reduction for prevention of ventilator-induced lung injury in acute respiratory distress syndrome. The Multicenter Trail Group on Tidal Volume reduction in ARDS. Am J Respir Crit Care Med 1998;158(6): 1831–8.

[22] Brower RG, Shanholtz CB, Fessler HE, et al. Prospective, randomized, controlled clinical trial comparing traditional versus reduced tidal volume ventilation in acute respiratory distress syndrome patients. Crit Care Med 1999;27(8):1492–8.

[23] Stewart TE, Meade MO, Cook DJ, et al. Evaluation of a ventilation strategy to prevent barotrauma in patients at high risk for acute respiratory distress syndrome. Pressure- and Volume-Limited Ventilation Strategy Group. N Engl J Med 1998;338(6):355–61.

[24] Ventilation with lower tidal volumes as compared with traditional tidal volumes for acute lung injury and the acute respiratory distress syndrome. The Acute Respiratory Distress Syndrome Network. N Engl J Med 2000;342(18):1301–8.

[25] Eichacker PQ, Gerstenberger EP, Banks SM, et al. Meta-analysis of acute lung injury and acute respiratory distress syndrome trials testing low tidal volumes. Am J Respir Crit Care Med 2002;166(11):1510–4.

[26] Parshuram CS, Kavanagh BP. Positive clinical trials: understand the control group before implementing the result. Am J Respir Crit Care Med 2004;170(3):223–6.

[27] Brower RG, Lanken PN, MacIntyre N, et al. Higher versus lower positive end-expiratory pressures in patients with the acute respiratory distress syndrome. N Engl J Med 2004; 351(4):327–36.

[28] Mercat A, Richard JC, Brochard L. Comparison of two strategies for setting PEEP in ARDS/ALI (ExPress study). Am J Respir Crit Care Med 2007;175:A507.

[29] Carlo W, Siner B, Chatburn R, et al. Early randomized intervention with high-frequency jet ventilation in respiratory distress syndrome. J Pediatr 1990;117:765–70.

[30] Keszler M, Modanlou H, Brudno D, et al. Multicenter controlled clinical trial of high-frequency jet ventilation in preterm infants with uncomplicated respiratory distress syndrome. Pediatrics 1997;100:593–9.

[31] Kercsmar C, Martin R, Chatburn R, et al. Bronchoscopic findings in infants treated with high-frequency jet ventilation versus conventional ventilation. Pediatrics 1988;82:884–7.

[32] Delafosse C, Chevrolet J, Suter P, et al. Necrotizing tracheobronchitis: a complication of high frequency jet ventilation. Virchows Arch A Pathol Anat Histopathol 1988;413:257–64.

[33] Wiswell T, Graziani L, Kornhauser M, et al. High-frequency jet ventilation in the early management of respiratory distress syndrome is associated with a greater risk for adverse outcomes. Pediatrics 1996;98:1035–43.

[34] Rimensberger PC, Beghetti M, Hanquinet S, et al. First intention high-frequency oscillation with early lung volume optimization improves pulmonary outcome in very low birth weight infants with respiratory distress syndrome. Pediatrics 2000;105(6):1202–8.

[35] Arnold J, Anas N, Luckett P, et al. High-frequency oscillatory ventilation in pediatric respiratory failure: a multicenter experience. Crit Care Med 2000;28(12):3913–9.

[36] Moriette G, Paris-Llado J, Walti H, et al. Prospective randomized multicenter comparison of high-frequency oscillatory ventilation and conventional ventilation in preterm infants of less than 30 weeks with respiratory distress syndrome. Pediatrics 2001;107(2):363–72.

[37] Johnson AH, Peacock JL, Greenough A, et al. High-frequency oscillatory ventilation for the prevention of chronic lung disease of prematurity. N Engl J Med 2002;347(9):633–42.

[38] Courtney SE, Durand DJ, Asselin JM, et al. High-frequency oscillatory ventilation versus conventional mechanical ventilation for very-low-birth-weight infants. N Engl J Med 2002; 347:643–52.

[39] Rimensberger PC, Cox PN, Frndova H, et al. The open lung during small tidal volume ventilation: concepts of recruitment and "optimal" PEEP. Crit Care Med 1999;27: 1946–52.

[40] Mehta S, Lapinsky SE, Hallett DC, et al. Prospective trial of high-frequency oscillation in adults with acute respiratory distress syndrome. Crit Care Med 2001;29(7):1360–9.

[41] Clark RH, Slutsky AS, Gerstmann DR. Lung protective strategies of ventilation in the neonate: what are they? Pediatrics 2000;105:112–4.

[42] Gattinoni L, Vagginelli F, Chiumello D, et al. Physiologic rationale for ventilator setting in acute lung injury/acute respiratory distress syndrome patients. Crit Care Med 2003;31: S300–4.

[43] Crotti S, Mascheroni D, Caironi P, et al. Recruitment and derecruitment during acute respiratory failure. A clinical study. Am J Respir Crit Care Med 2001;164(1):131–40.

[44] Carvalho CR, Barbas CS, Medeiros DM, et al. Temporal hemodynamic effects of permissive hypercapnia associated with ideal PEEP in ARDS. Am J Respir Crit Care Med 1997; 156:1458–66.

[45] Richard JC, Maggiore SM, Jonson B, et al. Influence of tidal volume on alveolar recruitment. Respective role of PEEP and a recruitment maneuver. Am J Respir Crit Care Med 2001;163:1609–13.

[46] Bollen C, Uiterwaal C, Vught AV. Cumulative meta-analysis of high-frequency versus conventional ventilation in premature neonates. Am J Respir Crit Care Med 2003;168:1105–55.

[47] Blumenthal I. Periventricular leucomalacia: a review. Eur J Pediatr 2004;163:435–42.

[48] Giannakopoulou C, Korakaki E, Manoura A, et al. Significance of hypocarbia in the development of periventricular leukomalacia in preterm infants. Pediatr Int 2004;46:268–73.

[49] Fessler HE, Derdak S, Ferguson ND, et al. A protocol for high frequency ventilation in adults: results from a roundtable discussion. Crit Care Med 2007;35:1649–54.

[50] Bryan A, Cox P. History of high frequency oscillation. Schweiz Med Wochenschr 1999;129:1613–6.

[51] Nobuhara K, Wilson J. Pathophysiology of congenital diaphragmatic hernia. Semin Pediatr Surg 1996;5:234–42.

[52] Arnold JH, Hanson JH, Toro-Figuero LO, et al. Prospective, randomized comparison of high-frequency oscillatory ventilation and conventional mechanical ventilation in pediatric respiratory failure. Crit Care Med 1994;22(10):1530–9.

[53] Duval EL, van Vught AJ. Status asthmaticus treated by high-frequency oscillatory ventilation. Pediatr Pulmonol 2000;30:350–3.

[54] Duval EL, Leroy PL, Gemke RJ, et al. High-frequency oscillatory ventilation in RSV bronchiolitis patients. Respir Med 1999;993:435–40.

[55] Wratney AT, Gentile MA, Hamel DS, et al. Successful treatment of acute chest syndrome with high-frequency oscillatory ventilation in pediatric patients. Respir Care 2004;49:263–9.

[56] Kaisers U, Busch T, Dhea M, et al. Selective pulmonary vasodilatation in acute respiratory distress syndrome. Crit Care Med 2000;31:s337–42.

[57] Dobyns EL, Anas NG, Fortenberry HD, et al. Interactive effects of high-frequency oscillatory ventilation and inhaled nitric oxide in acute hypoxemic respiratory failure in pediatrics. Crit Care Med 2002;30:2425–9.

[58] Fioretto JR, de Moraes MA, Bonatto RC, et al. Acute and sustained effects of early administration of inhaled nitric oxide to children with acute respiratory distress syndrome. Pediatr Crit Care Med 2005;5:469–74.

[59] Baldauf M, Silver P, Sagy M. Evaluating the validity of responsiveness to inhaled nitric oxide in pediatric patients with ARDS: an analytic tool. Chest 2001;119:1166–72.

[60] Kinsella JP, Cutter GR, Walsh WF, et al. Early inhaled nitric oxide therapy in premature newborns with respiratory failure. N Engl J Med 2006;355(4):354–64.

[61] Ballard RA, Truog WE, Cnaan A, et al. Inhaled nitric oxide in preterm infants undergoing mechanical ventilation. N Engl J Med 2006;355(4):343–53.

[62] Clark RH, Kueser TJ, Walker MW, et al. Low-dose nitric oxide therapy for persistent pulmonary hypertension of the newborn. Clinical Inhaled Nitric Oxide Research Group. N Engl J Med 2002;342:469–74.

[63] Davidson D, Barefield ES, Kattwinkel J, et al. Inhaled nitric oxide for the early treatment of persistent pulmonary hypertension of the term newborn: a randomized, double masked, placebo controlled, dose response, multicenter study. The I-NO/PPHN Study Group. Pediatrics 1998;101:325–34.

[64] Roberts JD Jr, Fineman JR, Morin FC III, et al. Inhaled nitric oxide and persistent pulmonary hypertension of the newborn. The Inhaled Nitric Oxide Study Group. N Engl J Med 1997;336:605–10.

[65] The Neonatal Inhaled Nitric Oxide Study. Inhaled nitric oxide in full-term and nearly full-term infants with hypoxic respiratory failure. N Engl J Med 1997;336:597–604.

[66] Hoffman GF, Nelin L. Mean airway pressure and response to inhaled nitric oxide in neonatal and pediatric patients. Lung 2005;183:441–53.

[67] Platt DR, Swanton D, Blackney D. Inhaled nitric oxide (iNO) delivery with high-frequency jet ventilation (HFJV). J Perinatol 2003;23:387–91.

[68] Chkaidze M, Kutubidze R, Tevzadze M, et al. Variation of inspired nitric oxide and nitrogen dioxide concentrate during mechanical ventilation. Georgian Med News 2005;118:35–9.

[69] Kohelet D. Nitric oxide inhalation and high frequency oscillator ventilation in hypoxemic respiratory failure in infants. Isr Med Assoc J 2003;5:19–23.

[70] Sieffert E, Ducros L, Losser MR, et al. Inhaled nitric oxide fraction is influenced by both the site and the mode of administration. J Clin Monit Comput 1999;15:509–17.

[71] Heinonen E, Merilainen P, Hogman M. Administration of nitric oxide into open lung regions: delivery and monitoring. Br J Anaesth 2003;90:338–42.

[72] Arabi Y, Kumar A, Wood K, et al. The feasibility of nitrate oxide delivery with high frequencey jet ventilation. Respirology 2005;10:673–7.

[73] Kissoon N. Treatment of Persistent Pulmonary Hypertension of the Newborn (PPHN) is in its infancy. J Crit Care 2006;21:223.

[74] Armerick C, Arno FJ, Brouwers M, et al. Abnormalities of coagulation related to the use of inhaled nitric oxide before extracorporeal membrane oxygenation. Pediatr Crit Care Med 2007;8:261–3.

[75] Datex-Ohmedia, Inc. Nitric oxide delivery system: PPHN clinical study manual. Madison (WI): BOC Health Care Inc.; 1994.

[76] National Institute for Occupational Safety and Health. NIOSH pocket guide to chemical hazards. Washington, DC: US Government Printing Office; 1997.

[77] Venkataraman ST. Heliox during mechanical ventilation. Respir Care 2006;51(6):632–9.

[78] Phillips ML, Hall TA, Krishnamurthy S, et al. Assessment of medical personnel exposure to nitrogen oxides during inhaled nitric oxide treatment of neonatal and pediatric patients. Pediatrics 1999;104(5):1095–100.

[79] Hess DR, Acosta FL, Ritz RH, et al. The effect of heliox on nebulizer function using a β-agonist bronchodilator. Chest 1999;115(1):184–9.

[80] Habib DM, Garner SS, Brandeburg S. Effect of helium-oxygen on delivery of albuterol in a pediatric, volume-cycled, ventilated lung model. Pharmacotherapy 1999;19:143–9.

[81] Goode ML, Fink JB, Dhand R, et al. Improvement in aerosol delivery with helium-oxygen mixtures during mechanical ventilation. Am J Respir Crit Care Med 2001;164:109–14.

[82] Chatmongkolchard S, Kacmaret RM, Hess DR. Heliox delivery with noninvasive positive pressure ventilation: a laboratory study. Respir Care 2001;46:248–54.

[83] Katz AL, Gentile MA, Craig DM, et al. Heliox does not affect gas exchange during high frequency oscillatory ventilation if tidal volume is held constant. Crit Care Med 2003;31: 2006–9.

[84] Abd-Allah SA, Rogers MS, Terry M, et al. Helium-oxygen therapy for pediatric acute severe asthma requiring mechanical ventilation. Pediatr Crit Care Med 2003;4:353–7.

[85] McGee DL, Wald DA, Hinchcliffe S. Helium-oxygen therapy in the emergency department. J Emerg Med 1997;15(3):291–6.

[86] Tassaux D, Jolliet P, Thouret JM, et al. Calibration of seven ICU ventilators for mechanical ventilation with helium-oxygen mixtures. Am J Respir Crit Care Med 1999;160(1):22–32.

[87] Oppenheim-Eden A, Cohen Y, Weissman C, et al. The effect of helium on ventilator performance: study of five ventilators and a bedside Pitot tube spirometer. Chest 2001; 120(2):582–8.

[88] Berkenbosch JW, Grueber RE, Dabbagh O, et al. Effect of helium-oxygen (heliox) gas mixtures on the function of four pediatric ventilators. Crit Care Med 2003;31(7):2052–8.

[89] Brown MK, Willms DC. A laboratory evaluation of 2 mechanical ventilators in the presence of helium-oxygen mixtures. Respir Care 2005;50(3):354–60.

[90] Stillwell PC, Quick JD, Munro PR, et al. Effectiveness of open-circuit and oxyhood delivery of helium-oxygen. Chest 1989;95(6):1222–4.

[91] Gross MF, Spear RM, Peterson BM. Helium-oxygen mixture does not improve gas exchange in mechanically ventilated children with bronchiolitis. Crit Care 2000;4:188–92.

[92] Winters JW, Willing MA, Sanfilippo D. Heliox improves ventilation during high-frequency oscillatory ventilation in pediatric patients. Pediatr Crit Care Med 2000;1:33–7.

[93] Gupta VK, Grayck EN, Cheifetz IM. Heliox administration during high-frequency jet ventilation augments carbon dioxide clearance. Respir Care 2004;49:1038–44.

[94] Stucki P, Scalfaro P, de Halleux, et al. Successful management of severe respiratory failure combining heliox with noninvasive high-frequency percussive ventilation. Crit Care Med 2002;30:692–4.

[95] Hill JD, O'Brien TG, Murray JJ, et al. Prolonged extracorporeal oxygenation for acute post-traumatic respiratory failure (shock-lung syndrome). Use of the Bramson membrane lung. N Engl J Med 1972;286(12):629–34.

[96] Gille JP, Bagniewski AM. Ten years of use of extracorporeal membrane oxygenation (ECMO) in the treatment of acute respiratory insufficiency (ARI). Trans Am Soc Artif Intern Organs 1976;22:102–9.

[97] Zapol WM, Snider MT, Hill JD, et al. Extracorporeal membrane oxygenation in severe acute respiratory failure. A randomized prospective study. JAMA 1979;242:2193–6.

[98] Bartlett RH, Andrews AF, Toomasian JM, et al. Extracorporeal membrane oxygenation for newborn respiratory failure: forty-five cases. Surgery 1982;92(2):425–33.

[99] ELSO Registry. Extracorporeal Life Support Organization 2007.

[100] Flori HR, Glidden DV, Rutherford GW, et al. Pediatric acute lung injury: prospective evaluation of risk factors associated with mortality. Am J Respir Crit Care Med 2005;171(9): 995–1001.

[101] Trachsel D, McCrindle BW, Nakagawa S, et al. Oxygenation index predicts outcome in children with acute hypoxemic respiratory failure. Am J Respir Crit Care Med 2005; 172(2):206–11.

[102] Green TP, Timmons OD, Fackler JC, et al. The impact of extracorporeal membrane oxygenation on survival in pediatric patients with acute respiratory failure. Pediatric Critical Care Study Group. Crit Care Med 1996;24(2):323–9.

[103] Haefner SM, Bratton SL, Annich GM, et al. Complications of intermittent prone positioning in pediatric patients receiving extracorporeal membrane oxygenation for respiratory failure. Chest 2003;123(5):1589–94.

[104] Dominguez TE, Mitchell M, Friess SH, et al. Use of recombinant factor VIIa for refractory hemorrhage during extracorporeal membrane oxygenation. Pediatr Crit Care Med 2005; 6(3):348–51.

[105] Horwitz JR, Cofer BR, Warner BW, et al. A multicenter trial of 6-aminocaproic acid (Amicar) in the prevention of bleeding in infants on ECMO. J Pediatr Surg 1998;33(11): 1610–3.

[106] Swaniker F, Kolla S, Moler F, et al. Extracorporeal life support outcome for 128 pediatric patients with respiratory failure. J Pediatr Surg 2000;35(2):197–202.

[107] Pettignano R, Heard M, Davis R, et al. Total enteral nutrition versus total parenteral nutrition during pediatric extracorporeal membrane oxygenation. Crit Care Med 1998;26(2): 358–63.

[108] Brown KL, Walker G, Grant DJ, et al. Predicting outcome in ex-premature infants supported with extracorporeal membrane oxygenation for acute hypoxic respiratory failure. Arch Dis Child Fetal Neonatal Ed 2004;89(5):F423–7.

[109] Kolovos NS, Schuerer DJ, Moler FW, et al. Extracorporeal life support for pulmonary hemorrhage in children: a case series. Crit Care Med 2002;30(3):577–80.

[110] Siden HB, Sanders GM, Moler FW. A report of four cases of acute, severe pulmonary hemorrhage in infancy and support with extracorporeal membrane oxygenation. Pediatr Pulmonol 1994;18(5):337–41.

[111] Kane TD, Greenhalgh DG, Warden GD. Pediatric burn patients with respiratory failure: predictors of outcome with the use of extracorporeal life support. J Burn Care Rehabil 1999;20(2):145–50.

[112] Pierre EJ, Zwischenberger JB, Angel C, et al. Extracorporeal membrane oxygenation in the treatment of respiratory failure in pediatric patients with burns. J Burn Care Rehabil 1998; 19(2):131–4.
[113] Fortenberry JD, Meier AH, Pettignano R, et al. Extracorporeal life support for posttraumatic acute respiratory distress syndrome at a children's medical center. J Pediatr Surg 2003;38(8):1221–6.
[114] Halasa NB, Barr FE, Johnson JE, et al. Fatal pulmonary hypertension associated with pertussis in infants: does extracorporeal membrane oxygenation have a role? Pediatrics 2003; 112(6 Pt 1):1274–8.
[115] Pooboni S, Roberts N, Westrope C, et al. Extracorporeal life support in pertussis. Pediatr Pulmonol 2003;36(4):310–5.
[116] Gow KW, Wulkan ML, Heiss KF, et al. Extracorporeal membrane oxygenation for support of children after hematopoietic stem cell transplantation: the Extracorporeal Life Support Organization experience. J Pediatr Surg 2006;41(4):662–7.
[117] Linden V, Karlen J, Olsson M, et al. Successful extracorporeal membrane oxygenation in four children with malignant disease and severe Pneumocystis carinii pneumonia. Med Pediatr Oncol 1999;32(1):25–31.

PEDIATRIC CLINICS
OF NORTH AMERICA

ELSEVIER
SAUNDERS

Pediatr Clin N Am 55 (2008) 735–755

Pharmacokinetics and Pharmacodynamics in the Critically Ill Child

Athena F. Zuppa, MD, MSCE, FAAP, FCP*,
Jeffrey S. Barrett, PhD, FCP

*The Children's Hospital of Philadelphia, Abramson Research Center,
3516 Civic Center Boulevard, Suite 916 H, Philadelphia, PA 19104, USA*

Pharmacology encompasses drug composition, drug properties, interactions, toxicology, and desirable effects that can be used in therapy of diseases. Underlying the discipline of pharmacology are the fields of pharmacokinetics and pharmacodynamics. Each of these disciplines can be further defined by the underlying processes that dictate specific pathways (eg, absorption, distribution, metabolism, elimination). Pharmacology is essential to our understanding of how drugs work and how to guide their administration. Pediatric pharmacotherapy can be challenging because of developmental changes that may alter drug kinetics, pathophysiologic differences that may alter pharmacodynamics, disease etiologies that may differ from adults, and other factors that may result in great variation in safety and efficacy outcomes. The situation becomes more difficult when one considers critically ill children and the paucity of well-controlled pediatric clinical trials in this vulnerable population. Prescribing caregivers of critically ill children must have some understanding of the basic processes that govern the current dosing recommendations for their patients. This article provides a review of the pharmacologic principles that guide pharmacotherapy in general, with a focus on pharmacotherapy frequently used in the pediatric critical care setting.

* Corresponding author.
E-mail address: zuppa@email.chop.edu (A.F. Zuppa).

0031-3955/08/$ - see front matter © 2008 Elsevier Inc.
doi:10.1016/j.pcl.2008.02.017 *pediatric.theclinics.com*

Pharmacokinetics

Absorption is the process of drug transfer from its site of administration to the bloodstream. The rate and efficiency of absorption depend on the route of administration. For intravenous administration, absorption is complete; the total dose reaches the systemic circulation. Drugs administered enterally may be absorbed by either passive diffusion or active transport. The bioavailability (F) of a drug is defined by the fraction of the administered dose that reaches the systemic circulation. If a drug is administered intravenously, then the bioavailability is 100% and F = 1.0. When drugs are administered by routes other than intravenous, the bioavailability is usually less. Bioavailability is reduced by incomplete absorption, first-pass metabolism, and distribution into other tissues. The volume of distribution (Vd) is a hypothetical volume of fluid through which a drug is dispersed. A drug rarely disperses solely into the water compartments of the body. Instead, most drugs disperse to several compartments, including adipose tissue and plasma proteins. The total volume into which a drug disperses is called the apparent volume of distribution. This volume is not a physiologic space, but instead a conceptual parameter. It relates the total amount of drug in the body to the concentration of drug (C) in the blood or plasma: Vd = Drug/C.

Fig. 1 represents the fate of a drug after intravenous administration. After administration, a maximal plasma concentration is achieved, and the drug is immediately distributed. The plasma concentration then decreases over time. This initial phase is called the alpha (α) phase of drug distribution, wherein the decline in plasma concentration is attributable to the

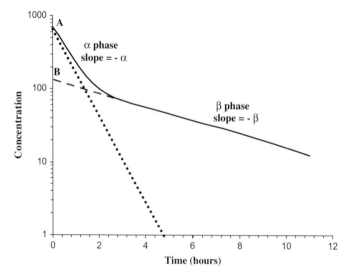

Fig. 1. Semilogarithmic plot of concentration versus time after an intravenous administration of a drug that follows two-compartment pharmacokinetics.

distribution of the drug. Once a drug is distributed, it undergoes metabolism and elimination. The second phase is called the beta (β) phase, wherein the decline in plasma concentration is attributable to drug metabolism and clearance. The terms A and B are intercepts with the Y axis. The extrapolation of the β phase defines B. The dotted line is generated by subtracting the extrapolated line from the original concentration line. This second line defines α and A. The plasma concentration can be determined using the formula: $C = Ae^{-\alpha t} + Be^{-\beta t}$. The distribution and elimination half-lives can be determined by: $t_{1/2\alpha} = 0.693/\alpha$ and $t_{1/2\beta} = 0.693/\beta$, respectively [1,2]. For drugs in which distribution is homogenous along the varied physiologic spaces, the distinction between the α and β phases may be subtle and essentially a single phase may best describe the decline in drug concentration.

The metabolism of drugs is catalyzed by enzymes, and most reactions follow Michaelis Menten kinetics: V(rate of metabolism) = (Vmax) (C)/(Km + C), where C is the drug concentration and Km is the Michaelis Menten constant. In most situations, the drug concentration is much less than Km and the equation simplifies to V = (Vmax) (C)/Km. In this case, the rate of drug metabolism is directly proportional to the concentration of free drug, and follows first-order kinetics. A constant percentage of the drug is metabolized over time, and the rate of elimination is proportional to the amount of drug in the body. Most drugs used in the clinical setting are eliminated in this manner. A few drugs, such as aspirin, ethanol, and phenytoin are used in higher doses, resulting in higher plasma concentrations. In these situations, C is much greater than Km, and the equation reduces to: V(rate of drug metabolism) = (Vmax) (C)/(C) = Vmax. The enzyme system becomes saturated by a high free-drug concentration, and the rate of metabolism is constant over time. This is called zero-order kinetics, and a constant amount of drug is metabolized per unit time. A large increase in serum concentration can result from a small increase in dose for drugs that follow zero-order elimination.

The liver is the principle organ of drug metabolism. Other tissues that display considerable metabolic activity include the gastrointestinal tract, the lungs, the skin, and the kidneys. Following oral administration, many drugs are absorbed intact from the small intestine and transported to the liver by way of the portal system, where they are metabolized. This process is called first-pass metabolism, and may greatly limit the bioavailability of orally administered drugs. In general, all metabolic reactions can be classified as either phase I or phase II biotransformations. Phase I reactions usually convert the parent drug to a polar metabolite by introducing or unmasking a more polar site ($-OH$, $-NH_2$). If phase I metabolites are sufficiently polar, they may be readily excreted. Many phase I metabolites undergo a subsequent reaction in which endogenous substances, such as glucuronic acid, sulfuric acid, or an amino acid, combine with the metabolite to form a highly polar conjugate. Many drugs undergo these sequential reactions. Phase II reactions may precede phase I reactions, however, as in the case of isoniazid. Phase I reactions are usually catalyzed by enzymes of the cyto-chrome P450 system. These drug-metabolizing enzymes are located in the lipophilic membranes of the endoplasmic reticulum of the liver and other tis-sues. Three families, CYP1, CYP2, and CYP3, are responsible for most drug biotransformations. The CYP3A subfamily accounts for greater than 50% of phase I drug metabolism, predominantly by the CYP3A4 subtype. CYP3A4 is responsible for the metabolism of drugs commonly used in the intensive care setting, including acetaminophen, cyclosporine, diazepam, methadone, midazolam, spironolactone, and tacrolimus. Most other drug biotransformations are performed by CYP2D6 (eg, clozapine, codeine, fle-cainide, haloperidol, oxycodone), CYP2C9 (eg, phenytoin, S-warfarin), CYP2C19 (eg, diazepam, omeprazole, propanolol), CYP2E1 (eg, acetamin-ophen, enflurane, halothane), and CYP1A2 (eg, acetaminophen, caffeine, theophylline, warfarin). Drug biotransformation reactions may be enhanced or impaired by multiple factors, including age, enzyme induction or inhibi-tion, pharmacogenetics, and the effects of other disease states [3,4]. For example, the metabolic pathways for acetaminophen have been well studied. Approximately 95% of the metabolism occurs by way of conjugation to glu-curonide (50%–60%) and sulfate (25%–35%). Most of the remainder of acetaminophen is metabolized by way of the cytochrome P450 forming N-acetyl-p-benzoquinone imine (NAPQI), which is believed to be responsi-ble for hepatotoxicity. This minor but important pathway is catalyzed by CYP2E1, and to a lesser extent, CYP1A2 and CYP3A4. NAPQI is detoxi-fied by reacting with either glutathione directly or through a glutathione transferase catalyzed reaction. When the hepatic synthesis of glutathione is overwhelmed, manifestations of toxicity appear producing centrilobular necrosis. In the presence of a potent CYP2E1 inhibitor, disulfiram, there was a 69% reduction in the urinary excretion of these 2E1 metabolic prod-ucts, which supports the assignment of a major role for 2E1 in the formation of NAPQI. Studies of inhibitors of other CYP pathways (eg, 1A2 and 3A4) have failed to document a significant effect on the urinary excretion of glu-tathione conjugates; thus 2E1 seems to be the primary pathway overwhelm-ingly responsible for NAPQI. CYP2E1 is unique among the CYP families in an ability to produce reactive oxygen radicals through a reduction of O_2 and is the only CYP system strongly induced by alcohol, which is itself a sub-strate. In addition to alcohol, isoniazid acts as inducer and a substrate. Ketoconazole and other imidazole compounds are inducers but not sub-strates. Barbiturates and phenytoin, which are nonspecific inducers, have no role as CYP2E1 inducers nor are they substrates for that system. Phenyt-oin in fact may be hepatoprotective because it is an inducer of the glucuro-nidation metabolic pathway for acetaminophen, thus shunting metabolism away from NAPQI production [5–8].

Elimination is the process by which a drug is removed or "cleared" from the body. Clearance (CL) is usually referred to as the amount of blood from which all drug is removed per unit time (volume/time). The main organs responsible for drug clearance are the kidneys and the liver. The total body clearance of a drug is equal to the sum of the clearances from all mechanisms. Typically, this is partitioned into renal and nonrenal clearance. Most elimination by the kidneys is accomplished by glomerular filtration. Glomerular integrity, the size and charge of the drug, water solubility, and the extent of protein binding determine the amount of drug that is filtered. Highly protein-bound drugs are not readily filtered. Estimation of the glomerular filtration rate, therefore, has traditionally served as an approximation of renal function. In addition to glomerular filtration, drugs may be eliminated from the kidneys by active secretion. Secretion occurs predominantly at the proximal tubule, where active transport systems secrete primarily organic acids and bases. Organic acids include most cephalosporins, loop diuretics, methotrexate, nonsteroidal anti-inflammatories, penicillins, and thiazide diuretics. Organic bases include ranitidine and morphine. As drugs move toward the distal convoluting tubule, the concentration increases. High urine flow rates decrease the concentration of drug in the distal tubule, decreasing the likelihood that a drug will diffuse from the lumen. For weak acids and bases, the non-ionized form of the drug is reabsorbed more readily. Altering the pH (ion trapping) can minimize reabsorption, by placing a charge on the drug and preventing its diffusion. For example, salicylate is a weak acid. In cases of salicylate toxicity, urine alkalinization places a charge on the molecule and increases its elimination. The liver also contributes to elimination through metabolism or excretion into the bile. After a drug is secreted in the bile it may then be either excreted into the feces or reabsorbed by way of enterohepatic recirculation [1,3,4]. The half-life of elimination is the time it takes to clear half of the drug from plasma. It is directly proportional to the Vd and inversely proportional to CL [1]: $t_{1/2\beta} = (0.693) (Vd)/CL$.

Physiologic differences in children that affect drug disposition

As children develop and grow, changes in body composition, development of metabolizing enzymes, and maturation of renal and liver function all affect drug disposition [1,2].

Renal

Renal function in the premature and full-term neonate, both glomerular filtration and tubular secretion, is significantly reduced compared with older children. Maturation of renal function is a dynamic process that begins during fetal life and is complete by early childhood. Maturation of tubular function is slower than that of glomerular filtration. The glomerular filtration rate is approximately 2 to 4 mL/min/1.73 m^2 in term neonates, but it may be as low as 0.6 to 0.8 mL/min/1.73 m^2 in preterm neonates. The glomerular filtration rate increases rapidly during the first two weeks of life and continues to increase until adult values are reached at 8 to 12 months of age. For drugs that are renally eliminated, impaired renal function decreases clearance, increasing the half-life. For drugs that are primarily eliminated by the kidney, therefore, dosing should be performed in an age-appropriate fashion that takes into account maturational changes in kidney function [1,2,9].

Hepatic

Hepatic biotransformation reactions are substantially reduced in the neo-natal period. At birth, the cytochrome p450 system is 28% that of the adult [1,2]. The expression of phase I enzymes, such as the P-450 cytochromes, changes markedly during development. CYP3A7, the predominant CYP isoform expressed in fetal liver, peaks shortly after birth and then declines rapidly to levels that are undetectable in most adults. Within hours after birth, CYP2E1 activity increases, and CYP2D6 becomes detectable soon thereafter. CYP3A4 and CYP2C appear during the first week of life, whereas CYP1A2 is the last hepatic CYP to appear, at 1 to 3 months of life. The ontogeny of phase II enzymes is less well established than the on-togeny of reactions involving phase I enzymes. Available data indicate that the individual isoforms of glucuronosyltransferase (UGT) have unique mat-urational profiles with pharmacokinetic consequences. For example, the glu-curonidation of acetaminophen (a substrate for UGT1A6 and, to a lesser extent, UGT1A9) is decreased in newborns and young children as compared with adolescents and adults. Glucuronidation of morphine (a UGT2B7 sub-strate) can be detected in premature infants as young as 24 weeks of gesta-tional age [9].

Gastrointestinal

Overall the rate at which most drugs are absorbed is slower in neonates and young infants than in older children. As a result, the time required to achieve maximal plasma levels is longer in the very young [9]. The effect of age on enteral absorption is not uniform and is difficult to predict [1,2]. Gastric emptying and intestinal motility are the primary determinants of the rate at which drugs are presented to and dispersed along the mucosal surface of the small intestine. At birth, the coordination of antral contrac-tions improves, resulting in a marked increase in gastric emptying during the first week of life. Similarly, intestinal motor activity matures throughout early infancy, with consequent increases in the frequency, amplitude, and duration of propagating contractions [9]. Changes in the intraluminal pH in different segments of the gastrointestinal tract can directly affect the sta-bility and the degree of ionization of a drug, thus influencing the relative amount of drug available for absorption. During the neonatal period, intra-gastric pH is relatively elevated (greater than 4). Oral administration of acid-labile compounds, such as penicillin G, produces greater bioavailability in neonates than in older infants and children [10]. In contrast, drugs that are weak acids, such as phenobarbital, may require larger oral doses in the very young to achieve therapeutic plasma levels. Other factors that impact the rate of absorption include age-associated development of villi, splanchnic blood flow, changes in intestinal microflora, and intestinal surface area [9].

Body composition

Age-dependent changes in body composition alter the physiologic spaces into which a drug may be distributed [9]. The percent of total body water drops from about 85% in premature infants to 75% in full-term infants to 60% in the adult. Extracellular water decreases from 45% in the infant to 25% in the adult. Total body fat in the premature infant can be as low as 1%, compared with 15% in the normal, term infant. Many drugs are less bound to plasma proteins in the neonate and infant than in the older child [1,2]. Limited data in neonates suggest that the passive diffusion of drugs into the central nervous system is age dependent, as reflected by the progressive increase in the ratios of brain phenobarbital to plasma phenobarbital from 28 to 39 weeks of gestational age, demonstrating the increased transport of phenobarbital into the brain [11].

Impact of critical illness

Renal dysfunction

Renal failure can affect the pharmacokinetics of drugs. In renal failure, the binding of acidic drugs to albumin is decreased because of competition with accumulated organic acids and uremia-induced structural changes in albumin that decrease drug binding affinity, altering the Vd [4]. Drugs that are more than 30% eliminated unchanged in the urine are likely to have significantly diminished CL in the presence of renal insufficiency [4].

Hepatic dysfunction

Drugs that undergo extensive first-pass metabolism may have a significantly higher oral bioavailability in patients who have liver failure than in normal subjects. Gut hypomotility may delay the peak response to enterally administered drugs in these patients. Hypoalbuminemia or altered glycoprotein levels may affect the fractional protein binding of acidic or basic drugs, respectively. Altered plasma protein concentrations may affect the extent of tissue distribution of drugs that are normally highly protein bound. The presence of significant edema and ascites may alter the Vd of highly water-soluble agents, such as aminoglycoside antibiotics. The capacity of the liver to metabolize drugs depends on hepatic blood flow and liver enzyme activity, both of which can be affected by liver disease. In addition, some p450 isoforms are more susceptible than others to liver disease, impairing drug metabolism [4,12].

Cardiac dysfunction

Circulatory failure, or shock, can alter the pharmacokinetics of drugs frequently used in the intensive care setting. Drug absorption may be impaired because of bowel wall edema. Passive hepatic congestion may impede first-pass metabolism, resulting in higher plasma concentrations. Peripheral edema inhibits absorption by intramuscular parenteral routes. The balance of tissue hypoperfusion versus increased total body water with edema may unpredictably alter Vd. In addition, liver hypoperfusion may alter drug-metabolizing enzyme function, especially flow-dependent drugs, such as lidocaine [4].

Pharmacodynamics

Pharmacodynamics, in general terms, seeks to define what the drug does to the body, or the effects or response to drug therapy. Pharmacodynamic response to drug therapy evolves only after active drug molecules reach their intended sites of action. The link between pharmacokinetic and pharmacodynamic processes is thus implicit. Differences in pharmacodynamic time course among drug entities can be broadly associated with the nature of the concentration–effect relationship as being direct (effect is directly proportional to concentration at the site of measurement, usually the plasma) or indirect (effect exhibits some type of temporal delay with respect to drug concentration either because of differences between site of action and measurement or because the effect of interest results after other physiologic or pharmacologic conditions are satisfied). Direct-effect relationships are easily observed with cardiovascular agents. Pharmacologic effects, such as blood pressure, angiotensin-converting enzyme inhibition, and inhibition of platelet aggregation, can be characterized by direct-response relationships. Other drugs exhibit an indirect relationship between concentration and response. In this case the concentration–effect relationship is time dependent. One explanation for such effects is hysteresis. Hysteresis refers to the phenomenon in which there is a time lapse between the cause and its effect. With respect to pharmacodynamics, this most often indicates a situation in which there is a delay in equilibrium between plasma drug concentration and the concentration of active substance at the effect site. Three conditions predominate this phenomenon: the active site is not in the central compartment, the mechanism of action involves protein synthesis, and active metabolites are present. More complicated models (indirect-response models) have been used to express the same observations but typically necessitate a greater understanding of the underlying physiologic process (eg, cell trafficking, enzyme recruitment, and so forth). The salient point is that pharmacodynamic characterization and likewise dosing guidance derived from such investigation stands to be more informative than drug concentrations alone.

Pharmacogenomics

Pharmacogenomics is the study of how an individual's genetic inheritance affects the body's response to drugs. Pharmacogenomics holds the promise that drugs might one day be tailored to individuals and adapted to each person's own genetic makeup. Environment, diet, age, lifestyle, and state of health all can influence a person's response to medicines, but understanding an individual's genetic composition is believed to be the key to creating personalized drugs with greater efficacy and safety. Pharmacogenomics combines traditional pharmaceutical sciences, such as biochemistry, with annotated knowledge of genes, proteins, and single nucleotide polymorphisms (SNPs). Genetic variations, or SNPs, in the human genome can be a diagnostic tool to predict a person's drug response. For SNPs to be used in this way, a person's DNA must be sequenced for the presence of specific SNPs. SNP screenings benefit drug development, and those people whose pharmacogenomic screening shows that the drug being tested would be harmful or ineffective for them would be excluded from clinical trials. Prescreening clinical trial subjects might also allow clinical trials to be smaller, faster, and therefore less expensive. Finally, the ability to assess an individual's reaction to a drug before it is prescribed increases confidence in prescribing the drug and the patient's confidence in taking the drug, which in turn should encourage the development of new drugs tested in a like manner. For example, the major enzyme responsible for tacrolimus metabolism is CYP3A. CYP3A5 genes have multiple SNPs. One study found that at 3, 6, and 12 months post heart transplantation, there was a significant difference in tacrolimus blood concentrations per dose/kg/d between the CYP3A5 *1/*3 (CYP3A5 expressor) and the *3/*3 (nonexpressor) genotypes, with the *1/*3 patients requiring larger tacrolimus doses to achieve the same blood concentration. It was concluded that specific genotypes of CYP3A5 in pediatric heart transplant patients require larger tacrolimus doses to maintain their tacrolimus blood concentration, and that this information could be used prospectively to manage patient's immunosuppressive therapy [13].

Medications used in pediatric intensive care

Benzodiazepines

Benzodiazepines are often used to provide sedation and amnesia. Benzodiazepines exert their anxiolytic, amnestic, anticonvulsant, and muscle-relaxing effects through interaction at specific binding sites on neuronal γ-aminobutyric acid (GABA) receptors [14]. Chronic administration of benzodiazepines can lead to decreased receptor activity and drug tolerance. Tolerance is a common finding in ICU patients receiving benzodiazepines or other sedative agents for periods longer than 24 hours. Withdrawal syndromes have been reported with cessation of midazolam and other benzodiazepine infusions. Risk factors for acute withdrawal include high infusion rates, prolonged duration, and abrupt cessation. For these reasons, gradual tapering of sedative infusions is suggested to reduce the chance of withdrawal reactions. Midazolam is rapidly absorbed after administration of the oral syrup formulation, with adolescents absorbing the drug at approximately half the rate observed in younger children (aged 2 to <12 years) [15]. Midazolam undergoes extensive metabolism by the cytochrome P450 3A subfamily to a major hydroxylated metabolite (1-OH-midazolam). 1-OH-midazolam is equipotent to midazolam, and is subsequently metabolized to 1-OH-midazolam-glucuronide by uridine diphosphate-glucuronosyltransferases (UGTs). 1-OH-midazolam-glucuronide also seems to have sedative properties when concentrations are high, as has been observed in adult patients who have renal failure [16]. The elimination half-life is prolonged and clearance reduced in adolescents as compared with younger children [15]. CYP3A activity reaches adult levels between 3 and 12 months of postnatal age [17]. Developmental differences in CYP3A activity may therefore alter the pharmacokinetics of midazolam in pediatric intensive care patients of different ages [16]. The elimination half-life of midazolam is 2 hours in young, healthy adults but increases rapidly in the elderly and following major surgery [18]. The most dramatic changes in the pharmacokinetics of midazolam in the critically ill may result from altered hepatic metabolism. Accumulation occurs in critically ill patients at the peak of their illness with low or absent concentrations of 1-OH-midazolam, suggesting the failure of liver metabolism [19]. Several drugs, including cimetidine, erythromycin, propofol, and diltiazem, have been reported to delay midazolam metabolism and therefore increase its duration of effect. The accumulation of the active metabolite also may be important in some ICU patients. Midazolam causes dose-related respiratory depression (as do other benzodiazepines) and in large doses can cause vasodilation and hypotension [18]. As with many highly lipid-soluble drugs, after continuous infusion for extended time periods drug accumulates in peripheral tissues and in the bloodstream rather than being metabolized. When the infusion is discontinued, peripheral tissue stores release midazolam back into the plasma, and the duration of clinical effect can be prolonged. Obese patients who have larger volumes of distribution and elderly patients who have decreased hepatic and renal function may be even more prone to prolonged sedation [20]. Diazepam is highly lipid soluble, highly protein bound, and distributes quickly into the brain. Diazepam administration results in antegrade but not retrograde amnesia. It reduces the cerebral metabolic rate for oxygen consumption and thus decreases cerebral blood flow in a dose-dependent manner. As do other benzodiazepines, diazepam raises the seizure threshold [18]. Diazepam is metabolized by hepatic microsomal enzymes (CYP2C19) to active compounds such as desmethyldiazepam and oxazepam. Desmethyldiazepam has a long elimination half-life of 100 to

200 hours and is eliminated by the kidneys. Oxazepam has an elimination half-life of 10 hours. The elimination half-life of diazepam averages 72 hours, varies widely, and is increased in the elderly, neonates, and patients who have liver disease. Metabolism also is affected by genetics, gender, endocrine status, nutritional status, smoking, and concurrent drug therapy [18]. Diazepam alone has minimal cardiovascular depressant effects, although systemic vascular resistance is reduced slightly, producing a small decline in arterial blood pressure. Respiratory drive is likewise minimally decreased by diazepam [18]. Lorazepam is the least lipid-soluble of the three benzodiazepines and traverses the blood–brain barrier most slowly, resulting in delayed onset and prolonged duration of effect [18]. Lorazepam is metabolized to inactive products by hepatic glucuronidation. The pharmacokinetics of lorazepam do not change significantly in the elderly or critically ill populations. The elimination half-life ranges from 10 to 20 hours but is prolonged by liver and end-stage kidney disease [18]. Because lorazepam is insoluble in water, it is manufactured with polyethylene glycol. This drug vehicle may be associated with lactic acidosis, hyperosmolar coma, and a reversible nephrotoxicity after high doses or prolonged infusions [18]. Flumazenil acts at the benzodiazepine binding site on the GABA receptor to antagonize the effects of benzodiazepine agonists. Flumazenil is chemically and structurally similar to other benzodiazepine receptor agonists. Flumazenil produces reversal of benzodiazepine-induced sedative and amnestic effects. Clinical effects are seen immediately after intravenous administration. Flumazenil does not reverse the effects of opioids, barbiturates, alcohol, or other GABA-mimetic agents [18]. Flumazenil is short acting, and careful clinical observation is crucial. Repeated administrations may be necessary to maintain its antagonistic action [21]. The elimination half-life of flumazenil is approximately 1 hour, which is significantly shorter than many of the benzodiazepine compounds used clinically [18]. Flumazenil can precipitate withdrawal or seizures in patients who have benzodiazepine dependence caused by chronic exposure [18].

Barbiturates

Barbiturates are weak acids that are absorbed and rapidly distributed to all tissues and fluids with high concentrations in the brain, liver, and kidneys. Lipid solubility of the barbiturates is the dominant factor in their distribution within the body. The more lipid soluble the barbiturate, the more rapidly it penetrates all tissues of the body. Thiopental is an ultra short-acting barbiturate. It is administered for brain hypoxic-ischemic injuries, and neurosurgical diseases, such as cerebral vascular diseases and intracranial hypertension. Another use of high-dose thiopental therapy is in the management of status epilepticus refractory to more conventional therapy. Following an intravenous dose, unconsciousness occurs within 10 to 20 seconds; the depth of anesthesia may increase for up to 40 seconds, and then decreases until consciousness returns in 20 to 30 minutes [22,23]. Thiopental produces a dose-related depression of respiration. Cardiac output is somewhat decreased. In the presence of hypovolemia, sepsis, or circulatory failure, however, therapeutic doses may result in circulatory collapse [22]. Pentobarbital has a potent effect on GABA-sensitive chloride channels, and is a potent central nervous system depressant. Following intravenous administration, the onset of action is almost immediate. Pentobarbital enters the brain more rapidly than phenobarbital or diazepam, and is a potent antiepileptic drug. High-dose pentobarbital infusions have been advocated as an effective adjunct in controlling persistent intracranial hypertension after severe head trauma in patients refractory to conventional therapy. Pentobarbital has also been recommended as a sedative agent for diagnostic imaging studies [24,25].

Opioids

Opioids are endogenous or exogenous substances that bind to receptors found in the central nervous system and peripheral tissue. Three classes of opiate receptors have been classified: mu (1 and 2), kappa (1–3), and delta (1 and 2). The mu1 (spinal) and mu2 (supraspinal) subtypes are present in the central nervous system. Stimulation of these receptors produces analgesia, respiratory depression, and miosis. Kappa1 receptors elicit spinal analgesia when stimulated. The pharmacologic properties of kappa2 receptors remain unknown. The analgesic effects of kappa3 receptors are exerted through supraspinal mechanisms [26]. Opioids lead to a dose-dependent, centrally mediated respiratory depression, mediated by the mu2 receptors in the medulla. Opioids have little hemodynamic effect on patients who have euvolemia whose blood pressure is not sustained by the sympathetic nervous system. Opiate side effects include nausea, vomiting, decreased gastrointestinal motility, urinary retention, and pruritus [20]. Morphine is a potent mu-receptor agonist with additional kappa-receptor activity [26]. Morphine's onset of action is relatively slow (5–10 minutes) because of low lipid solubility. The duration of action is dose dependent but is approximately 4 hours after a single dose [20]. Metabolism primarily occurs through the liver by glucuronide conjugation, and excretion occurs through the kidney. Morphine's predominant metabolite, morphine 6-glucuronide, is an active analgesic and may accumulate in patients who have renal failure. This active metabolite is several times more potent than morphine itself [26]. The pharmacologic effects of morphine-like agents include analgesia, respiratory depression, gastrointestinal effects (nausea and vomiting), orthostatic hypotension, sedation, and altered mentation [26]. Morphine administration may cause histamine release [20]. Hydromorphone is a morphine-like agonist and a semisynthetic opioid analgesic with roughly threefold to fourfold greater potency than morphine. Hydromorphone, like morphine, provides analgesic effects within 15 to 30 minutes of administration. Its metabolism primarily occurs by the liver to hydromorphone-3-glucuronide. Although it has been recommended as an alternative to morphine for patients in renal failure, hydromorphone's metabolite may accumulate in renal failure, resulting in neuroexcitability and cognitive impairment [26]. Meperidine is primarily a mu-receptor agonist and has approximately one tenth the potency of morphine. Analgesic effects of meperidine are detectable within 5 minutes of intravenous administration and 10 minutes after intramuscular or subcutaneous administration. Meperidine is useful for drug-induced rigors and pain, such as those that accompany administration of amphotericin B. It is metabolized through the liver to an active metabolite, normeperidine [26]. Normeperidine accumulates in renal failure and produces neurotoxicity, which may result in tremors, myoclonic jerks, and seizures. Case reports of seizures with meperidine have been noted with administration by patient-controlled analgesia pumps [27]. Risk for seizures also is reported in patients who have renal insufficiency, with sickle cell anemia, and in those receiving high-dose meperidine [26]. Fentanyl is a synthetic opioid commonly used in anesthesia and in the ICU for pain management and sedation. Fentanyl is 50 to 100 times as potent as morphine, and provides a relatively quick onset of action and short duration (approximately 0.5–1 hour). Fentanyl is more lipid soluble than morphine and has a more rapid onset of action because of quicker penetration of the central nervous system. Fentanyl may be administered by the intravenous, intramuscular, epidural, transdermal, intranasal, or intrathecal routes [26,28]. Long-term continuous infusions of fentanyl may result in a prolonged elimination half-life and duration of action as a result of drug accumulation in peripheral tissues. Unlike morphine, fentanyl is not associated with histamine release and may be preferred in patients susceptible to the cardiovascular effects of morphine [28]. Rapid administration has been associated with chest wall rigidity. Naloxone is an opiate antagonist. Small doses can result in prompt reversal of opiate-induced respiratory depression, sedation, analgesia, and hypotension. Naloxone can be administered endotracheally. The duration of action is 1 to 4 hours. Naloxone undergoes significant first-pass metabolism and is metabolized in the liver by conjugation with glucuronic acid. Caution must be used when treating opiate overdose in a patient who has pain.

Ketamine

Ketamine is a racemic mixture consisting of two optical enantiomers, R($-$) and S($+$). Administration produces a dose-dependent central nervous system depression that leads to a dissociative state, characterized by profound analgesia and amnesia but not necessarily loss of consciousness. Ketamine is a bronchodilator and causes minimal respiratory depression. Increased oral secretions can occur with its use, however. It is used clinically for indications such as induction of anesthesia in patients in hemodynamic shock or active asthmatic disease; intramuscular sedation of uncooperative patients; supplementation of incomplete regional or local anesthesia; sedation in the intensive care setting; and for analgesia for short, painful procedures, such as dressing changes in burn patients. Common side effects include emergence delirium and severe hallucinations. These effects can be reduced with concomitant administration of a benzodiazepine, such as midazolam. Although ketamine administration is generally associated with increases in heart rate, cardiac output, and blood pressure, hypotension from direct myocardial depression can occur [20].

Propofol

Propofol is an alkyl phenol intravenous anesthetic. Its exact mechanism of action is unclear, but it is believed to act at the GABA receptor. Propofol is highly lipid soluble and rapidly crosses the blood–brain barrier. Onset of sedation is rapid (1–5 minutes). The duration of action is dose dependent but is usually short (2–8 minutes) because of rapid redistribution to peripheral tissues. Propofol is a hypnotic agent that provides a suppression of awareness from mild depression of responsiveness to obtundation. It is a potent anxiolytic and a potent amnestic agent, but does not possess analgesic properties [20]. Apnea often occurs after a loading dose, and administration can cause significant decreases in blood pressure, especially in hypovolemic patients. This reaction is mainly a result of preload reduction from dilation of venous capacitance vessels. A lesser effect is mild myocardial depression. Because it is delivered in a lipid carrier, hypertriglyceridemia is a possible side effect of propofol [20]. Lactic acidosis has been associated with its use in the pediatric population [29]. Recent reports of dysrhythmia, heart failure, metabolic acidosis, hyperkalemia, and rhabdomyolysis have been described in adults treated with high doses of propofol (>80 µg/kg/min) [30].

Etomidate

Etomidate is an ultra–short-acting nonbarbiturate hypnotic agent without analgesic effects. Intravenous administration of 0.3 mg/kg induces sleep for approximately 5 minutes. Cardiovascular and respiratory adverse events are minimal [22]. Etomidate administration is associated with a transient 20% to 30% decrease in cerebral blood flow. Etomidate is rapidly metabolized in the liver to inactive metabolites. Approximately 75% of the administered dose is excreted in the urine during the first day after injection [3]. Involuntary muscle movements are a frequent occurrence. Etomidate may inhibit adrenal steroidogenesis, causing a decrease in cortisol plasma concentrations [22], which has led to controversy regarding its use in the care of critically ill patients [31].

Dexmedetomidine

Dexmedetomidine is a highly selective α_2-agonist with hypnotic and anxiolytic properties attributed to the α_{2A}-adrenoreceptors in the locus ceruleus. Analgesic properties are a result of stimulation of α_2-adrenoreceptors in the brain, spinal cord, and peripheral sites [32]. Dexmedetomidine is being increasingly used in the adult ICU setting because it allows postoperative patients to remain sedated but to arouse easily with gentle stimulation [33]. Although there is additional experience with dexmedetomidine in children, only limited pharmacokinetic data are currently available to help guide dosing. In clinical studies the significant treatment-emergent adverse events reported in dexmedetomidine patients compared with placebo patients were hypotension and bradycardia [34].

Neuromuscular blockers

During neurotransmission, the neurotransmitter acetylcholine is synthesized, stored in vesicles at the neuromuscular junction, released into the synapse, and bound to nicotinic receptors in the muscle end plate. The postsynaptic nicotinic receptor at the neuromuscular junction is the major site of action of depolarizing and nondepolarizing neuromuscular blockers [35]. Succinylcholine, a depolarizing muscle relaxant, is used because of its favorable pharmacokinetic profile, with quick onset and short duration [35]. Administration is followed by muscle fasciculations and subsequent neuromuscular blockade approximately 60 seconds after intravenous dosing. The blockade remains for approximately 5 to 10 minutes [2]. Succinylcholine is eliminated by plasma cholinesterase, has a short duration of action, and can be used independent of a patient's renal and hepatic status. Prolongation of blockade occurs in patients who have conditions associated with plasma cholinesterase deficiency and with high doses [35]. Succinylcholine can cause severe, although uncommon, adverse drug reactions, such as malignant hyperthermia, increased intraocular pressure, masseter muscle rigidity, rhabdomyolysis, bradycardia, and hyperkalemia [2,35]. Pancuronium is a nondepolarizing neuromuscular blocking agent. Onset of action occurs 4 to 6 minutes after administration and remains for 120 to 180 minutes [22]. Pancuronium is largely excreted unchanged in the urine, but a small percentage is metabolized to 3-desacetylpancuronium, which may accumulate after prolonged infusion. Although only 10% is eliminated by the liver, pancuronium also accumulates in fulminant hepatic failure [2,36]. Its administration causes tachycardia, largely because of the blocking of cardiac muscarinic cholinergic receptors [2]. Vecuronium, a steroid-based compound derived from pancuronium, is a nondepolarizing neuromuscular blocker [36]. The onset of action occurs 2 to 4 minutes after administration and remains for 30 to 40 minutes [22]. Even though it is primarily metabolized, cumulative effects of vecuronium are evident in renal transplant recipients and patients who have severe renal failure. This effect is attributable to its metabolite, 3-desacetyl vecuronium, which has 80% of the activity of the parent drug and reportedly accumulates to a greater degree in patients who have renal failure. Vecuronium may also accumulate in patients who have hepatic failure because of decreased biliary uptake [2]. Atracurium is a non-depolarizing neuromuscular blocker of intermediate action [36]. Onset of action occurs 2 to 4 minutes after administration and remains for 30 to 40 minutes [22]. Atracurium (and cisatracurium) are eliminated by Hofmann elimination, which is a spontaneous nonenzymatic degradation at physiologic pH and temperature. Atracurium is a good choice for patients who have multiorgan dysfunction [35]. Mivacurium is a nondepolarizing neuromuscular blocker [36]. Onset of action occurs 2 to 4 minutes after administration, similar to succinylcholine, and remains for 12 to 18 minutes [22]. Mivacurium is eliminated by plasma cholinesterase, has short duration of action, and can be used independent of a patient's renal and hepatic status [35]. Higher doses are associated with histamine release [22].

Sympathomimetics

Dopamine is the metabolic precursor to norepinephrine and epinephrine. It is a central neurotransmitter, also found in the sympathetic nervous system and in the adrenal medulla. Dopamine stimulates dopamine (D1 and D2) receptors in the brain and vascular beds in the kidneys, mesentery, and coronary arteries. By activating cyclic-AMP, D1-receptor activation leads to vasodilation. It also stimulates α and β receptors, although its affinity for these receptors is lower [37]. Low infusion rates (1–5 µg/kg/min) augment renal sodium excretion through dopamine receptor agonism. Intermediate dosing (5–10 µg/kg/min) results in chronotropic and inotropic effects through β-receptor agonism. Administration of these doses usually results in an increase in systolic blood pressure, minimal change in diastolic pressure, and a subsequent increase in pulse pressure. Systemic vascular resistance (SVR) is unchanged, secondary to the balance of dopamine's ability to reduce regional arteriolar resistance in the mesentery and kidneys with only a minor increase in other vasculature. Higher doses (10–20 µg/kg/min) result in increased vascular resistance secondary to a predominant α effect [22]. Dopamine toxicity includes tachycardia, hypertension, and dysrhythmias, and an increase in myocardial oxygen consumption. Dopamine depresses the ventilatory response to hypoxemia by as much as 60%. It can decrease PaO_2 by interfering with hypoxic vasoconstriction. Dopamine administration may suppress the release of thyrotropin [38]. Dobutamine resembles dopamine structurally and is delivered as a racemate. The (+) isomer is a strong β-agonist and α_1-antagonist. The (−) dobutamine isomer is a weak β-antagonist and a potent α_1-agonist. Dobutamine has somewhat greater selectivity for β_1 than β_2 receptors. As a result of opposing α_1 activities, dobutamine produces significant inotropic support, with less chronotropic and vasopressor activity [22]. Doses of 5 to 20 µg/kg/min are used for inotropic support. Dobutamine increases myocardial oxygen demand and may predispose to arrhythmias [22]. Acute high-dose dobutamine lowers thyroid stimulating hormone by an unknown mechanism [39].

Epinephrine is useful in treating shock associated with myocardial dysfunction and hypotension. Epinephrine activates α_1, β_1, and β_2 receptors. It is a principle hormone of stress and produces widespread metabolic and hemodynamic effects. β_1 receptors are affected by very low plasma concentrations of epinephrine, seen at doses of 0.05 to 0.1 $\mu g/kg/min$. The earliest effects of epinephrine are an increase in heart rate and inotropy. At these doses, stimulation of β_2 receptors promotes relaxation of resistance arterioles, promoting a decrease in systemic vascular resistance and diastolic blood pressure. Higher plasma concentrations result in activation of α_1 receptors, with a subsequent increase in systemic vascular resistance. At moderate doses (0.1–1 $\mu g/kg/min$) the α stimulation is often balanced by the improved cardiac output and relaxation of the arteriolar beds. High-dose infusions (1–2 $\mu g/kg/min$) are associated with significant vasoconstriction, with possible compromise of blood flow to individual organs. Epinephrine has many uses. It is commonly used in the treatment of respiratory diseases with elements of bronchospasm. It can also be used to treat the symptoms of hypersensitivity reactions to drugs and other allergens [22]. In the pediatric critical care environment the most frequent indications for intravenous epinephrine are cardiogenic shock and septic shock with reduced stroke volume. The septic patient who does not improve after aggressive volume repletion and treatment with dopamine or dobutamine may benefit from epinephrine. Norepinephrine differs from epinephrine by lacking the methyl substitution on the amino group. Norepinephrine has little β_2 activity, but is a potent α_1 and β_1 agonist. Infusions in normal subjects result in elevations of systemic vascular resistance because the α_1 effects are not opposed by β_2 stimulation. Reflex vagal activity reduces the heart rate, blunting the expected chronotropic effect of β_1 stimulation. Stoke volume increases, but there is minimal change in cardiac output. Peripheral vascular resistance increases in most vascular beds, including the kidney, liver, and skeletal muscle. Glomerular filtration is maintained unless the decrease in renal blood flow is substantial. Mesenteric vessels are also constricted, decreasing splanchnic and hepatic blood flow. Coronary blood flow increases because of direct coronary dilation and increase in blood pressure [22]. Isoproterenol is a potent, nonselective β-adrenergic agonist with very low affinity for α-adrenergic receptors. The principle cardiovascular effects relate to its inotropic, chronotropic peripheral vasodilator effects. Isoproterenol increases heart rate and enhances contractility. Peripheral vasodilatation produces a decrease in systemic vascular resistance. The increase in inotropy and chronotropy in the face of decreased SVR results in an increase in cardiac output. Isoproterenol relaxes almost all smooth muscle but has a significant impact on bronchial and gastrointestinal smooth muscle. If the patient is intravascularly fluid depleted, and not provided with fluid resuscitation, hypotension may occur with the institution of the drug [22]. Phenylephrine demonstrates predominantly α_1-adrenergic agonism. It causes marked vasoconstriction of the arterial and venous capacitance vessels, causing an increase in blood pressure and a sinus bradycardia attributable to vagal reflexes [40]. Vasopressin is an exogenous, parenteral form of antidiuretic hormone. Antidiuretic hormone is produced in the parvocellular and magnocellular neurons within the supraoptic and paraventricular nuclei of the hypothalamus. It is stored and released by the posterior pituitary gland in response to increases in plasma osmolality or as a baroreflex response to decreases in blood pressure or blood volume. The cellular effects of vasopressin are mediated by two major receptors, V_1 and V_2. V_1 receptors have been further subdivided as V_{1a} and V_{1b}. The V_{1a} receptor is the most widespread and is found in vascular smooth muscle, myometrium, the bladder, adipocytes, hepatocytes, platelets, renal medullary interstitial cells, vasa recta in the renal circulation, epithelial cells in the renal cortical collecting duct, spleen, testis, and many central nervous system structures. Only the adenohypophysis is known to contain V_{1b} receptors. V_2 receptors are predominantly found in the principal cells of the renal collecting duct system. V_2 receptors mediate the most predominant renal response to vasopressin, resulting in increased water permeability in the collecting duct. These V_2-mediated effects occur at much lower concentrations than are required to engage V_1-receptor–mediated actions. Other renal activities mediated by V_2 include increased urea and Na^+ transport, increasing the urine concentrating ability of the kidneys. The cardiovascular effects of vasopressin are complex. Vasopressin administration results in significant vasoconstriction, mediated by V_1 receptors. Vascular smooth muscle in the skin, skeletal muscle, fat, pancreas, and thyroid gland seem to be most sensitive, with vasoconstriction also occurring in gastrointestinal tract, coronary vessels, and brain. Activation of V_2 receptors increases circulating concentrations of procoagulant factor VIII and von Willebrand factor, and vasopressin is presumed to stimulate the secretion of these factors from storage sites in the vascular endothelium. Diabetes insipidus is a disease of impaired renal conservation of water, either secondary to an inadequate secretion of vasopressin (central diabetes insipidus), as seen with many patients who have sustained traumatic brain injury, or an insufficient renal response to vasopressin (nephrogenic diabetes insipidus). Vasopressin is most commonly indicated in the treatment of patients who have high urine flow because of central diabetes insipidus [22]. Because of its vasoactive effects, vasopressin therapy has also been evaluated in the specific setting of cardiac arrest and refractory hypotension in septic shock. It was recently recommended by the American Heart Association as an alternative to epinephrine for adult patients in ventricular fibrillation and it is used to control upper gastrointestinal hemorrhage given its ability to cause vasoconstriction of the mesenteric vasculature [41]. Vasopressin must be administered parenterally because it is degraded by trypsin in the gastrointestinal tract. The duration of antidiuretic effect following intramuscular or subcutaneous administration is approximately 2 to 8 hours. Approximately 5% of a subcutaneously administered dose is excreted unchanged in the urine within 4 hours.

Large doses can result in cardiac complications, such as arrhythmias and decreased cardiac output [22].

Vasodilators

Despite its widespread use, there is a paucity of information on the safety, efficacy, and pharmacokinetic/pharmacodynamic relationships of sodium nitroprusside in children. Nitroprusside dilates arterioles and venules. Its onset of action is within 30 seconds, with the peak hypotensive effect at approximately 2 minutes after the start of the infusion. Nitroprusside is metabolized to produce nitric oxide and cyanide. Cyanide is metabolized to thiocyanate by rhodanese using sulfur. The administration of thiosulfate with sodium nitroprusside, as an additional sulfur donor, can prevent the accumulation of cyanide in patients receiving sodium nitroprusside. Thiocyanate is renally cleared. Signs of thiocyanate toxicity include nausea, fatigue, and disorientation. The administration of sodium nitroprusside can worsen arterial hypoxemia because it hinders hypoxemic pulmonary vasoconstriction [22]. Hydralazine causes direct relaxation of arteriole smooth muscle. Venous capacitance vessels are not dilated, and postural hypotension is uncommon. Intravenous hydralazine may be used for hypertensive emergencies, but is rarely the sole agent to treat hypertension. Sympathetic stimulation can result in an increase in heart rate, increased renin activity, and subsequent fluid retention. Side effects also include headache, nausea, flushing, and palpitations. Administration can also result in a syndrome that resembles systemic lupus, serum sickness, hemolytic anemia, vasculitis, and glomerulonephritis [22]. Nicardipine is a calcium entry blocker (slow channel blocker or calcium ion antagonist) that inhibits the transmembrane influx of calcium ions into cardiac muscle and smooth muscle without changing serum calcium concentrations. The effects of nicardipine are more selective to vascular smooth muscle than cardiac muscle, and it produces a significant decrease in systemic vascular resistance. The degree of vasodilation and the resultant hypotensive effects are more prominent in hypertensive patients [42]. Milrinone, an inodilating and lusitropy agent [43], is primarily used for the treatment of congestive heart failure. It is commonly used to support cardiac output after congenital heart surgery in neonates, infants, and children. The drug is primarily cleared through renal secretion (85%), with 15% undergoing glucuronidation [44].

Summary

Pharmacology is an important discipline that underlies the management of pharmacotherapy or the safe and effective administration of pharmaceuticals. The understanding of pharmacologic principles is essential for application of pharmacotherapeutic treatment modalities in critically ill children. Although much of the pharmacologic knowledge used to derive dosing guidance for critically ill children is obtained from adult and other pediatric populations, research into understanding the dose requirements for critically ill children is more active than ever.

References

[1] Carruthers SG, Hoffman BB, Melmon KL, editors. Melmon and Morelli's clinical pharmacology. 4th edition. New York: McGraw-Hill; 2000. p. 14–33.

[2] Chernow B, editor. The pharmacologic approach to the critically ill patient. 3rd edition. Baltimore (MD): Williams and Wilkins; 1994. p. 1220.

[3] Katzung BG, editor. Basic and clinical pharmacology. 8th edition. McGraw Hill; 2001.

[4] Krishnan V, Murray P. Pharmacologic issues in the critically ill. Clin Chest Med 2003;24: 671–88.

[5] Makin AJ, Williams R. Acetaminophen-induced hepatotoxicity: predisposing factors and treatments. Adv Intern Med 1997;42:453–83.

[6] Manyike PT, Kharasch ED, Kalhorn TF, et al. Contribution of CYP2E1 and CYP3A to acetaminophen reactive metabolite formation. Clin Pharmacol Ther 2000;67:275–82.

[7] Prescott LF. Paracetamol: past, present, and future. Am J Ther 2000;7:143–7.

[8] Rumack BH. Acetaminophen hepatotoxicity: the first 35 years. J Toxicol Clin Toxicol 2002; 40:3–20.

[9] Kearns GL, Abdel-Rahman SM, Alander SW, et al. Developmental pharmacology—drug disposition, action, and therapy in infants and children. N Engl J Med 2003;349:1157–67.

[10] Huang NN, High RH. Comparison of serum levels following the administration of oral and parenteral preparations of penicillin to infants and children of various age groups. J Pediatr 1953;42:657–8.

[11] Painter MJ, Pippenger C, Wasterlain C, et al. Phenobarbital and phenytoin in neonatal seizures: metabolism and tissue distribution. Neurology 1981;31:1107–12.

[12] Rodighiero V. Effects of liver disease on pharmacokinetics. An update. Clin Pharmacokinet 1999;37:399–431.

[13] Zheng H, Webber S, Zeevi A, et al. Tacrolimus dosing in pediatric heart transplant patients is related to CYP3A5 and MDR1 gene polymorphisms. Am J Transplant 2003;3:477–83.

[14] Mendelson WB. Neuropharmacology of sleep induction by benzodiazepines. Crit Rev Neurobiol 1992;6:221–32.

[15] Reed MD, Rodarte A, Blumer JL, et al. The single-dose pharmacokinetics of midazolam and its primary metabolite in pediatric patients after oral and intravenous administration. J Clin Pharmacol 2001;41:1359–69.

[16] de Wildt SN, de Hoog M, Vinks AA, et al. Population pharmacokinetics and metabolism of midazolam in pediatric intensive care patients. Crit Care Med 2003;31:1952–8.

[17] Lacroix D, Sonnier M, Moncion A, et al. Expression of CYP3A in the human liver–evidence that the shift between CYP3A7 and CYP3A4 occurs immediately after birth. Eur J Biochem 1997;247:625–34.

[18] Young CC, Prielipp RC. Benzodiazepines in the intensive care unit. Crit Care Clin 2001;17: 843–62.

[19] Shelly MP, Mendel L, Park GR. Failure of critically ill patients to metabolise midazolam. Anaesthesia 1987;42:619–24.

[20] Gehlbach BK, Kress JP. Sedation in the intensive care unit. Curr Opin Crit Care 2002;8:290.

[21] Klotz U, Kanto J. Pharmacokinetics and clinical use of flumazenil (Ro 15-1788). Clin Pharmacokinet 1988;14:1–12.

[22] Hardman JG, Limbird LE. Goodman and Gilman's the pharmacologic basis of therapeutics. 9th edition. New York: McGraw-Hill; 1996.

[23] Russo H, Bressolle F. Pharmacodynamics and pharmacokinetics of thiopental. Clin Pharmacokinet 1998;35:95–134.

[24] Greenberg SB, Adams RC, Aspinall CL. Initial experience with intravenous pentobarbital sedation for children undergoing MRI at a tertiary care pediatric hospital: the learning curve. Pediatr Radiol 2000;30:689–91.

[25] Hubbard AM, Markowitz RI, Kimmel B, et al. Sedation for pediatric patients undergoing CT and MRI. J Comput Assist Tomogr 1992;16:3–6.

[26] Hall LG, Oyen LJ, Murray MJ. Analgesic agents. Pharmacology and application in critical care. Crit Care Clin 2001;17:899–923.

[27] Hagmeyer KO, Mauro LS, Mauro VF. Meperidine-related seizures associated with patient-controlled analgesia pumps. Ann Pharmacother 1993;27:29–32.

[28] Volles DF, McGory R. Pharmacokinetic considerations. Crit Care Clin 1999;15:55–75.

[29] Cray SH, Robinson BH, Cox PN. Lactic acidemia and bradyarrhythmia in a child sedated with propofol. Crit Care Med 1998;26:2087–92.

[30] Cremer OL, Moons KG, Bouman EA, et al. Long-term propofol infusion and cardiac failure in adult head-injured patients. Lancet 2001;357:117–8.

[31] Annane D. ICU physicians should abandon the use of etomidate! Intensive Care Med 2005; 31:325–6.

[32] Bhana N, Goa KL, McClellan KJ. Dexmedetomidine. Drugs 2000;59:263–70.

[33] Venn RM, Grounds RM. Comparison between dexmedetomidine and propofol for sedation in the intensive care unit: patient and clinician perceptions. Br J Anaesth 2001;87:684–90.

[34] Abbott: Precedex Product Label, 2003.

[35] McManus MC. Neuromuscular blockers in surgery and intensive care, Part 1. Am J Health Syst Pharm 2001;58:2287–99.

[36] Power BM, Forbes AM, van Heerden PV, et al. Pharmacokinetics of drugs used in critically ill adults. Clin Pharmacokinet 1998;34:25–54.

[37] Notterman DA, Greenwald BM, Moran F, et al. Dopamine clearance in critically ill infants and children: effect of age and organ system dysfunction. Clin Pharmacol Ther 1990;48: 138–47.

[38] Van den Berghe G, de Zegher F, Lauwers P. Dopamine suppresses pituitary function in infants and children. Crit Care Med 1994;22:1747–53.

[39] Lee E, Chen P, Rao H, et al. Effect of acute high dose dobutamine administration on serum thyrotrophin (TSH). Clin Endocrinol (Oxf) 1999;50:487–92.

[40] Cooper DW, Carpenter M, Mowbray P, et al. Fetal and maternal effects of phenylephrine and ephedrine during spinal anesthesia for cesarean delivery. Anesthesiology 2002;97: 1582–90.

[41] Holmes CL, Patel BM, Russell JA, et al. Physiology of vasopressin relevant to management of septic shock. Chest 2001;120:989–1002.

[42] Wyeth Laboratories. Product information: Cardene I.V., nicardipine; 1999.

[43] Shipley JB, Tolman D, Hastillo A, et al. Milrinone: basic and clinical pharmacology and acute and chronic management. Am J Med Sci 1996;311:286–91.

[44] Young RA, Ward A. Milrinone. A preliminary review of its pharmacological properties and therapeutic use. Drugs 1988;36:158–92.

Medical Errors Affecting the Pediatric Intensive Care Patient: Incidence, Identification, and Practical Solutions

Mark A. Nichter, MD[a,b,*]

[a]University of South Florida School of Medicine, St. Petersburg, FL 33701, USA
[b]Florida Pediatric Associates, LLP, 1033 Dr. Martin Luther King, Jr. Street,
Suite 103, St. Petersburg, FL 33701, USA

A 2-year old child presents to a referring emergency department 100 miles away with fever and lethargy. Meningitis is suspected, and laboratory data confirm the diagnosis. Transport is requested using the pediatric ICU (PICU)–based transport team. Departure from the regional tertiary care hospital is delayed because the only team available is 60 miles in the opposite direction retrieving another child. Four hours later, transport is initiated. In the interim, the child has developed respiratory compromise, and the trachea is intubated. Hypotension is noted, and vasoactive infusions are started via a peripheral intravenous line. The child arrives in the PICU 9 hours after the initial request, minimally responsive, hypotensive, volume depleted, and tachypneic.

The accepting nurse has been floated from the neonatal ICU. This is her third shift in the PICU. The respiratory therapist is just off orientation but seems competent. Both are assisted by their respective supervisors, who have patient care duties of their own. The pediatric intensivist is on the twenty-second hour of his shift and is distracted by another patient who has life-threatening dysrhythmias. Rapid assessment of the patient reveals a child in extremis. Heart rate is 190 beats/minute, respiratory rate is 42 breaths/minute, and the blood pressure is 60/30. The extremities are cold with a capillary refill time of more than 6 seconds. The endotracheal tube is two sizes too large, and the single intravenous line has malfunctioned.

An intraosseous needle is inserted, and a percutaneous central intravenous line is inserted. Difficulty is encountered placing an arterial catheter.

* Florida Pediatric Associates, LLP, 1033 Dr. Martin Luther King, Jr. Street, Suite 103, St. Petersburg, FL 33701.
E-mail address: marknicht@aol.com

0031-3955/08/$ - see front matter © 2008 Elsevier Inc. All rights reserved.
doi:10.1016/j.pcl.2008.02.014

One hour later, it is finally secured in the right femoral artery, but the distal perfusion is worse than on the contralateral side. The endotracheal tube is changed to a more appropriate size.

Two days later, the blood and cerebrospinal fluid cultures have identified streptococcus pneumonia as the offending organism, despite an initial Gram's stain report of gram-positive rods. Hypotension improves on an epinephrine infusion, and the intravascular volume has been normalized, but evidence of acute lung injury and renal insufficiency precludes the removal of life-sustaining therapies. The patient has been cared for by nine different nurses, 11 different respiratory therapists and five different pediatric intensivists.

After 1 week of hospitalization, now improved from a respiratory and cardiovascular standpoint, the child has survived a 10-fold bolus overdose of fentanyl and accidental dislodgement of his endotracheal tube. Morning laboratory studies are repeated, the first set obviously belonging to a neighboring child who has diabetic ketoacidosis. The chest radiograph shows signs of increased opacification of the right mid lung field, and *Klebsiella* species is isolated from the endotracheal secretions. Renal and respiratory functions worsen. The parents, an adult intensive care nurse and her attorney husband, are concerned about their only child's lack of progress.

By 3 weeks of hospitalization, respiratory, circulatory, and renal failure has resolved, and the child is transferred to the pediatric inpatient ward. Diarrhea is noted, and evidence of *Clostridium difficile* enteritis is found. Appropriate therapy is initiated, and the child is discharged to home on the twenty-fourth day.

Five years later, and after recurrent hospitalizations for stridor, subglottic stenosis is found, and the child responds favorably to laser therapy. School performance is at the fifth percentile for age, and the right foot is one shoe size smaller than the left. The mother secretly wonders whether her child's difficulties are the result of a single glass of Chardonnay she consumed before she knew she was pregnant.

Does the scenario seem plausible?

Does the scenario seem preventable?

Overt and clandestine medical errors occur with enough regularity in the pediatric ICU to warrant concern for the safety of any child admitted there. Efforts to describe, identify, analyze, and prevent medical errors are key to improving patient outcomes and diminishing avoidable patient harm and even death.

History

Perhaps the first description of systematic medical error in hospitalized patients was given by Alexander Gordon of Aberdeen, Scotland, in 1795, who suggested that puerperal fever is an infectious process, that physicians were the carriers, and that "I myself was the means of carrying the infection to a great number of women" [1]. Thomas Watson, Professor of Medicine at King's College Hospital, London, in 1842, recommended hand washing with chlorine solution to prevent puerperal fever "to prevent the practitioner becoming a vehicle of contagion and death between one patient and another" [2]. In 1843, Oliver Wendell Holmes incurred ridicule after publishing *The Contagiousness of Puerperal Fever*, controversially concluding that puerperal fever frequently was carried from patient to patient by physicians and nurses and suggesting that hand washing, clean clothing, and avoidance of autopsies by those aiding birth would prevent its spread [1].

In 1844, Ignaz Semmelweis, now widely recognized as the father of hospital antisepsis, was appointed assistant lecturer in the First Obstetric Division of the Vienna Hospital where medical students received their training. Semmelweis noticed that his ward's 16% mortality rate from fever was substantially higher than the 2% mortality rate in the Second Division where midwifery students were trained. He also noticed that puerperal fever was rare in women who gave birth before arriving at the hospital. Semmelweis noted that doctors in the First Division performed autopsies each morning on women who had died the previous day, but the midwives were not required to perform such autopsies.

Semmelweis began experimenting with various cleansing agents beginning in May, 1847, and ordered that all doctors and students working in the First Division wash their hands in chlorinated lime solution before starting ward work and later before each vaginal examination. The mortality rate from puerperal fever in the division fell from 18% in May, 1847 to less than 3% in June through November of the same year, an impressive result, even by today's standards [3]. Initially Semmelweis was ridiculed for his findings, but his efforts eventually led to changes in hospital hygiene that contributed significantly to a decrease in the rate of death during childbirth.

In spite of the overwhelming evidence of the effectiveness of hand washing in preventing nosocomial infections, and the intervening period of more than 150 years, clinicians today still struggle to implement fully the suggestions of Watson, Holmes, and Semmelweis [4]. Clearly, much work remains for those interested in reducing medical errors.

In the modern era, initial efforts at reducing medical errors in the PICU were limited largely to individual units, frequently based on seminal events. Publication of the results of local quality improvement efforts was unusual, much as it is today, for fear of unwanted scrutiny or litigation. Formal reporting of efforts to reduce medical errors began only in the early 1980s [5–7].

On a broader scale, the first large study of the impact of medical errors was Brennan and colleagues' [8] reporting the results of the Harvard Medical Practice Study in 1991. This seminal work described an incidence of adverse events of 3.7% in 51 New York hospitals caring for 30,000 admitted patients in 1984. Thomas and colleagues [9] reported similar findings in Colorado and Utah hospitals. A 2.9% incidence of adverse events was described in 15,000 patient discharges in 1992. In both studies more than

half of the adverse events were thought to be preventable. Death as a conse-
quence of medical error was estimated at 13.6% and 6.6%, respectively, in
the two studies. Similar reports in Australia [10] and Great Britain [11] confirmed the magnitude of medical error in health care systems.

In 1999, in the United States, based largely on these two studies, the
Institute of Medicine (IOM) reported that between 44,000 and 98,000 deaths
were caused by medical error in 1997, costing $37.6 billion annually, of which
$17 billion was preventable [12]. This study resulted in widespread public
reporting that "100,000" deaths were caused annually by medical error. Although the methodologies of the IOM report later were questioned [13], the
original report put the national spotlight on medical error and helped spur
the development of congressional initiatives to improve in-hospital care.

On a national level, The Patient Safety Act of 1999 required providers
under the Medicare program to disclose publicly nursing staffing levels
and outcome data. The Medical Error Reduction Act of 2000 mandated
that the Health Care Financing Administration establish medical error demonstration projects. The Medical Error Reduction and Improvement in Patient Safety Act of 2000 established a voluntary reporting system and
established a Center for Quality Improvement. The Patient Safety and Quality Improvement Act of 2005 defined data involved in safety programs as
"patient safety work product" (PSWP) and protected PSWP from discovery
in civil lawsuits [14].

These acts, and others, led to the prioritization of patient safety research
within the Agency for Health Care Research and Quality [15]. Subsequently,
specific national and state [16] reporting mechanisms and patient safety
goals have been developed, have been implemented [17], and have been successful [18–20]. In many hospitals, local, unit-directed quality improvement
projects have been supplanted by efforts to adhere to national or discipline-
specific patient safety referenda. The PICU has been identified as a specific
area of concern in child health safety [21–25], and a number of initiatives
have been targeted specifically at the PICU environment and its patients
[26–28].

Medical errors in the pediatric ICU

The 1999 IOM report defines medical errors as "the failure of a planned
action to be completed as intended or the use of a wrong plan to achieve an
aim" [12]. Variably, medical error has been described in terms of "adverse
events" or "adverse incidents." In Florida, an adverse incident has been
defined by statute as "an event over which health care personnel could ex-
ercise control and which is associated in whole or in part with medical intervention, rather than a condition for which such intervention occurred."
Specifically, Florida defines adverse incidents as those in which surgery
was performed on the wrong patient, a wrong procedure, wrong surgical
site, or an unnecessary procedure. Adverse incidents resulting in death,

brain damage, or permanent disfigurement and those requiring special medical attention are included, as are others. Florida statutes require reporting of these incidents to the State Department of Health [16].

To date, many efforts in reducing medical error focus on specific adverse events. In the PICU, current foci target reduction in medication errors, including those caused by errors in prescribing, admixture, administration, and monitoring. Additional efforts target the prevention of nosocomial infection, unintentional mishaps in airway and mechanical ventilation, and events related to the use of medical devices or procedures. Recently, the issues of caregiver fatigue and of communication patterns and their effects on specific adverse events have received scrutiny.

Unfortunately, this event-related approach has done little to change important aspects of care delivery which practical experience suggests may affect patient outcome significantly. These less tangible aspects of care include degree of caregiver education and training, unit staffing levels and the frequency of non–PICU-trained personnel use, the use of PICU-based versus traveling nursing personnel, the effects of locum tenens physician staffing, variable patient transport mechanisms, and the timeliness of patient transport. Other even more insidious aspects of quality remain unexplored, including the degree of institutional commitment to quality assurance, the impact of specific nurse training programs, and the effectiveness of dedicated quality control personnel.

Medication errors

Medications errors have been described as mistakes in drug ordering, transcribing, dispensing, administering, or monitoring. Adverse drug events (ADEs) are injuries that result from use of a drug. ADEs often are described as potential (an ADE that was intercepted before reaching the patient), actual (an ADE that was not intercepted before reaching the patient), preventable (an ADE that was associated with a medication error), or nonpreventable (an ADE not associated with a medication error). Nonpreventable ADEs may result from known or unknown complications of appropriate drug therapy.

The reported incidence of medication errors in the PICU ranges from 22 to 59/1000 doses [23,29]. ADEs have been reported in 3.1% of PICU days affecting 2.5% of children admitted [30]. In pediatric inpatients, Kaushal and colleagues [23], reported that 11% of ADEs were potentially life threatening and that the most common ADEs occurred at the stage of drug ordering. Most commonly, ADEs involved incorrect dosing, anti-infective drugs, and intravenous medications. The Institute for Safe Medication Practices has identified several "high alert" medications for targeting. The consequences of error involving these medications were thought to be more devastating to patients than those of other commonly used medications. Many of these medications (insulin, magnesium sulfate, nitroprusside sodium, injectable potassium chloride, and hypertonic sodium chloride) are used frequently in the PICU [31].

To prevent drug-ordering errors, the most effective strategy may be automating the ordering process. Most studies have shown that computerized provider order entry (CPOE) reduces medication prescribing errors in the PICU by 66% to 100% when compared with handwritten orders [29,32,33]. Benefits of CPOE include finding drug–drug interactions, checking ordered drugs against known patient allergies, checking the ordered drug dose and interval against known standards, prompting requests for therapeutic drug monitoring when appropriate, and the ability to track provider prescribing trends easily over time. Barriers to CPOE implementation include the initial cost of such systems and a perceived increase in provider time allocated to the ordering process. To date, little is known about whether CPOE implementation shifts the ordering process toward or away from senior members of the health care team (and little is known about the effect of this shift, if indeed it occurs) or the effectiveness of CPOE implementation in units with fewer physician extenders.

Medication admixture errors also have benefited from the effects of automation. In many institutions, parenteral alimentation solutions now are mixed by an automated process, although human interaction remains at the level of order entry. The development of standard drug concentrations and smart-pump technology has helped reduce continuous medication infusion errors in pediatric patients [31,34,35].

Errors in drug administration can be reduced by provider (usually nurse) education programs, by instituting double-check systems, and by minimizing floor stock medications such as intravenous potassium and calcium solutions [24,36]. To date, little has been written about the elimination of floor stock and its potential effect on timeliness of emergent or pre-emergent drug administration. This effect, if present, is likely to be demonstrated most easily in the most tenuous patients.

Finally, the effectiveness of clinical pharmacists in identifying and reducing medical errors in the intensive care environment is well demonstrated [37,38]. The American Academy of Pediatrics and the Society of Critical Care Medicine have published guidelines advocating the use of pharmacists in the health care team [39].

Laboratory and radiology errors

Little is known of the effects of laboratory and radiology errors on the care of PICU patients. For the practitioner, errors in patient identification, blood sampling, and "critical value" reporting are seen routinely in the PICU and may affect patient care both in terms of the appropriateness of clinical decisions made relying on such data and the timeliness of therapeutic decision making. Similarly, patient identification errors, image wrong-sidedness, and the timeliness of "critical finding" reporting remain potential areas of improvement in radiologic care.

The timeliness of critical value reporting has been improved in the operating suite by the use of point-of-care (POC) testing. POC testing has been available in some PICUs for several years. Recently, the development of more rapid and more complete blood analyzers has brought functional testing of electrolyte, blood cell count, and coagulation parameters to the bedside. As a result of POC testing, improvement in pediatric ICU laboratory error rates is expected but still unproven [40,41].

Similarly, improvements in radiologic equipment now allow real-time POC testing of many simple radiologic tests. In many institutions, around-the-clock radiologist interpretation reduces critical finding reporting times. The effects of these changes on PICU care remain unproven, although the functional utility of the radiologic testing system seems improved by these developments.

Nosocomial infection

The pediatric intensive care patient is at a heightened risk of nosocomial infection (Table 1). Brown and colleagues reported 7% of patients admitted to a PICU developed an ICU-related infection [42]. Richards and colleagues [43] reported a 6.1% overall PICU nosocomial infection rate. The very young PICU patient is at risk secondary to incomplete immune system development. Congenital and acquired immune-deficient children frequently are admitted to the PICU. Disease-specific conditions such as acute leukemia, short gut syndrome, and chronic disease place many PICU patients at heightened risk. Immune-modulating therapies and multiple or prolonged antibiotic use pose similar risks for the development of secondary infection. Finally, dependence on intravenous access, mechanical ventilators, and bladder catheters puts the PICU patient at particular risk for nosocomial infection.

Efforts to prevent and reduce nosocomial infection are important projects in any PICU. Once considered "routine" complications of care, nosocomial infections increasingly have been viewed as preventable results of medical

Table 1
Nosocomial infection rates in patients in the pediatric ICU

Type of infection	Number of pediatric ICUs	NNIS (mean, 1992–1997)	Number of pediatric ICUs	NNIS (mean, 2002–2004)
Bloodstream infections/ 1000 CVC days	61	7.9	54	6.6
Ventilator-associated pneumonia/1000 ventilator days	61	5.4	52	2.9
Urinary tract infection/ 1000 catheter days	61	5.4	52	4.0

Abbreviations: CVC, central venous catheter; NNIS, National Nosocomial Infection Surveillance.

error. National and international focus on the costs and morbidity of catheter-related bloodstream infections, ventilator-associated pneumonia, and surgical site infections has highlighted the importance of reducing nosocomial infections. Reduction of nosocomial urinary tract infection and otitis media/sinusitis remain important goals. The ICU has been identified as a central area for the identification and prevention of nosocomial infection.

The Joint Commission on Accreditation of Health care Organizations (JCAHO) has identified reduction of health care-associated infections as a National Patient Safety Goal for hospitals in 2008 [44]. The Institute for Health Care Improvement (IHI) has identified catheter-related bloodstream infections, ventilator-associated pneumonia, and surgical site infection as Strategic Improvement Initiatives with specific strategies for improvement [45]. The Children's Health Corporation of America (CHCA) has identified these three nosocomial infections as child-specific targets for quality improvement [46]. The National Initiative for Children's Health care Quality (NICHQ) similarly has identified catheter-related bloodstream infections, ventilator-associated pneumonia, and surgical site infection as topics for improvement of child health care and has offered a specific change package for each [47].

Bloodstream infection

The IHI, the JCAHO, the CHCA, and the NICHQ have all identified similar bundles or packages for the prevention of bloodstream infections in ICUs [44–47]. At central venous line insertion, each has recommended hand hygiene and the use of maximal sterile barrier precautions. These precautions include strict compliance with hand washing and wearing a cap, mask, sterile gown, and gloves. Chlorhexidine 2% is recommended for skin preparation during line insertion and change of dressing. Optimal catheter site selection with regard to risk of infection leads to a recommendation that favors the subclavian approach in adults and the femoral approach in many children. Routine line replacement is discouraged. Daily assessment of the continued need for central lines and discontinuation at the earliest opportunity is advocated. When this "central line bundle" has been instituted, favorable results have been noted in children.

All Children's Hospital is a 216-bed freestanding specialty children's hospital in St. Petersburg, Florida. The 46-bed intensive care complex is comprised of a 15-bed pediatric cardiovascular ICU, a 10-bed acute medical-surgical PICU (PICU-1), and a 21-bed transitional PICU (PICU-2). The intensive care complex cares for 2000 children annually. Twenty percent of patients are pre- or postcardiovascular surgery patients, 25% are other surgical subspecialty patients, and 55% are general and subspecialty medical patients. Children who have had heart, kidney, and bone marrow transplantations are cared for routinely, as are children who have congenital and acquired heart disease and those who have general oncologic and neuro-oncologic conditions, congenital and acquired immunodeficiency, sepsis, and other general medical and surgical conditions. Extracorporeal membrane oxygenation, mechanical heart support, intermittent and continuous renal replacement therapy, and a variety of respiratory, cardiac, and neurologic support programs are provided.

In 2003, the central line injection ports were changed to a new vendor hospital wide. Thereafter, an increase in central line–associated blood stream infections was noted. In 2004, multiple national consortia recommended standardized central line insertion and maintenance practices. At All Children's Hospital, in April, 2005 a standardized vascular line insertion bundle (maximal sterile barrier precautions, chlorhexidine 2% skin preparation) was instituted hospital wide. Little change was noted in the rate of central line infections following this change. In December, 2005 needleless injection caps were changed back to a split-septum variety. In January 2006, a standardized central line maintenance bundle was instituted with an education and skills fair. Education, monitoring, and competencies on central venous line dressing, cap changes, and laboratory specimen procurement from central lines was emphasized. The project was supported by an administrative mandate to reduce central line infections by 50% hospital wide, a dedicated infection control coordinator, two PICU nurse educators, the intravenous team, and the combined surgical, anesthesiology, and PICU medical and nursing staffs.

Following education and institution of this central line bundle, catheter-associated bloodstream infections decreased dramatically hospital wide (Fig. 1). Before intervention, the combined PICU (pediatric cardiovascular, acute PICU, and transitional PICU) infection rates were 13.7 per 1000 catheter days. Following the institution and adoption of the central line bundle, the combined infection rate was 4.4 per 1000 catheter days. Similar results were achieved in the neonatal ICU and in the bone marrow transplant unit. Education of new and existing staff as well as compliance monitoring is ongoing.

Ventilator-associated pneumonia

Ventilator-associated pneumonia is defined as pneumonia occurring 48 hours or more after tracheal intubation, which was not incubating at the time of admission. Ventilator-associated pneumonia is a common cause of nosocomial infection in the PICU. Stockwell [44] reported an incidence of 2.9/1000 ventilator days with the highest rates occurring in the population aged 2 to 12 months. Richards and colleagues [44] reported an incidence of 2.9/1000 ventilator days in PICU patients. A greater than fourfold increase in PICU length of stay (27.5 days) was noted in patients who had ventilator-associated pneumonia compared with those who did not (5.9 days). A similar increase in hospital length of stay was noted

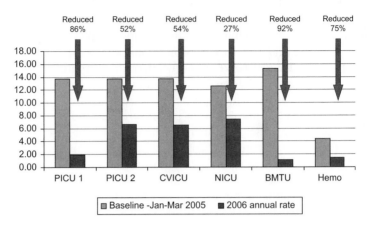

Fig. 1. All Children's Hospital central venous line–associated bloodstream infection rates. Comparison of baseline rates from January through March, 2005, with rates from January through December, 2006, after adoption of central line bundle. BMTU, bone marrow transplant unit; CVICU, pediatric cardiovascular ICU; Hemo, hematology/oncology unit; NICU, neonatal ICU; PICU 1, acute medical/surgical PICU; PICU 2, transitional PICU. (*Data courtesy of* JoEllen Harris, RN, Infection Control Coordinator, All Children's Hospital, St. Petersburg, FL.)

(52.6 days versus 14.8 days). Zar and Cotton [48] reported 73% of all bacterial isolates in pediatric nosocomial pneumoniae were gram-negative bacilli, with *Escherichia coli*, *Klebsiella pneumoniae*, and *Pseudomas aeruginosa* the most prevalent. *P aeruginosa* has been found to be the most prevalent organism in PICU cases of pediatric ventilator-associated pneumonia, accounting for 25.5% and 29.4% of isolates [49,50].

The PICU is an ideal setting for the development of nosocomial pneumonia. The primary risk factor for the development of nosocomial pneumonia is tracheal intubation and mechanical ventilation. Multiple factors favor colonization of the oropharynx and stomach, including administration of antibiotics, admission to the PICU, and underlying chronic lung disease. Factors that favor aspiration of oropharyngeal or refluxed gastric secretions into the respiratory tract include supine placement, the presence of a nasogastric tube, reintubation, immobilization, and surgery of the head, neck, thorax, or upper abdomen. Host factors that favor the development of nosocomial pneumonia include some underlying disease processes, extremes of age, malnutrition, and immunosuppression.

As it did for the prevention of bloodstream infection, the IHI has introduced a bundle of interventions aimed at preventing ventilator-associated pneumonia [45]. These interventions include elevation of the head of the bed, daily sedation holiday and assessment of readiness to extubate the trachea, prophylaxis for peptic ulcer disease, and deep venous thrombosis prophylaxis. Prophylaxis for peptic ulcer disease and for deep venous thrombosis are designed to prevent complications seen in mechanically ventilated patients rather than primarily for the prevention of ventilator-associated pneumonia.

In adults, the change from the supine to semirecumbent position has been shown to contribute to a decrease in the incidence of ventilator-associated pneumonia from 23% to 5% [51]. Also in adults, a sedation holiday until the patient was awake was associated with a reduction in duration of ventilation from 7.3 days to 4.9 days [52]. In the PICU, Deshpande and Curley [53] recommend a variation of the suggested adult regimen for children. This regimen includes strict adherence to hand-washing guidelines, elevation of the head of the bed to at least 30°, monitoring gastric residual every 4 hours, oral cleansing and suctioning the endotracheal tube every 2 hours with hypopharyngeal suctioning before suctioning or repositioning the endotracheal tube, and before repositioning the patient. Additionally, a closed suctioning system is recommended. At Vanderbilt, using these methods, an increase in days before the onset of ventilator-associated pneumonia has been noted [54].

Surgical site infection

Surgical site infection is a frequently preventable cause of PICU morbidity and mortality. In children, surgical site infections complicate 6.6% of surgical procedures [55,56], and 3.2 surgical site infections have been noted per 100 patients undergoing surgery. Among surgical site infections, intra-abdominal infections have been identified more frequently in children older than 2 months of age than in younger children (79/330 [23.9%] versus 8/116 [6.9%]; $P < .001$), and mediastinitis has been noted more commonly in children age 5 years or younger than in older children (44/341 [12.9%] versus 3/105 [2.9%]; $P = .001$) [42]. The NICHQ has targeted cardiac surgery, ventriculoperitoneal shunt procedures, and spinal instrumentation as high-volume surgical procedures in which site infection is costly, catastrophic, and preventable [47]. Site infections have been found in 6.0% of spinal procedures [57], 2.3% of cardiovascular procedures [58], and 3.4% of open-heart procedures [59]. Because surgical site infection sometimes is related to preoperative and operative factors, this parameter may not be simply a reflection of ICU care.

Most preventative strategies for surgical site infection are aimed at the preoperative and operative phase. These strategies include strict adherence to hand-washing guidelines, appropriate preparation of the patient, appropriate and timely use of prophylactic antibiotics, and surgical instrument preparation.

Suggested methods of decreasing surgical site infection once the patient arrives in the ICU include protecting the surgical site for 24 to 48 hours postoperatively with a sterile dressing, use of hand washing and sterile technique during dressing changes, and limiting perioperative prophylactic use of antibiotics to 48 hours [60].

Although studies of the appropriateness of several surgical site prevention bundle measures are available in adults, demonstration of the effectiveness of the application of a bundle in the pediatric population remains
limited.

Airway errors

Protection and maintenance of the natural airway, placement and maintenance of artificial airways, and transition back to the natural airway are
mainstays of pediatric intensive care. Patient instability during maintenance
of the natural airway, during placement of artificial airways, and during
unintended dislodgement of artificial airway may lead to significant, even
life-threatening consequences.

Safe placement of an endotracheal tube in critically ill children is a difficult task for the inexperienced. White and colleagues [61] noted that
although 97% of pediatric housestaff successfully ventilated a mannequin
using a bag-mask, only 53% used the correct bag, and only 80% used the
correct mask size. Only 27% checked that suction functioned before intubation, and the success rate for endotracheal tube placement in a mannequin
was 87%. Nadel and colleagues [62] found that although pediatric house
staff achieved high scores on the standardized pediatric life-support written
test, no resident was able to perform basic and advanced airway maneuvers,
and only 18% performed ancillary airway maneuvers properly. Falck and
colleagues [63] described only a 65% ultimate success rate in neonatal tracheal intubation by pediatric housestaff. Successful tracheal intubation
was achieved on the first or second attempt by only 50% of postgraduate
year 1 (PGY-1) residents, 55% of postgraduate year 2 (PGY-2) residents,
and 62% of postgraduate year 3 (PGY-3) residents. Adams and colleagues
[64] described a higher rate of successful tracheal intubation among pediatric respiratory care practitioners than pediatric housestaff in the interfacility
transport environment. Among emergency medicine staff in the United
States and Canada, Sagarin and colleagues [65] found the pediatric tracheal
intubation success rates by the first attempting physician were as follows:
PGY-1, 80%; PGY 2, 89%; PGY 3, 94%; PGY 4+, 93%; and attending
physician, 98%. Pitetti and colleagues [66] found that for children who presented in prehospital cardiac arrest there was no significant difference in
pediatric survival to hospital discharge between those children managed
with bag-valve-mask devices in the prehospital setting and those who underwent tracheal intubation attempts. This finding, along with recognition of
the significant morbidity and potential lethality of failure to place an endotracheal tube properly, contributed to the American Heart Association's
(AHA) diminishment of the importance of placing an endotracheal tube
as part of the Pediatric Advanced Life Support curriculum. The latest
AHA recommendations include caution that endotracheal intubation may
not be indicated early in pediatric resuscitation and that consideration

should be given to limiting its use to providers who have had adequate training and opportunities to practice and perform tracheal intubations [67].

These studies support the experience with endotracheal intubation in the PICU at All Children's Hospital. In 1994, 52 consecutive children undergoing tracheal intubation were studied. The time from initial laryngoscopy to endotracheal tube placement, the number of separate laryngoscopies during tube placement, the initial and lowest pulse oximeter reading, the initial and lowest heart rate, and practitioner experience were studied. Pediatric house officers successfully placed an endotracheal tube in 11% of laryngoscopic attempts (7 of 64); PICU respiratory therapists were successful in 60% of attempts (30 of 50); and attending physicians were successful in 75% of attempts (15 of 20). Successful tracheal intubation ultimately was achieved by pediatric house officers in 17% of patients attempted (7 of 41), by PICU respiratory therapists in 88% of patients attempted (30 of 34), and by attending physicians in 100% of patients attempted (15 of 15). Strikingly, the incidence of hypoxemia (pulse oximeter reading < 60) during attempts at tracheal intubation by house officers was 83%, and the incidence of bradycardia (heart rate < 60) was 15%. These preliminary findings led to a halt of the study and a change in practice. Subsequently, and especially since a change to in-house attending physician PICU coverage, pediatric tracheal intubation increasingly has been viewed as an attending-level procedure with back-up from the PICU respiratory therapist in the event of an emergency. Pediatric house officers attempt tracheal intubation in the presence of the attending physician, and then only on selected patients.

Unintended tracheal extubation remains a vexing and frequently preventable problem in most ICUs. Children are at increased risk for unintended tracheal extubation because of difficulty in securing the tube, increased oral and nasal secretions, the short intratracheal length of the tube, and difficulties with sedation. Kinking and obstruction of the endotracheal tube occur more frequently in children and may be affected by the relatively heavier weight of ventilator tubing and capnographic equipment.

Age less than 1 year has been identified as a contributing factor for airway events [68]. Scott and colleagues [69] described a 13% incidence of spontaneous tracheal extubation in a PICU and noted four independent risk factors: younger age, increased secretions, degree of endotracheal tube slippage, and increased state of consciousness. Baisch and colleagues [70] described a 4.1% incidence of tracheal extubation failure (endotracheal reintubation within 48 hours of removal) and noted that those who failed were younger than those who tolerated tracheal extubation (median age, 6.5 months versus 21.3 months). Patients who experienced failed extubation had a longer PICU and hospital stay, longer duration of mechanical ventilation, and a higher tracheostomy rate than patients who did not experience failed extubation. Similarly, Edmunds and colleagues [71] described a 4.9% incidence of failed planned tracheal extubation (endotracheal reintubation within 72 hours of removal) and noted that the median age of those who experienced failed extubation was younger than that of patients who tolerated tracheal extubation. The rate of failed extubation was higher (6.0%) among patients whose trachea was intubated for more than 24 hours and was higher still (7.9%) among those whose trachea was intubated for more than 48 hours.

Kurachek and colleagues [72], in a multicenter study, found a tracheal extubation failure rate of 6.2% among 2794 children in PICUs. They described several risk factors for pediatric unintended tracheal extubation: age of 24 months or younger, dysgenetic condition, syndromic condition, chronic respiratory disorder, chronic neurologic condition, medical or surgical airway condition, chronic noninvasive positive pressure ventilation, the need to replace the endotracheal tube on admission to the PICU, and the use of racemic epinephrine, steroids, helium-oxygen therapy (heliox), or noninvasive positive pressure ventilation within 24 hours of extubation. Patients experiencing failed extubation had longer pre-extubation intubation time (failed, 148.7 hours, SD ± 207.8, versus success, 107.9 hours, SD ± 171.3), longer PICU length of stay (17.5 days, SD ± 15.6, versus 7.6 days, SD ± 11.1; $P < .001$), and a higher mortality rate than patients not experiencing failed extubation (4.0% versus 0.8%; $P < .001$).

Descriptions of proven procedures for the prevention of airway events in PICU patients remain limited. At All Children's Hospital, three separate quality improvement efforts targeting reduction of airway events have been undertaken since 1990. Each resulted in PICU-wide systems changes and has led to the current view of each airway event as a seminal event. Each comprehensive study has led to the conclusion that the primary causes of airway events in intubated children are unwanted patient movement, insufficient patient monitoring (human or electronic), inadequate pre-extubation preparation, and inappropriate tracheal tube size, position, or fixation. Attention to each of these underlying causes led to the current PICU "airway bundle" listed in Table 2.

Pediatric ICU staffing

To date, most attention aimed at the identification and reduction of medical error in PICUs has been event driven. Medication errors, laboratory and radiologic errors, nosocomial infections, and airway events are definable and can be attributed to individual patients. Typical remedies involve changes in technology, monitoring, individual patient care, and event-specific education. Frequently, these changes result in increased initial expense and practitioner time. Other, more insidious factors related to PICU design, staffing, and education remain poorly studied. These factors may have a significant effect on overall PICU error and its reduction.

Significant evidence supports the importance of ICU staffing for patient safety and outcome. In adults, Tarnow-Mordi and colleagues [73] have shown a twofold increase in ICU severity-adjusted mortality in patients

Table 2
All Children's Hospital pediatric ICU airway bundle

Cause of targeted airway event	Intervention
Unwanted patient movement	Continuous intravenous sedation for all patients with an endotracheal tube
	Neuromuscular blockade for selected mechanically ventilated patients
	Appropriate use of patient restraints when necessary
	Nurse must be at bedside and respiratory therapist in the pediatric ICU during any radiographic procedure
	No routine patient weights. Patient is weighed only as needed.
Insufficient patient monitoring	Nurse staffing limited to two ventilated patients per nurse
	Grouping of nursing assignments for ventilated patients
	Continuous pulse oximetry of all pediatric ICU patients
	Capnograph immediately available for and used immediately after all tracheal intubations
	Continuous capnography of all pediatric ICU patients who have an endotracheal tube in place
	Transcutaneous partial pressure of CO_2 monitoring of patients receiving high-frequency oscillatory ventilation
	Preference for volume-preset modes of ventilation
	Tidal volume, minute ventilation, and peak inflating pressure alarms checked every hour
Inappropriate tracheal tube size, location, or fixation	Measure airway leak pressure every shift per respiratory therapy protocol
	Notify pediatric ICU attending physician when leak pressure > 40 cm H_2O
	Assess endotracheal tube position using cm marking and breath sounds every shift and chest radiograph every morning
	Use cloth tape to fix endotracheal tube position. Affix to skin overlying maxilla and spiral up the endotracheal tube.
Inadequate pre-extubation preparation	Dexamethasone 0.25 mg/kg administered every 8 hours for 24 hours before planned endotracheal tube removal
	Pre-oxygenate with 100% oxygen for 3 minutes before endotracheal tube removal
	Suction endotracheal tube and oropharynx before endotracheal tube removal
	Attending intensivist present in unit at time of endotracheal tube removal

exposed to higher nursing workloads compared with those exposed to a lower nursing workload. Also in adults, Binnekade and colleagues [74] demonstrated that the addition of nurses without specific ICU training decreased nursing-related incidents. This effect was explained primarily by the increase in available nursing time. In neonates, Tucker [75] demonstrated an approximate 50% increase in severity-adjusted neonatal ICU mortality for infants admitted when the unit was at full capacity versus those admitted when the unit was at half capacity. Mortality was raised in all neonatal ICUs with increasing workload. In the United Kingdom, Hamilton and colleagues [76] demonstrated that very low birth weight risk-adjusted mortality was related inversely to the provision of nurses with specific neonatal qualifications. Increasing the ratio of nurses with neonatal qualifications to 1:1 for high-acuity patients decreased risk-adjusted mortality by 48%.

In the PICU, Marcin and colleagues [77] demonstrated a fourfold increase in the odds ratio of unplanned tracheal extubation with a nurse-to-patient ration of 1:2 relative to a nurse-to-patient ratio of 1:1. Ream and colleagues [28] demonstrate a higher risk of unintended tracheal extubation in PICU patients with higher patient/nurse ratios. They also found a higher likelihood of unintended extubation with higher patient acuity/nurse ratios.

Although optimal patient-to-nurse staffing ratios in the PICU remain undefined, the interpolation of adult and neonatal studies, as well as the limited available PICU-specific data, indicates that nursing staffing ratios and patient acuity levels relative to staffing levels can effect the PICU error rate and, ultimately, patient outcome. Although the premise remains untested, if the adult and neonatal ICU experience translates to the PICU, one might infer that optimal nursing staffing ratios are a key factor in ICU error reduction and, ultimately, patient outcome. Although specific data are again limited, practical experience suggests that nursing staffing levels must be weighed against the effect on staff retention and burnout as well as staff availability and cost.

In adult ICUs, Pronovost and colleagues [78] demonstrated a beneficial correlation between high-intensity intensivist staffing (mandatory intensivist consultation or all care directed by an intensivist) when compared with units with low-intensity staffing (no intensivist or elective intensivist consultation). High-intensity staffing was associated with a relative risk of ICU mortality of 0.61 (95% confidence interval, 0.50–0.75) and decreased ICU length of stay. The effect of pediatric intensivists on PICU patient outcome is less well demonstrated. Current high-intensity intensivist staffing of most large PICUs makes an independent analysis of pediatric intensivist effect on outcome difficult.

Other errors and opportunities

If one accepts the premise that suboptimal design, implementation, and integration of PICU systems are, in themselves, medical errors, multiple other areas of concern and their effects on outcome become evident. In the pre-PICU environment, pediatric transport mechanisms may have an effect on ultimate PICU outcome. Pediatric transport teams often have significant PICU team composition and deliver a disproportionate number of children to the PICU. To the extent that transport team management, composition, experience, and deployment times affect PICU outcome, failure to meet optimum transport team goals may be viewed as medical error or

Table 3
Event-specific and systems factor areas for improvement of pediatric ICU outcomes

Medical error	Intervention
Medication prescription	Computerized provider order entry
	Clinical pharmacist
Medication admixture	Automated parenteral alimentation admixture
	Standardized medication infusion concentration
Medication administration	Provider education
	Double checks
	Limiting floor stock
	Use of "smart pumps"
Laboratory error	Automating patient identification
	Point-of-care testing
Radiologic error	Automating patient identification
	Point-of-care testing
	Enhance radiologist feedback mechanisms and timeliness
Nosocomial bloodstream infection	Institute IHI, CHCA, NICHQ bundle items
Nosocomial ventilator-associated pneumonia	Institute IHI, CHCA, NICHQ bundle items
Surgical site infection	Hand washing
	Sterile dressing changes
	Limit duration of postoperative prophylactic antibiotics
Airway events	Institute airway bundle (see Table 2)
Staffing	Optimize patient-to-nurse ratio
	High-intensity pediatric intensivist staffing
Other	Study effect of pediatric transport team on pediatric ICU outcome
	Study effect of institutional commitment to quality on pediatric ICU outcome
	Study the impact of specific nurse training programs on pediatric ICU outcome
	Study effect of dedicated quality control personnel on pediatric ICU outcome

Abbreviations: CHCA, Child Health Corporation of America; IHI, Institute for Health care Improvement; NICHQ, National Initiative for Children's Health care Quality.

opportunity for improvement. Other even more insidious aspects of quality improvement or error reduction remain unexplored. Among these are the degree of institutional commitment to quality assurance, the impact of specific nurse training programs, and the effectiveness of dedicated quality control personnel. Formal studies of these factors, although largely unavailable at present, may reveal significant effects on error reduction.

Summary

The complexity of patient care and the potential for medical error make the PICU environment a key target for improvement of outcomes in hospitalized children. To date, several event-specific errors as well as proven and potential solutions have been described (Table 3). Analysis of pediatric intensive care staffing, education, and administration systems, although a less "traditional" manner of thinking about medial error, may reveal further opportunities for improved PICU outcome.

References

[1] Holmes O. The contagiousness of puerperal fever. The Harvard classics. Vol. 38, Part 5. New York: P.F. Collier & Son; 1909–14.
[2] DeCosta C. The contagiousness of childbed fever: a short history of puerperal sepsis and its treatment. Med J Aust 2002;177(11/12):668–71.
[3] Raju TN. Ignaz Semmelweis and the etiology of fetal and neonatal sepsis. J Perinatol 1999; 19(4):307–10.
[4] Trick W, Vernon M, Welbel S, et al. Multicenter intervention program to increase adherence to hand hygiene recommendations and glove use and to reduce the incidence of antimicrobial resistance. Infect Control Hosp Epidemiol 2007;28(1):42–9.
[5] Perlstein PH, Callison C, White M, et al. Errors in drug computations during newborn intensive care. Am J Dis Child 1979;133(4):376–9.
[6] Schollenberg E, Albritton W. Antibiotic misuse in a pediatric teaching hospital. Can Med Assoc J 1980;122(1):49–52.
[7] Tisdale J. Justifying a pediatric critical-care satellite pharmacy by medication-error reporting. Am J Hosp Pharm 1986;43(2):368–71.
[8] Brennan T, Leape L, Laird N, et al. Incidence of adverse events and negligence in hospitalized patients. Results of the Harvard Medical Practice Study I. N Engl J Med 1991;324(6):370–6.
[9] Thomas E, Studdert D, Burstin H, et al. Incidence and types of adverse events and negligent care in Utah and Colorado. Med Care 1999;38(3):261–71.
[10] Wilson R, Runciman W, Gibberd B, et al. The quality in Australian healthcare study. Med J Aust 1995;163(9):458–71.
[11] National Health Service. Report of an expert group on learning from adverse events in the NHS chaired by the Chief Medical Officer. An organization with a memory. Available at: http://www.doh.gov.uk/orgmemreport/index.htm. Accessed October 15, 2007.
[12] Kohn L, Corrigan J, Donaldson M, Institute of Medicine (U.S.) Committee on Quality of Health Care in America. To err is human: building a safer health system. Washington, DC: National Academy Pr.; 2000.
[13] Sox H, Woloshin S. How many deaths are due to medical error? Getting the number right. Eff Clin Pract 2006;6:277–83.
[14] Clancy T. Medication error prevention. Progress on initiatives. JONAS Healthc Law Ethics Regul 2004;6(1):3–12.
[15] Meyer G, Battles J, Hart J, et al. The US Agency for Healthcare Research and Quality's activities in patient safety research. Int J Qual Health Care 2003;15(Suppl 1):i25–30.
[16] Rapp C, Putz J, Strickland S. Prevention of medical errors. Available at: http://www.fmaonline.org/education/onlinecme/premederrors.pdf. Accessed October 15, 2007.
[17] Krein S, Hofer T, Kowalski C, et al. Use of central venous catheter-related bloodstream infection prevention practices by US hospitals. Mayo Clin Proc 2007;82(6):672–8.
[18] Albuali W, Singh R, Fraser D, et al. Have changes in ventilation practice improved outcome in children with acute lung injury. Pediatr Crit Care Med 2007;8(4):324–30.
[19] Tsuchida T, Makimoto K, Toki M, et al. The effectiveness of a nurse-initiated intervention to reduce catheter-associated bloodstream infections in an urban acute hospital: an intervention study with before and after comparison. Int J Nurs Stud 2006; [Epub ahead of print].

[20] Warren D, Cosgrove S, Diekema D, et al, Prevention Epicenter Program. A multicenter intervention to prevent catheter-associated bloodstream infections. Infect Control Hosp Epidemiol 2006;27(7):662–9 [Epub 2006 Jun 9].

[21] Stambouly J, McLaughlin L, Mandel F, et al. Complications of care in a pediatric intensive care unit: a prospective study. Intensive Care Med 1996;22:1098–104.

[22] Larson G, Donaldson A, Parker H, et al. Preventable harm occurring to critically ill children. Pediatr Crit Care Med 2007;8(4):331–6.

[23] Kaushal R, Bates D, Landrigan C, et al. Medication errors and adverse drug events in pediatric inpatients. JAMA 2001;285:2114–20.

[24] Fernandez C, Gillis-Ring J. Strategies for the prevention of medical error in pediatrics. J Pediatr 2003;143:155–62.

[25] Fortenberry J. Making the pediatric intensive care unit a safe haven. Pediatr Crit Care Med 2007;8(2 Suppl):S1–2.

[26] Sowan A, Gaffoor M, Soeken K, et al. A comparison of medication administration errors using CPOE orders vs. handwritten orders for pediatric continuous drug infusions. AMIA Annu Symp Proc 2006;1:1105.

[27] Milliken J, Tait G, Ford-Jones L, et al. Nosocomial infections in a pediatric intensive care unit. Crit Care Med 1988;16(3):233–7.

[28] Ream R, Mackey K, Leet T, et al. Association of nursing workload and unplanned extubation in a pediatric intensive care unit. Pediatr Crit Care Med 2007;8(4):366–71.

[29] Potts A, Barr F, Gregory D, et al. Computerized physician order entry and medication errors in a pediatric critical care unit. Pediatrics 2004;113(1):59–63.

[30] Holdsworth M, Fichtl R, Behta M, et al. Incidence and impact of adverse drug events in pediatric inpatients. Arch Pediatr Adolesc Med 2003;157:60–5.

[31] Institute for Safe Medication Practices. ISMP's list of high alert medications. Available at: http://www.ismp.org/Tools/highalertmedications.pdf. Accessed October 15, 2007.

[32] Vaidya V, Sowan A, Maills M, et al. Evaluating the safety and efficiency of a CPOE system for continuous medication infusions in a pediatric ICU. AMIA Annu Symp Proc 2006;1128.

[33] Vardi A, Efrati O, Matok I, et al. Prevention of potential errors in resuscitation medication orders by means of a computerized physician order entry in pediatric critical care. Resuscitation 2007;73:400–6.

[34] Apkon M, Leonard J, Probst L, et al. Design of a safer approach to intravenous drug infusions: failure mode effects analysis. Qual Saf Health Care 2004;13:265–71.

[35] Roman N. Standardized concentrations facilitate the use of continuous infusions for pediatric intensive care unit at a community hospital. Dimens Crit Care Nurs 2005;24(6):275–8.

[36] White J, Veltri M, Fackler J. Preventing adverse event is the pediatric intensive care unit: prospectively targeting factors that lead to intravenous potassium chloride errors. Pediatr Crit Care Med 2005;6(1):25–31.

[37] Leape L, Cullen D, Clapp M, et al. Pharmacist participation on physician rounds and adverse drug events in the intensive care unit. JAMA 1999;282:267–70.

[38] Costello J, Torowicz D, Yeh T. Effects of a pharmacist-led pediatrics medication safety team on medication-error reporting. Am J Health Syst Pharm 2007;64:1422–6.

[39] American Academy of Pediatrics Committee on Hospital Care and Pediatric Section of the Society of Critical Care Medicine. Guidelines and level of care for pediatric intensive care units. Pediatrics 2004;114:1114–25.

[40] Kalra J. Medical errors: impact on clinical laboratories and other critical areas. Clin Biochem 2004;37:1052–62.

[41] Kavsak P, Zielinski N, Patrick D, et al. Challenges of implementing point-of-care (POCT) glucose meters in a pediatric acute care setting. Clin Biochem 2004;37:811–7.

[42] Brown RB, Stechenberg B, Sands M, et al. Infections in a pediatric intensive care unit. Am J Dis Child 1987;141(3):267–70.

[43] Richards M, Edwards J, Culver D, et al. Nosocomial infections in pediatric intensive care units in the United States. Pediatrics 1999;103:1–7.

[44] Stockwell J. Nosocomial infections in the pediatric intensive care unit: affecting the impact on safety and outcome. Pediatr Crit Care Med 2007;8(2):S21–37.

[45] Institute for Healthcare Improvement. Available at: http://www.ihi.org/IHI/Topics/Critical Care/IntensiveCare/Changes/. Accessed October 15, 2007.

[46] Child Health Corporation of America. Available at: http://www.chca.com/index_flash. html. Accessed October 15, 2007.

[47] National Initiative for Children's Healthcare Quality (NICHQ). Available at: http://www. nichq.org/nichq. Accessed October 15, 2007.

[48] Zar H, Cotton M. Nosocomial pneumonia in pediatric patients. Paediatr Drugs 2002;4(2): 73–83.

[49] Urrea M, Pons M, Serra M, et al. Prospective incidence of nosocomial infections in a pediatric intensive care unit. Pediatr Infect Dis J 2003;22:490–4.

[50] Elward A, Warren K, Fraser V. Ventilator-associated pneumonia in pediatric intensive care patients. Pediatrics 2002;109:758–64.

[51] Drakulovic M, Torres A, Bauer T, et al. Supine body position as a risk factor for nosocomial pneumonia in mechanically ventilated patients: a randomised trial. Lancet 1999;354:1851–8.

[52] Kress J, Rubin A, Pohlman A, et al. Daily interruption of sedative infusions in critically ill patients undergoing mechanical ventilation. N Engl J Med 2000;342:1471–7.

[53] Deshpande J, Curley M. Reducing morbidity and mortality from ventilator associated pneumonia. Available at: http://www.chca.com/mm/webcasts/2005/20050720_vap_webcast.pdf. Accessed October 15, 2007.

[54] Curley MA, Schwalenstocker E, Deshpande JK, et al. Tailoring the Institute for Health Care Improvement 100,000 Lives Campaign to pediatric settings: the example of ventilator-associated pneumonia. Pediatr Clin North Am 2006;53(6):1231–51.

[55] Uludag O, Rieu P, Niessen M, et al. Incidence of surgical site infections in pediatric patients: a 3-month prospective study in an academic pediatric surgical unit. Pediatr Surg Int 2000; 16(5-6):417–20.

[56] Muhlemann K, Franzini C, Aebi C, et al. Prevalence of nosocomial infections in Swiss children's hospitals. Infect Control Hosp Epidemiol 2004;25:765–71.

[57] Labbé AC, Demers AM, Rodrigues R, et al. Surgical-site infection following spinal fusion: a case-control study in a children's hospital. Infect Control Hosp Epidemiol 2003;24(8): 591–5.

[58] Allpress AL, Rosenthal GL, Goodrich KM, et al. Risk factors for surgical site infections after pediatric cardiovascular surgery. Pediatr Infect Dis J 2004;23(3):231–4.

[59] Nateghian A, Taylor G, Robinson JL. Risk factors for surgical site infections following open-heart surgery in a Canadian pediatric population. Am J Infect Control 2004;32(7): 397–401.

[60] Kato Y, Shime N, Hashimoto S, et al. Effects of controlled perioperative antimicrobial prophylaxis on infectious outcomes in pediatric cardiac surgery. Crit Care Med 2007; 35(7):1763–8.

[61] White JR, Shugerman R, Brownlee C, et al. Performance of advanced resuscitation skills by pediatric housestaff. Arch Pediatr Adolesc Med 1998;152(12):1232–5.

[62] Nadel FM, Lavelle JM, Fein JA, et al. Assessing pediatric senior residents' training in resuscitation: fund of knowledge, technical skills, and perception of confidence. Pediatr Emerg Care 2000;16(2):73–6.

[63] Falck AJ, Escobedo MB, Baillargeon JG, et al. Proficiency of pediatric residents in performing neonatal endotracheal intubation. Pediatrics 2003;112(6 Pt 1):1242–7.

[64] Adams K, Scott R, Perkin RM, et al. Comparison of intubation skills between interfacility transport team members. Pediatr Emerg Care 2000;16(1):5–8.

[65] Sagarin MJ, Barton ED, Chng YM, et al. Airway management by US and Canadian emergency medicine residents: a multicenter analysis of more than 6,000 endotracheal intubation attempts. Ann Emerg Med 2005;46(4):328–36.

[66] Pitetti R, Glustein JZ, Bhende MS. Prehospital care and outcome of pediatric out-of-hospital cardiac arrest. Prehosp Emerg Care 2002;6(3):283–90.

[67] Highlights of the 2005 American Heart Association guidelines for cardiopulmonary and emergency cardiovascular care. Currents in emergency cardiovascular care. American Heart Association 2005;16(4):19.

[68] Needham D, Thompson D, Holzmueller C, et al. A system factor analysis of airway events from the Intensive Care Unit Safety Reporting System (ICUSRS). Crit Care Med 2004; 32(11):2227–33.

[69] Scott P, Eigen H, Moye L, et al. Predictability and consequences of spontaneous extubation in a pediatric ICU. Crit Care Med 1985;13(4):228–32.

[70] Baisch SD, Wheeler WB, Kurachek SC, et al. Extubation failure in pediatric intensive care. Incidence and outcomes. Pediatr Crit Care Med 2005;6(3):312–8.

[71] Edmunds S, Weiss I, Harrison R. Extubation failure in a large pediatric ICU population. Chest 2001;119(3):897–900.

[72] Kurachek SC, Newth CJ, Quasney MW, et al. Extubation failure in pediatric intensive care: a multiple-center study of risk factors and outcomes. Crit Care Med 2003;31(11):2657–64.

[73] Tarnow-Mordi WO, Hau C, Warden A, et al. Hospital mortality in relation to staff workload: a 4-year study in an adult intensive-care unit. Lancet 2000;356(9225):185–9.

[74] Binnekade JM, Vroom MB, de Mol BA, et al. The quality of intensive care nursing before, during, and after the introduction of nurses without ICU-training. Heart Lung 2003;32(3): 190–6.

[75] Tucker J. Patient volume, staffing, and workload in relation to risk-adjusted outcomes in a random stratified sample of UK neonatal intensive care units: a prospective evaluation. Lancet 2002;359(9301):99–107.

[76] Hamilton KE, Redshaw ME, Tarnow-Mordi W. Nurse staffing in relation to risk-adjusted mortality in neonatal care. Arch Dis Child Fetal Neonatal Ed 2007;92(2):F99–103 [Epub 2006 Nov 6].

[77] Marcin JP, Rutan E, Rapetti PM, et al. Nurse staffing and unplanned extubation in the pediatric intensive care unit. Pediatr Crit Care Med 2005;6(3):254–7.

[78] Pronovost PJ, Angus DC, Dorman T, et al. Physician staffing patterns and clinical outcomes in critically ill patients: a systematic review. JAMA 2002;288(17):2151–62.

ELSEVIER
SAUNDERS

PEDIATRIC CLINICS

OF NORTH AMERICA

Pediatr Clin N Am 55 (2008) 779–790

Parent Satisfaction in the Pediatric ICU

Jos M. Latour, RN, MSN[a],*,
Johannes B. van Goudoever, MD, PhD[b],
Jan A. Hazelzet, MD, PhD, FCCM[c]

[a]Department of Pediatrics, Division of Pediatric Intensive Care, Erasmus MC – Sophia
Children's Hospital, Sp 1539, P.O. Box 2060, 3000 CB Rotterdam, The Netherlands
[b]Department of Pediatrics, Division of Neonatology, Erasmus MC – Sophia Children's
Hospital, Sp-3432, P.O. Box 2060, 3000 CB Rotterdam, The Netherlands
[c]Department of Pediatrics, Division of Pediatric Intensive Care, Erasmus MC – Sophia
Children's Hospital, Sk-3228, P.O. Box 2060, 3000 CB Rotterdam, The Netherlands

Various strategies and models have been developed to improve the quality of health care. Initiatives such as evidence-based medicine and evidence-based nursing [1,2], quality improvement circles [3], and clinical performance indicators [4] have been found valuable. Less attention has been given to the empowerment of patients and families as a means of increasing health care standards based on their needs.

Despite the efforts to improve quality in health care, the American Institute of Medicine (IOM) identified six areas in today's health care system that still are below standard: safety, effectiveness, timeliness, patient centeredness, efficiency, and equity [5]. A major challenge for health care workers is putting patients in the center of care, giving them autonomy, and accepting them as partners in care. Professionals therefore need to find methods to empower patients. In pediatric intensive care most children may be unable to express their needs and experiences. Here the experiences of parents are recognized as being fundamental for the definition of quality [6]. In this perspective the principles of family-centered care mandate incorporation of parents in daily care. Subsequently, measures of parent satisfaction become a valuable tool in establishing a family-centered and parent-driven care model that would benefit quality of care.

Satisfaction surveys are suggested to be relevant for patient-driven care models [7]. Although patient satisfaction is studied widely in various medical services, most surveys take a medical or nursing perspective rather than

* Corresponding author.
 E-mail address: j.latour@erasmusmc.nl (J.M. Latour).

0031-3955/08/$ - see front matter © 2008 Elsevier Inc. All rights reserved.
doi:10.1016/j.pcl.2008.02.013   *pediatric.theclinics.com*

focusing on the patients' needs and experiences. Thus, parental input in developing a comprehensive pediatric ICU (PICU) satisfaction survey is indispensable [8]. Action for rigorous assessment of parent's needs and experiences of the perceived care and consequently the integration of their views in satisfaction surveys is warranted. So far, only a few studies have demonstrated this method [9,10]. This article analyzes and discusses a parental satisfaction framework for action toward quality improvement in pediatric intensive care by parental empowerment through the use of parent satisfaction measures.

Method

The authors performed a PubMed literature search focusing on three themes: parent satisfaction; parental needs and experiences; and family-centered care. For parent satisfaction and family-centered care a time limit was set between January 1990 and June 2007. No time limit was used for parental needs, because the authors were aware of some relevant references published before 1990. Search terms for parent satisfaction and parental needs were "parent(s)," "satisfaction," "pediatric," "intensive care," "needs," and "experience(s)". Search terms for family-centered care were "respect," "information," "education," "coordination of care," "physical," "emotional," "involvement," "parents," and "family-centered care." Besides these terms, all searches included the term "quality." References of the identified articles were screened to account for omissions in the electronic search. The literature on family-centered care provided particularly extensive references. For the purpose of this article, only key references supporting the rationale of the framework are used.

Family-centered care

The principles of family-centered care in the PICU should be grounded in collaborative relationships between health care professionals and parents. Six domains have been identified in the literature [5,11,12]:

- Respect
- Information and education
- Coordination of care
- Physical support
- Emotional support
- Involvement of parents

These domains relate to the roles of the professionals and the parents. Although the principles of family-centered care are well known by health care professionals, current practice seems not to be consistent with these concepts [13,14]. Evidence demonstrates that health care professionals find it difficult to build up a relationship with the family or parents and to meet their needs [15]. PICU physicians and nurses need to develop interventions to improve family-centered care [16].

Respect

The global attention to equity in health care for all children and parents has increased awareness of the need to safeguard the outcome of critically ill children and the well being of the parents unrelated to their background. Inconsistencies in the unequivocal approach to children and parents are related to discrimination in health care access and treatment based on personal characteristics [4,17]. A recent study in the United States provides data that children from ethnic minorities experience significant difficulties in accessing health care compared with white children [18]. National insurance policies often are to blame for this discrepancy. In Europe, the health care systems provide access to medical treatments for all children. Health care professionals, however, need to be aware of the needs and preferences of each individual child and its parents, regardless of their ethnic background and beliefs [19,20]. Respect and understanding must come from knowledge of different cultural and religious perspectives.

Information and education

Providing information and education to parents is a major challenge for professionals. It is within the realm of information where professionals and parents come together and collaborate in the care of the critically ill child. Effective and understandable communication between parents and professionals benefits the child, decreases parental stress and anxiety levels, and is the basis for trust [21,22]. Increasing attention is paid to interventions aimed at improving communication. Most intervention studies, however, originate from neonatology, general pediatrics, and anesthesiology; contributions from pediatric intensive care still are scarce.

Coordination of care

PICUs by nature are mostly transitional units. The critically ill child usually is admitted from an emergency department or a pediatric ward. Discharge often is planned to a pediatric ward. Transfers must be coordinated carefully between services. Transitional care, however, also encompasses other aspects, such as consultations, procedures, tests, and basic daily care. For parents, these processes become clear only when communication by the professionals is timely and accurate. Documented effective interventions to improve admission or discharge planning in PICU settings are limited [23].

Physical support

By nature, parents are concerned about their child's pain and comfort. The child's pain and discomfort may influence parental stress. In a multicenter study, parents reported that their infants had experienced more pain than they had expected; they also worried about the long-term effects of pain [24]. These worries were predictors of increased parental stress levels. Although validated pain and comfort assessment instruments are available in the PICU [25,26], professionals may not always be willing to use these instruments in daily practice. Improving the attitude of the health care professionals might benefit the recovery of the critically ill child and enhance parental well being.

Emotional support

Symptoms of traumatic stress are common among parents of PICU patients and may persist long after discharge [27]. The pioneering work of Carter and Miles [28], who developed and tested the Parental Stressor Scale: PICU, has contributed much to the identification of parental stress and coping strategies. The instrument was designed to measure the overall parental stress response during the admission of their child in the PICU. The 37 items were grouped in seven dimensions (Box 1). Despite many studies examining parental stress, effective interventions to reduce stress are limited in scope. In a randomized, controlled trial, the Creating Opportunities for Parent Empowerment (COPE) program, an educational-behavioral intervention, was tested on its positive effects on coping up to 12 months after hospital

---

Box 1. Dimensions of the Parental Stressor Scale: pediatric ICU

Child's appearance
Descriptions of the child's appearance (three items)
Sights and sounds
Alarms of equipment and surroundings near the child (three items)
Procedures
Tests and procedures that may have been done (six items)
Staff behavior
Behavior of physicians and nurses as experienced by parents (four items)
Alterations in parental role
Parents' perception of being unable to care for the child (six items)
Staff communication
How physicians and nurses communicate with the parents (five items)
Child's behavior and emotions
Behavioral and emotional responses of the child (10 items)

discharge [29]. The 87 mothers in the COPE group reported significantly less stress after the child was transferred from the PICU to the pediatric ward than the 76 mothers in the control group. Symptoms of depression also were significantly fewer in the COPE group 1 and 6 months after discharge. After 12 months the mothers in the COPE group reported significantly fewer posttraumatic stress disorders. These findings suggest that parenting programs may be valuable in long-term improvement of children's and parents' mental health after PICU admission. A systematic review of 26 parenting programs in pediatrics provides data covering mainly short-term effects [30]. Most programs are effective and seem to contribute significantly to the psychosocial health of the mothers.

Involvement of parents

PICUs provide open visiting hours, participation in care, parental presence during invasive procedures, and involvement in (critical) decision making, and some units even allow parental presence during medical rounds. The focus is on reaching partnership between PICU professionals and parents. The current multicultural changes in societies require health care professionals to be aware of the cultural diversity of the functioning family [16].

Despite the general agreement on the dimensions of family-centered care, evidence suggests that nurses may find it difficult to build up a relationship with parents and to meet their needs [31]. Physicians also need to invest in providing support to parents. As suggested by Azoulay and Sprung [32], assessment of intervention outcomes in family members would elucidate the extent to which family-centered care matches family expectations.

Family-centered care in the PICU setting is not a new concept, but there still is room for improvement. Knowledge of parental needs and perceived care is essential to achieve improvement. Parent satisfaction surveys that include a core set of items related to the dimensions of family-centered care eventually might provide interventions to improve family-centered care.

Parental needs and experiences

Pediatric intensive care staff should take a leading role by changing their attitudes, gaining in-depth understanding of parents' experiences, and acting on the parental needs. Parental needs in the PICU setting have been studied by various methods. The quantitative studies on this subject [33–36] used modified versions of the 45-item Critical Care Family Needs Inventory, originating from the adult intensive care setting [37]. The rankings of top 20 needs do not differ extensively among these studies (Table 1). Although the intensive care settings focus predominantly on the critically ill child's health status, the interpersonal interactions should be taken into account to meet the needs and preferences of both the child and parents. These studies have a few possible limitations. First, they generally leave out

Table 1
Ranking top 20 needs of parents in pediatric intensive care

Need	Ranking[a] Kirschbaum [35] 41 parents	Farrell and Frost [33] 27 parents	Fisher [34] 15 mothers 15 fathers	Scott [36] 21 mothers
Knowing how child is treated medically	1	3	4	1
Feeling there is hope	1	6	2	n.m.
Assured the best possible care is given	1	5	6	1
Knowing specific facts concerning progress	2	n.m.	4	n.m.
Having questions answered honestly	2	1	4	1
Knowing exactly what is being done	2	n.m.	5	n.m.
Being called at home about changes	3	1	5	1
Feeling the personnel care about my infant	3	n.m.	5	1
Knowing the prognosis/ outcome	4	2	1	1
Receive information once a day	4	n.m.	5	2
Knowing what is wrong with the child	n.m.	1	n.m.	n.m.
Understandable explanations	7	3	n.m.	n.m.
Talking with the doctor	9	4	6	n.m.
Talking with the nurse	20	5	n.m.	n.m.
Have a nurse with me at the bedside	n.m.	5	n.m.	n.m.
Knowing why things were done for the child	5	n.m.	2	n.m.
Knowing the child is being treated for pain and/or is comfortable	n.m.	n.m.	2	n.m.
Knowing the child may still be able to hear me if she/he is not awake	n.m.	n.m.	3	n.m.
Seeing the child frequently	6	n.m.	4	1
To visit at any time	8	n.m.	n.m.	1

Abbreviation: n.m, not mentioned.
[a] Ranking numbers can appear more than once because they have the same values in the results (mean or percentages).

multicultural issues and differences among the parents. These omissions could affect the identification of issues important for individual parent-centered care. Second, these studies date from the 1990s. Parental needs and preferences might have changed since then. Items related to the provision of information have ranked high over the years, however (see Table 1). Finally, Noyes [38] raised methodologic issues regarding the validity of the instruments, sample sizes, and the defined variables. It was suggested that the questionnaires used were inadequate to explore the parents' experiences. Indeed, although needs and experiences are two related concepts, different strategies should be used to explore each of them.

Several studies focused on parents' experiences during admission. A recent study interviewed 20 parents whose children had been hospitalized, either in the PICU (n = 11) or in the pediatric ward (n = 9) [39]. Experiences explored regarded illness onset, actual admission, stay, and the discharge process. In the PICU group, parents were less reassured at admission because of the child's severity of illness and the start of medical interventions. Interaction with the medical team during the PICU stay was a barrier for some parents and could turn into a source of stress and anxiety. Minor failings in the PICU discharge process generated a greater anxiety in the parents, although parents generally were satisfied with the aftercare by the pediatric outpatient departments. Similar findings were found in a study among fathers who had a child in the PICU (n = 15) and in a general pediatric ward (n = 10) using two stressor scales to identify specific sources of stress and stress symptoms [40]. Fathers whose children were in the PICU reported the technical procedures on the child and the parental role as most stressful to them. Surprisingly, professional staff communication was experienced as less stressful. These findings differ from the previous study [39], showing that parents who had children in the PICU were less content with the provision of information during admission and at discharge. These contrasting findings might result from differences in PICU environment and staff. Therefore, every PICU should assess carefully its own professional approaches toward parental guidance.

Combining the findings from the parental needs studies with those of the parental experiences studies may instill a fundamental understanding of means to ensure the empowerment of parents in critical care settings. Parent satisfaction measures based on both the needs and experiences of parents could provide comprehensive results that eventually might steer the professionals toward family-centered care improvement.

Framework for action

The PICU is a complex setting, particularly for the child and parents. Professionals involved in PICU probably do their utmost to provide the child and parents a safe passage through this critical period. Whether these efforts are well received by the parents usually is not documented. It is not known whether many PICUs measure parental satisfaction. So far, only two satisfaction studies have documented how parents perceive PICU care [9,10]. Both studies developed a parent satisfaction questionnaire based on literature reviews, parent consultation, and multidisciplinary input. Despite this rigorous instrument development, a gap remains between a framework and assumptions on the research topic. Furthermore, Haines and Childs [10] found the tool developed by McPherson and colleagues [9] insufficient in covering all areas of their PICU service. They therefore developed their own instrument for local use. Based on the results of the satisfaction survey of 110 families, Haines and Childs were able to identify strategies to optimize the service (Box 2).

Patient centeredness in particular focuses on the patient's experience and perceived care. The uniqueness of the PICU, with parents serving as proxies for their critically ill child, necessitates a clear distinction between the concepts of patient centeredness and family-centered care. The domains of family-centered care, as described previously, have in common the IOM goals of time, equity, effectiveness, efficiency, and safety. The synergy of these aims within family-centered care provides this concept with a comprehensive basis for health care improvement.

Family-centered care, parental needs, and parental experiences seem to be the core concepts that reflect the nature of multidisciplinary care for parents in the PICU. Extensive work on various care aspects of family-centered care has been done. A recent review identified 43 evidence-based guidelines to support family members in critical care [41]. Because satisfaction usually

---

Box 2. Identified strategies to improve practice by Haines and Childs

- Review timing and opportunities of preadmission visits
- Standardize planned PICU admissions
- Provide assistance for novice PICU nursing staff in bedside support of parents
- Improve communication with parents about unit routines and closure practices
- Improve availability of written communication
- Optimize the role of senior nurses in providing verbal information for parents
- Clarify communication channels when multiple medical teams are involved
- Optimize continuity in nursing allocations
- Improve the preparation of parents for the transition from PICU to wards
- Improve teamwork and communication during the discharge process

---

Data from Haines C, Childs H. Parental satisfaction with paediatric intensive care. Paediatr Nurs 2005;17(7):37–41.

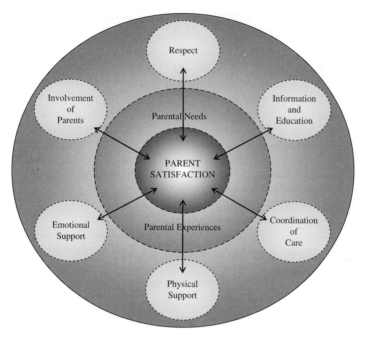

Fig. 1. Framework for parent satisfaction in pediatric intensive care.

was not an outcome variable, the question remains whether these guidelines will be well received by the parents.

The framework shown in the Fig. 1 puts parent satisfaction in the center line, because this concept can include measurable items. Parental needs and experiences are placed in the middle ring, impacting both the outer ring's six domains of family-centered care and the inner circle's parent satisfaction outcomes. During and after a PICU admission, parents build up a certain degree of understanding of the complexity of intensive care. This framework reflects the underlying philosophy of taking the parent's preferences into account. The satisfaction framework provides action toward research that crosses borders between professionals and parents and works toward partnership in pediatric intensive care. Eventually, the results of satisfaction studies need to trigger professionals to develop and test new interventions to meet the needs and preferences of the parents in the PICU.

Summary

The IOM's six aims to improve health care in the twenty-first century provide a useful framework for pediatric intensive care professionals. It is particularly the aim of patient centeredness that encompasses quality of compassion, empathy, and responsiveness to the needs, values, and expressed preferences of the individual patient. For the pediatric intensive care setting this concept can be translated into family-centered care because the parents and the critically ill child constitute one family unit with the right to the best possible care in relation to the best possible outcome for the child and parents.

Incorporating the concept of family-centered care, parental needs, experiences, and parent satisfaction surveys into the development of a parent satisfaction instrument may achieve a fundamental improvement in quality of care based on the empowerment of parents. Parent satisfaction survey can become quality performance indicators and may facilitate the evaluation of quality initiatives.

- The principles of family-centered care are well known but are not consistently implemented into practice.
- Parent satisfaction outcomes are not widely accepted as quality performance indicators.
- Empowerment of parents in the development of parent satisfaction instruments can provide accepted quality performance indicators.
- Measuring parent satisfaction requires involvement and participation of parents as well as partnership between parents and health care professionals.

References

[1] Lang NM. Discipline-based approaches to evidence-based practice: a view from nursing. Jt Comm J Qual Improv 1999;25(10):539–44.
[2] Murillo H, Reece EA, Snyderman R, et al. Meeting the challenges facing clinical research: solutions proposed by leaders of medical specialty and clinical research societies. Acad Med 2006;81(2):107–12.
[3] Wilson T, Berwick DM, Cleary PD. What do collaborative improvement projects do? Experience from seven countries. Jt Comm J Qual Saf 2003;29(2):85–93.
[4] Slonim AD, Pollack MM. Integrating the Institute of Medicine's six quality aims into pediatric critical care: relevance and applications. Pediatr Crit Care Med 2005;6(3):264–9.
[5] Committee on Quality Health Care in America Institute of Medicine. Crossing the quality chasm. a new health system for the 21st century. Washington, DC: National Academy Press; 2001.
[6] Berwick DM. A user's manual for the IOM's 'quality chasm' report. Health Aff (Millwood) 2002;21(3):80–90.
[7] Grol R. Improving the quality of medical care: building bridges among professional pride, payer profit, and patient satisfaction. JAMA 2001;286(20):2578–85.
[8] Latour JM, Hazelzet JA, van der Heijden AJ. Parent satisfaction in pediatric intensive care: a critical appraisal of the literature. Pediatr Crit Care Med 2005;6(5):578–84.
[9] McPherson ML, Sachdeva RC, Jefferson LS. Development of a survey to measure parent satisfaction in a pediatric intensive care unit. Crit Care Med 2000;28(8):3009–13.
[10] Haines C, Childs H. Parental satisfaction with paediatric intensive care. Paediatr Nurs 2005; 17(7):37–41.
[11] Hutchfield K. Family-centered care: a concept analysis. J Adv Nurs 1999;29(5):1178–87.
[12] American Academy of Pediatrics CoHC. Family-centered care and the pediatrician's role. Pediatrics 2003;112(3):691–7.
[13] Latour JM. Is family-centered care in critical care units that difficult? A view from Europe. Nurs Crit Care 2005;10(2):51–3.

[14] Latour JM, Haines C. Families in the ICU: do we truly consider their needs, experiences and satisfaction? Nurs Crit Care 2007;12(4):173–4.

[15] Holden J, Harrison L, Johnson M. Families, nurses and intensive care patients: a review of the literature. J Clin Nurs 2002;11(2):140–8.

[16] Schor EL. Family pediatrics: report of the Task Force on the Family. Pediatrics 2003; 111(6 Pt 2):1541–71.

[17] Flores G, Olson L, Tomany-Korman SC. Racial and ethnic disparities in early childhood health and health care. Pediatrics 2005;115(2):e183–93.

[18] Shi L, Stevens GD. Disparities in access to care and satisfaction among U.S. children: the roles of race/ethnicity and poverty status. Public Health Rep 2005;120(4):431–41.

[19] Bouwhuis CB, Kromhout MM, Twijnstra MJ, et al. [Few ethnic differences in acute pediatric problems: 10 years of acute care in the Sophia Children's Hospital in Rotterdam]. Ned Tijdschr Geneeskd 2001;145(38):1847–51 [in Dutch].

[20] Bengi-Arslan L, Verhulst FC, van der Ende J, et al. Understanding childhood (problem) behaviors from a cultural perspective: comparison of problem behaviors and competencies in Turkish immigrant, Turkish and Dutch children. Soc Psychiatry Psychiatr Epidemiol 1997;32(8):477–84.

[21] Co JP, Ferris TG, Marino BL, et al. Are hospital characteristics associated with parental views of pediatric inpatient care quality? Pediatrics 2003;111(2):308–14.

[22] Studdert DM, Burns JP, Mello MM, et al. Nature of conflict in the care of pediatric intensive care patients with prolonged stay. Pediatrics 2003;112(3):553–8.

[23] Bouve LR, Rozmus CL, Giordano P. Preparing parents for their child's transfer from the PICU to the pediatric floor. Appl Nurs Res 1999;12(3):114–20.

[24] Franck LS, Cox S, Allen A, et al. Parental concern and distress about infant pain. Arch Dis Child Fetal Neonatal Ed 2004;89(1):71–5.

[25] Ista E, van Dijk M, Tibboel D, et al. Assessment of sedation levels in pediatric intensive care patients can be improved by using the COMFORT "behavior" scale. Pediatr Crit Care Med 2005;6(1):58–63.

[26] Lebovits AH, Florence I, Bathina R, et al. Pain knowledge and attitudes of healthcare providers: practice characteristic differences. Clin J Pain 1997;13(3):237–43.

[27] Balluffi A, Kassam-Adams N, Kazak A, et al. Traumatic stress in parents of children admitted to the pediatric intensive care unit. Pediatr Crit Care Med 2004;5(6):547–53.

[28] Carter MC, Miles MS. The Parental Stressor Scale: Pediatric Intensive Care Unit. Matern Child Nurs J 1989;18(3):187–98.

[29] Melnyk BM, Alpert-Gillis L, Feinstein NF, et al. Creating opportunities for parent empowerment: program effects on the mental health/coping outcomes of critically ill young children and their mothers. Pediatrics 2004;113(6):e597–607.

[30] Barlow J, Coren E. Parent-training programmes for improving maternal psychosocial health. Cochrane Database Syst Rev 2004;(1):CD002020.

[31] Petersen MF, Cohen J, Parsons V. Family-centered care: do we practice what we preach? J Obstet Gynecol Neonatal Nurs 2004;33(4):421–7.

[32] Azoulay E, Sprung CL. Family-physician interactions in the intensive care unit. Crit Care Med 2004;32(11):2323–8.

[33] Farrell MF, Frost C. The most important needs of parents of critically ill children: parents' perceptions. Intensive Crit Care Nurs 1992;8(3):130–9.

[34] Fisher MD. Identified needs of parents in a pediatric intensive care unit. Crit Care Nurse 1994;14(3):82–90.

[35] Kirschbaum MS. Needs of parents of critically ill children. Dimens Crit Care Nurs 1990;9(6): 344–52.

[36] Scott LD. Perceived needs of parents of critically ill children. J Soc Pediatr Nurs 1998;3(1): 4–12.

[37] Leske JS. Internal psychometric properties of the Critical Care Family Needs Inventory. Heart Lung 1991;20(3):236–44.

[38] Noyes J. A critique of studies exploring the experiences and needs of parents of children admitted to paediatric intensive care units. J Adv Nurs 1998;28(1):134–41.

[39] Diaz-Caneja A, Gledhill J, Weaver T, et al. A child's admission to hospital: a qualitative study examining the experiences of parents. Intensive Care Med 2005;31(9): 1248–54.

[40] Board R. Father stress during a child's critical care hospitalization. J Pediatr Health Care 2004;18(5):244–9.

[41] Davidson JE, Powers K, Hedayat KM, et al. Clinical practice guidelines for support of the family in the patient-centered intensive care unit: American College of Critical Care Medicine Task Force 2004–2005. Crit Care Med 2007;35(2):605–22.

ELSEVIER
SAUNDERS

Pediatr Clin N Am 55 (2008) 791–804

PEDIATRIC CLINICS
OF NORTH AMERICA

Forgoing Life-Sustaining or Death-Prolonging Therapy in the Pediatric ICU

Denis Devictor, MD, PhD[a],*,
Jos M. Latour, RN, MSN[b], Pierre Tissières, MD[a]

[a]Pediatric Intensive Care, Hôpital de Bicêtre, AP-HP,
Department of Research on Ethics, Paris-Sud 11 University, Bicêtre 94275, France
[b]Division of Pediatric Intensive Care, Department of Pediatrics,
Erasmus MC – Sophia Children's Hospital, Sp 1539,
P.O. Box 2060, 3000 CB Rotterdam, The Netherlands

Advances in pediatric critical care medicine have led to ethical issues of profound concern to all pediatric intensivists and nurses. One of the most striking changes is that most children admitted to a pediatric intensive care unit (PICU) die after a decision is made to withhold or withdraw life-sustaining treatments. Although severity of illness of hospitalized children has progressively increased over the past decades, advanced techniques have allowed such patients to survive. At the same time, it is increasingly accepted that continued aggressive care may not always be beneficial. This notion has given rise to frequent limitation of life-sustaining treatments. Consequently, we have been obliged to expand the mission of pediatric intensive care to include provision of the best possible care to dying children and their families. It is important that all health care professionals in pediatric intensive care be competent in end-of-life decision making and palliative care.

The decision to forgo life-sustaining treatment is made for 20% to 55% of terminally ill children in North American and European PICUs [1–6]. There is a large variability, however, in the modes of death among countries (Table 1) [7–10]. Diverse cultural, religious, philosophic, legal, and professional attitudes may help to explain this variability [9–14]. Differences have been documented in all aspects of decision making, including the practices, the decision makers, and the frequencies of limitations of

---

* Corresponding author.

E-mail address: denis.devictor@bct.ap-hop-paris.fr (D. Devictor).

0031-3955/08/$ - see front matter © 2008 Elsevier Inc. All rights reserved.
doi:10.1016/j.pcl.2008.02.008

Table 1
Mode of death in the pediatric intensive care units (recent data)

First authors	Study	Year	Origin	Number of patients	CPR failure (%)	FLS (%)	DNR order (%)	Brain death (%)
Burns [1]	Retro, MC	2000	Boston	97	30	55	—	15
Devictor [2]	Prosp, MC	2001	France	264	—	40	—	—
Garros [3]	Retro, MC	2003	Toronto	99	27	39	20	13
Althabe [4]	Retro, UC	2003	Argentina	457	52	20	16	11
Devictor [5]	Prosp, MC	2004	North Europe	68	32	47	—	21
Devictor [5]	Prosp, MC	2004	South Europe	282	48	30	—	22
Zawistowski [6]	Retro, UC	2004	Pittsburgh	125	16	40	25	19
Kiper [7]	Retro, MC	2005	Brazil	509	73	18	—	8

Abbreviations: CPR, cardiopulmonary resuscitation; DNR, do not resuscitate; FLS, forgoing life support; MC, multicentric; Prosp, prospective study; Retro, retrospective study; UC, unicenter.

life-sustaining therapies. For example, in a study from North America, the time elapsed from decision to withdraw life-sustaining treatment to actual withdrawal was a median of 30 minutes compared with 2 days in Europe [6,15].

Actually, the most salient international difference touches on the question of who should be responsible for decision making. In North America, parents are the main decision makers, which is in contrast to some European and South American countries, where doctors fulfill this role [7,16,17]. This latter paternalistic attitude is firmly contested, however, by North American intensivists [18,19]. The review of the literature shows that the ethical climate is rapidly evolving and that a convergence of opinion about good practice seems to be developing among professional societies in Europe and in the United States [20,21].

The decision-making process

The decision-making process could be divided into three steps: the deliberation leading to the decision, the implementation of the decision, and the evaluation of the decision and its application. During the deliberation, the caregivers and family consider the pros and cons of medical interventions. Then they come to a decision; in this case, to continue or forgo life-sustaining treatment. Finally, the decision is implemented and its consequences are evaluated. Several guidelines have been published on these different steps [22–27]. In the following sections relevant issues pertaining to these steps are elaborated.

The deliberation leading to the decision

During the deliberation phase, the decision makers weigh the benefits and burdens of medical treatments and take into account numerous factors, some of which are medical, such as factors that influence the prognosis (eg, the cause of the disease). Other factors are organizational, such as professional guidelines, training staff, and communicating with the staff, the patient, and the patient's family. There are factors with regards to patient and family wishes, their religion, and social interaction. Finally, societal factors may interfere, such as cultural background or legal framework. This nonexhaustive list shows that the decision is multifactorial, with the relative importance of each factor being weighed in each individual case.

The decision makers

Controversy persists regarding the roles of parents and physicians in the decision-making process. Schematically, two extreme scenarios are opposed. The first scenario emphasizes that parents—as surrogates of their child—should be the main decision makers [27,28]. The second scenario argues that parents may not have full decision-making capacities when, for example, under pressure as a result of the child's critical illness. In this case, physicians bear the sole responsibility of the final decision. Between these extremes, many countries have adopted the concept of shared decision (Fig. 1). The purpose is to reach consensus on a process that is in accordance with family's values and builds a collaborative relationship with the family. The shared decision paradigm allows for variations in family wishes regarding participation in the decision-making process. This feature points out the crucial role of communication within the health care team and with the family.

In fact, the concept of information and communication remains a central component of the shared decision model. To make decisions for their children, parents must acquire, process, and organize information. Assuming they have appropriate decision-making capacity, parents need clear

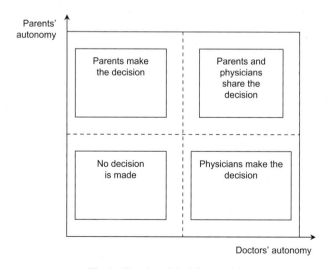

Fig. 1. The shared decision model.

information from the doctors about their child's condition, prognosis, and alternative treatments. Ethical and legal considerations require that the information be understandable and transparent. Regrettably, research suggests that physicians routinely overestimate what patients and family members understand [29,30]. Should a physician use excessive medical jargon or the child or family be ignorant of basic medical concepts, good understanding is unlikely. Similarly, parents may not fully comprehend what is said when struck by the realization that their child is severely ill. There may be only limited time to consider alternatives. Time limitations might influence the decision and invalidate full consent.

Parents' perspectives

Factors that influence parents' decisions are their possible previous experiences with death and end-of-life decision making for others, personal observations of their child's suffering, perceptions of their child's will to survive, their need to protect and advocate for their child, and the family's financial resources and concerns regarding life-long care [31]. Meyer and colleagues [32] showed that parents place the highest priorities on quality of life, likelihood of improvement, and perception of their child's pain when considering withdrawal of life support. The recommendations of physicians, the nature of the illness, the expected neurologic recovery, and quality of life are also important to parents when making end-of-life decisions for their child [33]. All these reports underline that establishing trust is crucial in guiding parents through the decision-making process.

Physicians' perspectives

Factors that influence physicians' perspectives mainly regard outcome prediction, the balance between burdens and benefits, and the concept of futility [34,35].

Predicting outcomes. Two scores are available to predict the risk of death for children receiving intensive care: the Pediatric Risk of Mortality (PRISM and PRISM III) and the Pediatric Index of Mortality (PIM and PIM2) [36,37]. Regrettably, both scores have several drawbacks. First, they make predictions based on hospital outcomes at the time of their creation. It seems that they need to be updated as medical treatments improve. Second, they derive their predictions from factors present at admission and do not provide updated mortality estimates as the patient's condition changes. Perhaps the most obvious problem is that they say nothing about morbidity, disability, quality of life, or survival after hospitalization.

The use of published data—an essential tool for clinicians in predicting the course of illness—also has drawbacks. One is that the population studied for a particular illness may not have the same characteristics as an individual patient. Another drawback is the rapidity with which therapies can change and improve.

The balance between burdens and benefits. One of the most commonly used justifications for withholding "high-tech" therapy from patients is the belief that "extraordinary" treatments are not ethically justified. Clinicians should understand that the distinction between ordinary and extraordinary treatments is not considered to be helpful when attempting to reason through the ethical aspects of difficult decisions [38]. A much more legitimate and useful approach to deliberating about whether a procedure is ethically required is to inquire about the benefit–burden balance for a particular procedure in a particular patient. In other words, rather than relying on such terminology as ordinary and extraordinary to decide whether a treatment should be offered, the physician should consider whether the proposed benefits outweigh the burdens. For example, a child's family might accept a 30% chance of survival if it were followed by high quality of life but not accept a 70% chance of survival if it were likely to entail poor quality of life.

The concept of futility. Who should determine that treatment is futile? This question remains largely unresolved for several reasons. First, the concept of futility is difficult to define. In 1990, Schneiderman and colleagues [39] provided the following definition: "When physicians conclude (either through personal experience, experiences shared with colleagues, or consideration of published empiric data) that in the last 100 cases a medical treatment has been useless, they should regard that treatment as futile. If a treatment merely preserves permanent unconsciousness or cannot end dependence on intensive care, the treatment should be considered futile." This definition is highly arguable, however, because each patient's situation is unique and cannot be compared with the 100 previous cases. Opinions on the value of life may differ. For instance, although some individuals may value the preservation of life at all costs, others may conclude that the foreseeable quality of life is so poor that death is the preferred outcome. Others may see hope in a small chance of success ("hoping for a miracle"), whereas others see a prolongation of the dying process. Another definition was provided by the Society for Critical Care Medicine. It states that treatments should be defined as futile only when they will "not accomplish their intended goal" [40]. This definition seems to be more pragmatic and useful.

Nurses' perspectives

The involvement of nurses in end-of-life decisions is crucial [41]. The role of nurses can be described as managing the process and care of the dying child and guiding the parents in these difficult times. Besides the caring components of care, nurses usually build a close relationship with the parents. Having not only expertise but also knowledge of the child's and parents' background, nurses are still not always involved in multidisciplinary end-of-life discussions. In a qualitative study using group interviews, 14 critical care nurses unveiled discrepancies between nursing and medical perspectives and their interactions [42]. The nurses felt that the physicians were more interested in their colleagues' views rather than the nurses' holistic knowledge.

Physicians usually make the ultimate decision on life and death in the ICU. Such a decision always should be based on the complete overview of the patient's status and the family perspectives, however. In this respect it seems logical that nurses should take part in any end-of-life care discussion, even from the first discussion session onwards. Unfortunately, this collaborative practice is often a far cry from reality. For example, a recent survey among nurses and physicians in the adult ICU revealed that nurses reported lower collaboration with physicians, resulting in higher moral distress and less satisfaction with care [43]. In a study from New Zealand among adult, pediatric, and neonatal critical care nurses, 88% of the 611 participating nurses felt that nurses should always be involved in end-of-life decisions [44]. Only 292 (48%) nurses reported that they were always or most of the time involved in the decision-making process. Regardless of who has to make the ultimate end-of-life decision, interdisciplinary collaboration is a must in any preliminary and ongoing discussions toward an end-of-life care decision. Giving all the PICU staff a role in this process can eventually improve the competencies of all professionals and safeguard judicious end-of-life decisions. Consequently, this collaboration benefits the complex care of the dying child and parents.

The implementation of the decision

The second step in the end-of-life decision making process concerns the actions that are taken once a decision has been made to forgo life-sustaining treatments. This issue raises different ethical questions and moral dilemmas.

Withholding and withdrawing life support: are they ethically different?

Is there a difference between stopping a treatment once it is started and not starting it in the first place? In a survey that included 110 physicians and 92 nurses from 31 pediatric hospitals in the United States, the statement that withholding and withdrawing life support is unethical was not endorsed by any of the physicians or nurses [41]. More physicians (78%) than nurses (58%) agreed or strongly agreed that withholding and withdrawing are ethically the same. This survey showed that physicians are much more comfortable with withholding treatments than withdrawing them [41]. The underlying reasoning is psychologic in part. Physicians feel more responsible for the death of a patient when it results from withdrawing a therapy than they do when it results from withholding a therapy.

Nutrition and hydration: are they natural or artificial?

Should techniques for providing medical nutrition and hydration be considered medical treatments? In other words, if it is ethically acceptable to withdraw a ventilator from a terminally ill child, would it also be ethically acceptable to withdraw medically provided nutrition and hydration? A gradually emerging consensus answers these questions in the affirmative [45]. Many clinicians have been reluctant to accept the withdrawal of medical nutrition and hydration, however, at least in part because "feeding" seems to be such a basic and fundamental aspect of the care they provide. Pediatricians have been particularly reluctant to acknowledge this emerging consensus for several reasons [46]. First, prognoses are often more uncertain in children because of their remarkable ability to recover from injury. Second, even healthy newborns need assistance with feedings, so pediatricians are less likely to see artificial feedings as a "medical" treatment. Third, although the hospice experience shows that elderly patients who are dying a natural death often refuse food and water, the death of a child is never a "natural" event, and caregivers are reluctant to accept it with apparent passivity.

Sedatives and analgesics: what is the real intention?

One crucial issue is the doctrine of double effect. This doctrine states that when an action has two effects—one of which is inherently good and the other inherently bad—it can be justified if certain conditions are met. For example, the administration of morphine to a dying patient produces a good effect (relief of pain and suffering) and the potential for a bad effect (hastening the patient's death through respiratory depression). Despite the beliefs of many clinicians, no moral, legal, or religious reasons justify withholding adequate pain relief from dying patients. Pain and suffering always should be treated adequately, even if the treatment results in a foreseen but unintended hastening of death. The key difference between this practice and euthanasia lies in the intention of the physician. When the physician's intention is to hasten the patient's death, then the line between accepted practice and euthanasia is crossed.

The goals of care: where is the border between curative and palliative care?

The clinician's responsibility to the child and family does not end with a decision to forgo life-sustaining treatment but continues throughout the dying process. The emerging perspective is that palliative care and intensive care are not mutually exclusive options but rather should be coexistent [25]. When physicians focus solely on extending the duration of life, as opposed to maximizing the quality of life, their goal can drive futile interventions that prohibit the patient from receiving optimal comfort care. This is especially true when the institution of palliative care is viewed as an abrupt all-or-nothing change from life-prolonging to symptom-oriented care [25,41]. Thinking in terms of the goals of care for an individual patient can aid physicians in discussions with the health care team and the family when making or revising a management plan [25,41]. The question then becomes how to best manage a patient during the dying process. Recommendations on this issue have been published by the Ethics Committee of the Society of Critical Care Medicine [25].

Needs of the dying child and family

Preparation of the patient and family is based on the knowledge of their needs. One can easily imagine the fundamental needs of a dying child, such as being with his or her parents and family, having no pain, having tender loving care, respecting his or her body, and respecting his or her parents' wishes.

Meyer and colleagues [47] recently reported on the specific needs of parents whose children had died after the forgoing of life-sustaining treatment. It seems that in practice, pediatric intensivists do not always satisfy these needs. As an example, 86.5% of parents ($n = 52$) of a dying child agreed or strongly agreed that they had obtained information regarding their child's condition, but only 48.1% agreed that they were informed about the persons to whom they could go with their questions [32]. The child and family should know the identity of the attending physician, understand that this individual is ultimately responsible for the care, and be assured of his or her involvement. Most families consider clinicians' communication skills equally or more important than clinical skills.

On that note, the critical care nurse plays a central role in addressing families' needs: she or he is able to explain various treatments the patient is receiving and assess the family's spiritual and cultural needs. Eventually the multidisciplinary team should consider jointly their communications with the parents. Strategies to improve communication with the family have been studied in the adult ICU. A French study implemented an intervention by which ICU staff took more time to converse with the family and provided a bereavement brochure [30]. The intervention group ($n = 56$) was compared with a control group ($n = 52$) approached in the customary way. Persons in the intervention group experienced less stress, anxiety, and depression 3 months after the death of their beloved relative. Similarly, meeting the parental needs and giving enough time to parents to express their emotions might help them cope with the loss of their child.

Family-centered care

Family-centered care is an approach to the planning, delivery, and evaluation of health care that is grounded in mutually beneficial partnerships among health care providers, patients, and families [48,49]. Family is acknowledged as expert in the care of the child, and the perspectives and information provided by the family are important to clinical decision making. This concept is demanding because it means recognizing the family as a constant in the child's life, facilitating collaboration between parents and professionals, sharing complete and unbiased information with families, and satisfying the child's and family's needs. Parents should be viewed as partners in care rather than visitors [49]. Parents are better able to cope when their roles as caregivers are recognized. Still, providing care can be alienating for parents who feel incompetent or too stressed. Parents may feel frightened by their child's appearance or overwhelmed by the technology. Staff, especially nurses, can help delineate the kind of care the parents can provide. Critical care nurses play an essential role in providing and facilitating the communication between health care workers and the family [50]. Parents' participation may be as simple as holding their child's hand. They also can participate more actively, such as by assisting with bathing, positioning, or massage.

Parental presence during medical rounds is encouraged in some institutions. On the other hand, many institutions are concerned that this practice will significantly increase the time spent conducting rounds and disrupt the usual workflow. There are also concerns that rounds may not be the best avenue to convey information and solicit family input in decision making. Conversely, there is a fear that the presence of parents might inhibit open discussion among staff [51,52].

The presence of family members during cardiopulmonary resuscitation is also a controversial issue. Concerns in the literature focus mainly on three points. The first is the potential for family members' presence to affect the performance of resuscitation staff. The second is that witnessing a traumatic event may have negative emotional and psychologic consequences. Third, many studies have identified that members of the public would like to be given the choice of whether to be present. The ethical principle is that all patients have the right to have family members present and that the patients' family members should have the opportunity to be present during resuscitation of a relative [53].

The philosophy of family-centered care reflects the nature of the concept of multidisciplinary care for parents in the PICU. A complete overview of related issues of family-centered care, including clinical practice guidelines, was recently published by the American College of Critical Care Task Force [54]. The Task Force reviewed the literature of the past two decades. The work was divided in ten subheadings related to the care of the family in the intensive care unit (Box 1).

Among these subheadings were also the issues of decision-making processes and palliative care. Basically the guidelines address partnership of family and the health care team. Six of the 43 recommendations are directed toward staff training and education—specifically toward communication, assessment of family needs and stress levels, cultural care, religious issues, family presence during resuscitation, and palliative care. Continuing education is needed to improve the clinical competency of health care workers to provide patient-driven care based on their needs [55].

Palliative care

In the curative model, the benefits of care are related to the degree to which the procedure will contribute to the patient's recovery from illness. In the palliative model, the benefits are related to whether the intervention

---

Box 1. Subheading of family-centered care

- Decision making
- Family coping
- Staff stress related to family visitation
- Cultural support
- Spiritual/religious support
- Family visitation
- Family presence on rounds
- Family presence at resuscitation
- Family environment of care
- Palliative care

Data from Davidson JE, Powers K, Hedayat KM, et al. Clinical practice guidelines for support of the family in the patient-centered intensive care unit: American College of Critical Care Medicine Task Force 2004–2005. Crit Care Med 2007;35(2):605–22.

---

will improve symptom relief, improve functional status, or ameliorate emotional, psychologic, or spiritual concerns [25]. The goal is to achieve the best possible quality of life for patients and their families [56,57]. Palliative care and curative care are not mutually exclusive options but rather should coexist. The palliative care objectives (Box 2) have the most relevance for patients whose goals of care have been redirected from life-sustaining curative goals to palliative goals. These patients are usually children with terminal illnesses or other conditions for which the benefits of further life-sustaining therapy are in question. Implicit in the phrase "redirecting the goals of care" is that care—apart from life-sustaining treatment—is never withdrawn.

Box 2. Objectives of palliative care

- To provide relief from pain and other distressing symptoms
- To intend neither to hasten nor postpone death
- To affirm life and regard dying as a normal process
- To integrate the psychologic and spiritual aspects of care for the patient and his/her family
- To offer a support system to help patients live as actively as possible until death
- To offer a support system to help family cope during the patient's illness and in their bereavement

---

The evaluation

Quality improvement procedures are important for evaluating the process of dying, just as they are for other hospital procedures. The concept of a "good" death has received substantial consideration. The Institute of Medicine defines a good death as "one that is free from avoidable distress and suffering for patients, families, and caregivers; in general accord with patients' and families' wishes; and reasonably consistent with clinical, cultural and ethical standards" [58]. Initially focused on adults, the Institute of Medicine later also focused the concept on children, with a publication called "When Children Die: Improving Palliative and End of Life Care for Children and their Families" [59]. Little research has been conducted on interventions to improve end-of-life care in the PICU setting. Two recent publications are available, based on a conference hosted by the Robert Wood Johnson Foundation and the Society of Critical Care Medicine: "Improving the Quality of End-of-Life Care in the ICU: Interventions That Work" [60,61]. At least six relevant domains were identified:

1. Strong interdisciplinary collaboration and communication within the critical care team and palliative care specialists.
2. Good communication skills of the team members.
3. Excellence in symptom assessment and management, including pain, dyspnea, delirium, anxiety, and a host of other symptoms.
4. Patient-centered care that focuses on patients' values and treatment preferences.
5. Family-centered care, including regular communication, psychologic, spiritual, and social support, and open visiting hours.
6. Regular interdisciplinary family meetings focused on shared decision making and support for family members.

Bereaved parents are in a unique position to comment on current practice in end-of-life care. Gaining an understanding of the perspectives of the family on the dying process is an essential step in understanding the quality of care provided.

Summary

For a long time, the research regarding end-of-life care in the PICU was descriptive and based on observational studies and surveys. Currently, we are entering a new era: the objective evaluation of health care professional's efforts to provide appropriate care to dying pediatric patients. This step is mandatory in efforts of health care staff to improve the quality of care for critically ill and dying children in the PICU.

References

[1] Burns JP, Mitchell C, Outwater KM, et al. End-of-life care in the pediatric intensive care unit after the forgoing of life-sustaining treatment. Crit Care Med 2000;28(8):3060–6.

[2] Devictor DJ, Nguyen DT. Forgoing life-sustaining treatments: how the decision is made in French pediatric intensive care units. Crit Care Med 2001;29(7):1356–9.

[3] Garros D, Rosychuk RJ, Cox PN. Circumstances surrounding end of life in a pediatric intensive care unit. Pediatrics 2003;112(5):e371.

[4] Althabe M, Cardigni G, Vassallo JC, et al. Dying in the intensive care unit: collaborative multicenter study about forgoing life-sustaining treatment in Argentine pediatric intensive care units. Pediatr Crit Care Med 2003;4(2):163–9.

[5] Devictor DJ, Nguyen DT. Forgoing life-sustaining treatments in children: a comparison between Northern and Southern European pediatric intensive care units. Pediatr Crit Care Med 2004;5(3):211–5.

[6] Zawistowski CA, DeVita MA. A descriptive study of children dying in the pediatric intensive care unit after withdrawal of life sustaining treatment. Pediatr Crit Care Med 2004;5(3):216–23.

[7] Kipper DJ, Piva JP, Garcia PC, et al. Evolution of the medical practices and modes of death on pediatric intensive care units in southern Brazil. Pediatr Crit Care Med 2005;6(3):258–63.

[8] Cuttini M, Nadai M, Kaminski M, et al. End-of-life decisions in neonatal intensive care: physicians' self reported practices in seven European countries. Lancet 2000;355(9221): 2112–8.

[9] Sprung CL, Eidelman LA. Worldwide similarities and differences in the forgoing of life-sustaining treatments. Intensive Care Med 1996;22(10):1003–5.

[10] Yaguchi A, Truog RD, Curtis R, et al. International differences in end-of-life attitudes in the intensive care unit. Arch Intern Med 2005;165(17):1970–5.

[11] Miccinesi G, Fischer S, Paci E, et al. Physicians' attitudes towards end-of-life decisions: a comparison between seven countries. Soc Sci Med 2005;60(9):1961–74.

[12] Vincent JL. Forgoing life support in western European intensive care units: the results of an ethical questionnaire. Crit Care Med 1999;27(8):1626–33.

[13] Sprung CL, Cohen SL, Sjokvist P, et al. End-of-life practices in European intensive care units: the ETHICUS study. JAMA 2003;290(6):790–7.

[14] Young RJ, King A. Legal aspects of withdrawal of therapy. Anaesth Intensive Care 2003; 31(5):501–8.

[15] Devictor DJ. Toward an ethics of communication among countries. Pediatr Crit Care Med 2004;5(3):290–1.

[16] American Academy of Pediatrics Committee on Bioethics. Informed consent, parental permission, and assent in pediatric practice. Pediatrics 1995;95(2):314–7.

[17] American Academy of Pediatrics Committee on Bioethics. Ethics and the care of critically ill infants and children. Pediatrics 1996;98(1):149–52.

[18] Hoehn KS, Nelson RM. Parents should not be excluded from decisions to forgo life-sustaining treatments! Crit Care Med 2001;29(7):1480–1.

[19] Frader JE. Forgoing life support across borders: who decides and why? Pediatr Crit Care Med 2004;5(3):289–90.

[20] Carlet J, Thijs LG, Antonelli M, et al. Challenges in end-of-life care in the ICU: statement of the 5th International Consensus Conference in Critical Care. Brussels, Belgium, April 2003. Intensive Care Med 2004;30(5):770–84.

[21] Singer PA, Bowman KW. Quality end-of-life care: a global perspective. BMC Palliat Care 2002;1(1):4.

[22] American Academy of Pediatrics. Committee on Bioethics: guidelines on forgoing life-sustaining medical treatment. Pediatrics 1994;93(3):532–6.

[23] Burns JP, Rushton CH. End-of-life in the pediatric intensive care unit: research review and recommendations. Crit Care Clin 2004;20(3):467–85.

[24] Solomon MZ, Sellers DE, Heller KS, et al. New and lingering controversies in pediatric end-of-life care. Pediatrics 2005;116(4):872–83.

[25] Truog RD, Cist AFM, Brackett SE, et al. Recommendations for end-of-life care in the intensive care unit: the Ethics Committee of the Society of Critical Care Medicine. Crit Care Med 2001;29(12):2332–48.

[26] Truog R, Burns J, Mitchell C, et al. Pharmacologic paralysis and withdrawal of mechanical ventilation at the end of life. N Engl J Med 2000;342(7):508–11.
[27] Nyman DJ, Sprung CL. End-of-life decision making in the intensive unit. Intensive Care Med 2000;26(10):1414–20.
[28] Burns JP, Truog RD. Ethical controversies in pediatric critical Care. In: Fink M, Abraham E, Vincent JL, editors. Textbook of critical care. 5th edition. Philadelphia: Elsevier Saunders; 2005. p. 2163–8.
[29] Azoulay E, Chevret S, Leleu G, et al. Half the families of intensive care unit patients experience inadequate communication with physicians. Crit Care Med 2000;28(8):3044–9.
[30] Lautrette A, Darmon M, Megarbane B, et al. A communication strategy and brochure for relatives of patients dying in the ICU. N Engl J Med 2007;356(5):469–78.
[31] Sharman M, Meert K, Sarnaik A. What influences parents' decisions to limit or withdraw life support? Pediatr Crit Care Med 2005;6(5):513–8.
[32] Meyer EC, Burns JP, Griffith JL, et al. Parental perspectives on end-of-life care in the pediatric intensive care unit. Crit Care Med 2002;30(1):226–31.
[33] Meert KL, Thurston CS, Sarnaik AP. End-of-life decision-making and satisfaction with care: parental perspectives. Pediatr Crit Care Med 2000;1(2):179–85.
[34] Randolph AG, Zollo MB, Egger MJ, et al. Variability in physician opinion on limiting pediatric life support. Pediatrics 1999;103(4):e43.
[35] Burns JP, Mitchell C, Griffith JL, et al. End-of-life care in the pediatric intensive care unit: attitudes and practices of pediatric critical care physicians and nurses. Crit Care Med 2001; 29(3):658–63.
[36] Slater A, Shann F, the ANZICS Paediatric Study Group. The suitability of the Pediatric Index of Mortality (PIM), PIM2, the Pediatric Risk of Mortality (PRISM), and PRISM III for monitoring the quality of pediatric intensive care in Australia and New Zealand. Pediatr Crit Care Med 2004;5(5):447–53.
[37] Gemke RJ, van Vught AJ. Scoring systems in pediatric intensive care: PRISM III versus PIM. Intensive Care Med 2002;28(2):204–7.
[38] Shaw A, Randolph JG, Manard B. Ethical issues in pediatric surgery: a national survey of pediatricians and pediatric surgeons. Pediatrics 1977;60(4):588–99.
[39] Schneiderman LJ, Jecker NS, Jonsen AR. Medical futility: its meaning and ethical implications. Ann Intern Med 1990;112(12):949–54.
[40] Ethics Committee of the Society of Critical Care Medicine. Consensus statement of the Society of Critical Care Medicine's Ethics Committee regarding futile and other possibly inadvisable treatments. Crit Care Med 1997;25(5):887–91.
[41] Puntillo KA, McAdam JL. Communication between physicians and nurses as a target for improving end-of-life care in the intensive care unit: challenges and opportunities for moving forward. Crit Care Med 2006;34(Suppl 11):S332–40.
[42] Hov R, Hedelin B, Athlin E. Being an intensive care nurse related to questions of withholding or withdrawing curative treatment. J Clin Nurs 2007;16(1):203–11.
[43] Hamric AB, Blackhall LJ. Nurse-physician perspectives on the care of dying patients in intensive care units: collaboration, moral distress, and ethical climate. Crit Care Med 2007;35(2):422–9.
[44] Ho KM, English S, Bell J. The involvement of intensive care nurses in end-of-life decisions: a nationwide survey. Intensive Care Med 2005;31(5):668–73.
[45] Quill TE. Terri Schiavo: a tragedy compounded. N Engl J Med 2005;352(16):1630–3.
[46] Frader J. Forgoing life-sustaining food and water: newborns. In: Lynn J, editor. By no extraordinary means: the choice to forgo life-sustaining food and water. Bloomington: Indiana University Press; 1989. p. 180–5.
[47] Meyer EC, Ritholz MD, Burns JP, et al. Improving the quality of end-of-life care in the pediatric intensive care unit: parents' priorities and recommendations. Pediatrics 2006;117(3):649–57.
[48] Shields L, Pratt J, Davis LM, et al. Family-centred care for children in hospital. Cochrane Database Syst Rev 2007;(1):CD004811.

[49] Riling DA, Hofmann KH, Deshler J. Family-centered care in the pediatric intensive care unit. In: Fuhrman BP, Zimmerman J, editors. Pediatric critical care. 3rd edition. Philadelphia: Mosby Elsevier; 2006. p. 106.

[50] Latour JM. Is family-centred care in critical care units that difficult? A view from Europe. Nurs Crit Care 2005;10(2):51–3.

[51] Muething SE, Kotagal UR, Schoettker PJ, et al. Family-centered bedside rounds: a new approach to patient care and teaching. Pediatrics 2007;119(4):829–32.

[52] Phipps LM, Bartke CN, Spear DA, et al. Assessment of parental presence during bedside pediatric intensive care unit rounds: effect on duration, teaching, and privacy. Pediatr Crit Care Med 2007;8(3):220–4.

[53] Fulbrook P, Latour J, Albarran J, et al, and the Presence of Family Members During Cardiopulmonary Resuscitation Working Group. The presence of family members during cardiopulmonary resuscitation: European Federation of Critical Care Nursing Associations, European Society of Paediatric and Neonatal Intensive Care and European Society of Cardiology Council on Cardiovascular Nursing and Allied Professions Joint Position Statement. Paediatr Nurs 2008;5(4):86–8.

[54] Davidson JE, Powers K, Hedayat KM, et al. Clinical practice guidelines for support of the family in the patient-centered intensive care unit: American College of Critical Care Medicine Task Force 2004–2005. Crit Care Med 2007;35(2):605–22.

[55] Latour JM, Haines C. Families in the ICU: do we truly consider their needs, experiences and satisfaction? Nurs Crit Care 2007;12(4):173–4.

[56] Kang T, Hoehn KS, Licht DJ, et al. Pediatric palliative, end-of-life, and bereavement care. Pediatr Clin North Am 2005;52(4):1029–46.

[57] Sahler OJ, Frager G, Levetown M, et al. Medical education about end-of-life care in the pediatric setting: principles, challenges, and opportunities. Pediatrics 2000;105(3):575–84.

[58] Institute of Medicine. Approaching death. Washington, DC: National Academies Press; 1997.

[59] Institute of Medicine. When children die: improving palliative and end of life care for children. Washington, DC: National Academies Press; 2003.

[60] Levy M, Curtis R. Improving end-of-life care in the intensive care unit. Crit Care Med 2006;34(Suppl):S301.

[61] Truog RD, Meyer EC. Toward interventions to improve end-of-life care in the pediatric intensive care unit. Crit Care Med 2006;34(Suppl):S373–9.

ELSEVIER
SAUNDERS

PEDIATRIC CLINICS
OF NORTH AMERICA

Pediatr Clin N Am 55 (2008) 805–833

Endocrine Issues in the Pediatric Intensive Care Unit

Lowell Clark, MD[a,e,*], Catherine Preissig, MD[b],
Mark R. Rigby, MD, PhD[c,d], Frank Bowyer, MD[a,e]

[a]Mercer University School of Medicine, Macon, GA, USA
[b]Emory University School of Medicine, Children's Healthcare of Atlanta at Egleston,
5105 WMB, 101 Woodruff Circle, Atlanta, GA 30322, USA
[c]Departments of Pediatrics and Surgery, Emory University School of Medicine,
Children's Healthcare of Atlanta at Egleston, 5105 WMB, 101 Woodruff Circle,
Atlanta, GA 30322, USA
[d]Critical Care Medicine, Emory University School of Medicine, Children's Healthcare
of Atlanta at Egleston 5105 WMB, 101 Woodruff Circle, Atlanta, GA 30322, USA
[e]Medical Center of Central Georgia, 777 Hemlock Street, Box 130, Macon,
GA 31201, USA

Critical illness threatens homeostasis, the internal milieu that must be maintained within a critical range for the machinery of life. Homeostasis is achieved by negative feedback loops that include sensors and effectors. The sensor responds to changes in a regulated parameter (such as the volume of intravascular fluid) by producing a signaling molecule. The effector responds to the signaling molecule by restoring the regulated parameter to the physiologic range. The specialized signaling molecules carried in the extracellular fluid are hormones, neurotransmitters, and cytokines.

Illness, injury, and shock activate survival mechanisms that are performed primarily by the autonomic nervous and endocrine systems (Fig. 1). Volume loss and shock are sensed through pressure and volume receptors in the vascular system, which communicates the threat by the vagus and glossopharyngeal afferents to the brainstem and hypothalamus. Breaches in barrier membranes result in foreign antigen access to sterile tissues, stimulating the immune system to signal the brain via cytokines. Central integration of these and other signals of homeostatic threat result in profound neurohumoral responses effected by adrenergic outflow and

* Corresponding author. Medical Center of Central Georgia, 777 Hemlock Street, Box 130, Macon, GA 31201.
E-mail address: clark.lowell@mccg.org (L. Clark).

0031-3955/08/$ - see front matter © 2008 Elsevier Inc. All rights reserved.
doi:10.1016/j.pcl.2008.03.001   pediatric.theclinics.com

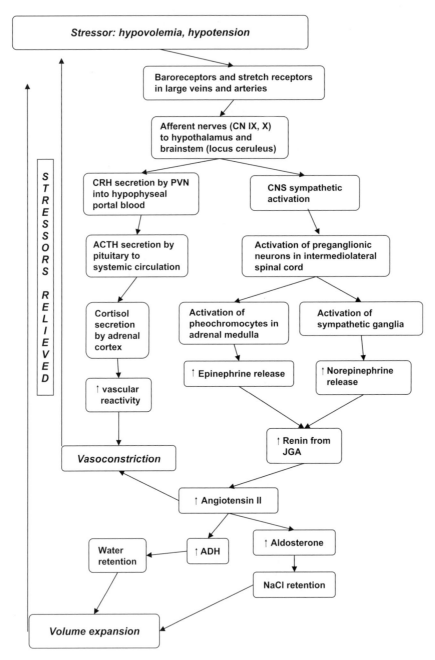

Fig. 1. Sympathoadrenergic system. ACTH, adrenocorticotrophic hormone; ADH, antidiuretic hormone; CNS, central nervous system; CRH, corticotrophin-releasing hormone; JGA, juxtaglomerular apparatus; NaCl, sodium chloride; PVN, paraventricular and supraoptic nuclei. (*Courtesy of* Balint Kacsoh, MD, PhD, Macon, GA.)

hypothalamic-pituitary-adrenal (HPA) activation. Stress-induced increase in output of cortisol results in marked changes in substrate mobilization, resulting in a ready supply of energy sources for use by brain, heart, muscles, hematopoitic elements, and the viscera. A surge in ADH results in water retention to maintain operating ranges of volume and osmolality. Glucose mobilization and synthesis not only provide energy, but also result in osmotic changes that temporarily recruit volume from the intracellular fluid (ICF). Catecholamines not only augment vascular tone but also liberate free fatty acids (FFAs) to fuel the heart and skeletal muscles, hepatic gluconeogenesis, and serve as substrates for hepatic ketone body production. Amino acids derived from muscle protein catabolism via the proteosome pathway become available for hepatic gluconeogenesis, the synthesis of hemostatic factors, and other acute phase reactants. Potent transcriptional systems become activated to marshal the immune system even as cortisol induces a temporary state of immune tolerance. If sustained, however, these profound responses come with substantial costs. Substrate mobilization via proteolysis results in unsustainable losses of structural (eg, extracellular matrix, such as collagen) and muscle proteins that manifest as easy bruising, cutaneous atrophy, muscle wasting and, ultimately, death. Unbalanced stress metabolism leads to sustained hyperglycemia with far reaching effects on immune competence and neurologic morbidities. Immune suppression or misdirection results in infectious complications. Wounds fail to heal. Exogenous substrates absorbed from the gut are misappropriated.

In this brief survey of endocrine issues in the intensive care unit, the authors review and describe the stress response, and then discuss a selected set of the more common endocrine scenarios in the pediatric intensive care unit (PICU).

The stress response

Stress is derived from the Latin *stringere*, "to draw tight," and has been defined as a condition of extreme difficulty, pressure, or strain. Physiologist Walter Cannon first described the "fight or flight" sympathoadrenal response in 1915 and later coined the term "homeostasis." Hans Selye described the generalized adaptation syndrome in 1936 [1]. As described [2], this "stress response" includes the pituitary-adrenocortical axis and consists of three phases: stage one, alarm as the organism senses and responds with a fight or flight reaction; stage two, resistance as the organism attempts to adapt to the ongoing demands of continued stress; and stage three, exhaustion and decompensation as all reserves are depleted and organ systems fail. At the time this process was described, patients either survived or succumbed without the benefit of modern intensive care. The generalized adaptation response evolved over eons as a short-lived survival technique meant to spend itself quickly. However, modern intensive care routinely prolongs life beyond "natural" boundaries, and practitioners are left with a complex clinical scene of "neuroendocrine-immune disarray," as described by Felmet and Carcillo [3].

The stress response is now recognized as a stereotypic neuroendocrine phenomenon. A system of sensors includes monitors of pain, heat, cold, barrier or visceral disruption, hypovolemia and hypotension, hypoglycemia, hypoxia, and invasion of sterile compartments by foreign antigen. Such homeostatic threats may alert the central nervous system either directly (eg, hypothalamic osmotic sensors, and cortical or limbic recognition) or by means of afferent nerves, especially cranial nerves IX and X, and blood-born molecules, especially cytokines. Central integration occurs in the hypothalamus and brainstem. The response triggers activation of the locus ceruleus, the central switch of the sympathetic nervous system, which signals via the sympathetic ganglionic chain and the adrenal medulla, releasing catecholamines into the general circulation. The other major arm of response is the hypothalamic-pituitary axis, with hypothalamic-releasing hormones acting through the pituitary to profoundly alter peripheral metabolism by actions on the adrenocortical, somatotropic, thyroidal, gonadal, and lactotropic axes [4]. The sum total is the rapid mobilization of energy reserves for use by vital organs, and rapid adaptation of respiratory, circulatory, and metabolic systems for maximal energy processing and function.

Hormonal response begins in the hypothalamus, a nest of nuclei concerned with vital function and homeostasis [5]. Most of the releasing and inhibiting hormones are small peptides expressed by hypothalamic neurons. The magnocellular neurons of the paraventricular and supraoptic nuclei produce ADH that reaches the posterior pituitary (neurohypophysis) by direct axonal transport, where it is released to the general circulation by the process of neurosecretion, with resulting retention of free water, enhancement of pituitary ACTH secretion, and in extreme states, rescue vasoconstriction. The parvocellular neurons in the hypophysiotrophic area of the hypothalamus produce corticotrophin-, somatotropin-, thyrotropin-, and gonadotropin-releasing hormones, which are secreted into the pituitary portal system and are delivered to the anterior pituitary. ACTH, growth hormone (GH), thyroid stimulating hormone (TSH), and gonadotropins—follicle stimulationg hormone and luteinizing hormone—are then delivered by the general circulation to distant target glands.

A general feature of releasing hormones is their rhythmic, intermittent, and circadian patterns, implying crucial influences from photic cues and the molecular circadian clock in the suprachiasmic nucleus, reinforced and entrained by melatonin secreted from the pineal gland. Releasing hormones and end-organ hormones, such as steroids, are also produced in tissues other than hypothalamus and adrenal, and outside the usual hypothalamic-pituitary-end organ axes; their regulation and physiologic functions are often poorly understood. Existing, but incompletely characterized and understood, are receptors for the releasing hormones, such as CRH in peripheral tissues, which may have opposite effects from HPA activation [6].

The HPA axis consists of CRH stimulating the release of ACTH from the anterior pituitary, which circulates to the adrenals and stimulates the synthesis of cortisol and adrenal androgens from the zona fasciculata and reticularis of the adrenal cortex [7]. ACTH induces the rate-limiting steroidogenic regulatory protein, which regulates the transport of cholesterol from the cytoplasm to the mitochondrial matrix. There, with ready availability of energy from the matrix and in the smooth endoplasmic reticulum, a series of P450 enzymes with location specificity synthesize cortisol and other steroids from a common pool of pregnenolone-derived precursors. The zona glomerulosa synthesizes only mineralocorticoids (mainly aldosterone), whereas the zona fasciculata and reticularis synthesize glucocorticoids (mainly cortisol), mineralocorticoids (mainly 11-deoxycorticosterone or 11-DOC), and androgens (dehydroepiandrosterone, dehydroepiandrosterone sulfate, and androstenedione). The ratio of glucocorticoid to androgen production is tilted in favor of androgens in the zona fasciculata. In contrast to the neurosecretory process for releasing hormones that are stored in secretory granules, cortisol, once synthesized, penetrates lipid membranes readily and passes from the cell into the circulation to become distributed bodywide, with approximately 90% bound to cortisol binding protein (vide infra).

The sympathetic arm of the stress response begins in the locus ceruleus, the dorsal pontine "blue spot" on the floor of the fourth ventricle, which receives a broad range of external and internal sensory input signaling homeostatic threat. Norepinephrine is the primary neurotransmitter of the locus ceruleus, and its efferent projections arborize widely through the CNS. The locus ceruleus also activates the HPA axis by stimulating the production of CRH. Descending activation of the paraspinal sympathetic chain occurs via the intermediolateral columns of the spinal cord, from which emerge preganglionic neurons to the paravertabral and prevertebral sympathetic ganglia, (eg, the organ of Zuckerkandl). Embryologically, the adrenal medulla may be thought of as a specialized sympathetic ganglion populated by pheochromocytes (anagolous to sympathetic ganglion cells) of neural crest origin, which has become invested by mesodermally derived cortex. Whereas sympathetic ganglia project either cholinergic or norepinephrinergic postganglionic axons directly to target organs and tissues, the medulla has no axonal extensions, but rather exerts its effects humorally, in part by norepinephrine and mostly by epinephrine, an N-methylated derivative of norepinephrine.

The particular anatomy of the adrenal gland allows a bimodal adrenergic effect through both norepinephrine from the sympathetic ganglia and epinephrine from the medulla [7]. Cortical arterial supply is derived from the outer surface of the gland, with perfusion draining through the sinusoids of the zona fasiculata toward the medulla. This allows the medulla to be bathed in blood enriched by the secretory products of the cortex. Norepinephrine synthesis by the medulla begins with active transport of L-tyrosine from the plasma into the cytosol of the pheochromocyte. Rate-limiting and pre-existing tyrosine hydroxylase is activated by protein kinase systems and preganglionic sympathetic nerves. Synthesis proceeds through dihydroxyphenylalanine and dopamine, after which the process enters the secretory and synaptic vesicles for conversion of dopamine to norepinephrine, where it is stored and ready for release. However, norepinephrine then leaks from the secretory vesicles back into the cytosol, where the enzyme phenylethanolamine-N-methyltransferase (PNMT) converts norepinephrine to epinephrine. PNMT activity is dependent on the rich concentration of cortisol perfusing the medulla from the cortical sinusoidal system. By this anatomic mechanism, cortisol strongly influences the elaboration of epinephrine from norepinephrine, giving considerable nuance to adrenergic expression. Cortisol and catecholamines are also linked by the permissive effects of cortisol on catecholamine receptor and downstream G-protein expression. In adults, plasma concentrations of norepinephrine normally exceed epinephrine by nine to one. Because most norepinephrine in the adrenal is converted to epinephrine, the bulk of circulating catecholamines is derived from sympathetic nerves and the paraganglia.

The integrated stress response thus provides an immediate jolt from the sympathoadrenergic system by catecholamines with half lives of less than 2 minutes, followed by more sustained adrenocortical mechanisms, which affect nuclear transcription and potent anti-inflammatory pathways, such as inhibition of nuclear factor kappa-B. The sum total of physiologic effects of the stress response primes the respiratory, cardiovascular, and metabolic systems for maximal oxygen delivery to the cells and energy processing. Cognitive awareness is peaked and afferent sensory input is sharpened. The airways are dried and opened. Bronchodilitation occurs to match alveolar delivery of oxygen to increased lung perfusion. Cardiac output and blood pressure increase. Blood is diverted from the skin and the splanchnic circulation, and digestion slows. Glycogenolysis and gluconeogenesis are stimulated in the liver to provide glucose, along with lipolysis in adipocytes to provide free fatty acids.

The stress response extends far beyond these mechanisms. Indeed, not only the HPA but the somatotropic, thyroid, and lactotropic axes are profoundly affected by the stress response [8]. There is a surge of GH, but a state of peripheral GH resistance develops, mediated partially by cytokines. Even though GH levels remain elevated, pulsatile release, upon which somatotropic effects depend, is severely disturbed, contributing to the wasting syndrome of chronic critical illness. In the thyroid axis, triiodothyronine (T_3) levels fall rapidly and reverse T_3 (rT_3) increases because of altered peripheral conversion of thyroxine (T_4). With time, T_4 and TSH normalize, but T_3 remains low ("low T_3 syndrome"). In the lactotropic axis, prolactin is a potent immune agonist that is activated in stress [9] and counterbalances the immune suppression induced by the HPA axis. With continued stress, and as with other axes, the pulsatile secretory pattern of prolactin is disturbed, and levels fall. Endogenous dopamine from the hypothalamus normally inhibits the release of prolactin from the anterior pituitary. Therapeutically administered dopamine for shock states has the same effect, and may therefore induce immune suppression [10].

Critical illness hyperglycemia

Hyperglycemia is a normal and important physiologic response to stress that, not surprisingly, is common in critically ill patients, who by nature of severe illness are undergoing significant body stresses because of their disease processes. Furthermore, the degree of hyperglycemia in these patients is heightened by the iatrogenic (albeit necessary) life-saving therapies that health care providers employ, many of which are prodiabetogenic (steroids, vasoactive infusions). This acute hyperglycemia may be advantageous, as increased glucose delivery, and thus energy to stressed organs and tissues during times of illness, is likely a positive evolutionary response to stress [11]. However, studies have shown that this "normal" physiologic response of hyperglycemia tends to go awry in patients with critical illness. In these patients, the normal mechanisms that counteract hyperglycemia are overwhelmed, leading to a persistent and unchecked state of high blood glucose. And while acute hyperglycemia may be beneficial to the stressed organism, prolonged hyperglycemia has been shown to be detrimental in this setting [12].

The cause of this unchecked hyperglycemia in critical illness is multifactorial and not completely understood, but likely represents a stress response secondary to insulin resistance, absolute insulin deficiency, glycogenolysis, and increased hepatic gluconeogenesis from release of catecholamines, cortisol, and glucagon [11]. In patients with sepsis, this hyperglycemic response is further promoted by the production of inflammatory mediators and cytokines. The relative contributions of these factors is unknown, but the effect of increased catecholamines, counter-regulatory hormones, and proinflammatory mediators in the setting of critical illness is thought to impair insulin signaling in target cells, leading to peripheral insulin resistance and high blood glucose. Concurrently, these same conditions of increased hormones, proinflammatory cytokines, and lipid derangements directly and adversely effect pancreatic β-cell function, leading to decreased insulin production with resultant high blood glucose [11]. In response to stress, glucagon is increased, likely because of stimulation of pancreatic cells by cortisol and epinephrine, while catecholamines, somatostatin, FFAs, and proinflammatory cytokines, such as tumor necrosis fatctor alpha (TNF-α), suppress insulin, leading to a relative hypoinsulinemia. TNF-α is a lipolytic cytokine that increases FFA levels, and is a potent inhibitor of glucose-induced release of insulin. Taken together, this leads to increased glucagon/insulin ratios and favors gluconeogenesis, resulting in increased hepatic glucose production [7]. At the same time, epinephrine, FFAs, and cytokines blunt the target cell response to insulin, leading to peripheral and hepatic insulin resistance. The combination of increased glucagon, suppression of insulin secretion, and insulin resistance results in hyperglycemia and inability of the organism to use substrate at the tissue level [7,12].

Indeed, it has been shown in multiple settings in both critically ill adults and children that prolonged hyperglycemia is associated with worse outcomes, including increased length of hospital stay, prolonged need for mechanical ventilation, worse neurologic sequelae in brain trauma, and even increased mortality [13–17]. Even more impressively, it has been shown in adults that goal-directed glycemic control with infused insulin reduces morbidity and mortality in this population. The landmark study in this field was Van den Berghe's 2001 report, which reviewed 1,548 adult patients in a surgical intensive care unit (ICU). Their findings suggested that maintaining blood glucose levels between 80 mg/dL and 110 mg/dL decreased ICU length of stay, number of mechanical ventilator days, reduced rates of septicemia, and reduced mortality [17]. Because of these and others' findings, multiple professional societies now recommend tight glucose control as standard practice in adults [18,19], and a recent consensus report endorsed by 11 professional societies recommended maintaining blood glucose at 80 mg/dL to 110 mg/dL in an effort to reduce mortality in patients with severe sepsis [20].

The reasons why prolonged hyperglycemia may be injurious in critically ill patients (and thus why treatment with insulin may be beneficial) are unclear, but may have to do with both glucose toxicity and the nonglycemic protective effects of insulin. Hyperglycemia causes free-radical formation and damage, promotes injury to hepatic mitochondria and other cellular structures, leads to apoptosis and cell death in certain organs, and can impair the innate and humoral immune response to infection. Insulin treatment may impart protective effects by inhibiting some of these pathologic processes caused by high blood glucose, as well as providing nonglycemic protection by its anabolic effects on lipid and protein metabolism, modulation of counter-regulatory hormones and catecholamines commonly increased during stress, and its direct anti-inflammatory properties [7,11,12,21].

Insulin itself is the most potent anabolic hormone in the body and is a key player in the control of intermediary metabolism. It has profound effects on both carbohydrate and lipid metabolism, and significant influences on protein and mineral metabolism. Consequently, derangements in insulin signaling have widespread and devastating effects on many organs and tissues. Signaling through the insulin pathway is critical for the regulation of intracellular and blood glucose levels and the avoidance of hyperglycemia. The insulin receptor is a tyrosine kinase in a family of enzymes that transfers phosphate groups from ATP to tyrosine residues on intracellular target proteins. Binding of insulin to the α-subunits of its receptor leads to autophosphorylation of the β-subunits and the tyrosine phosphorylation of insulin receptor substrates, leading to eventual downstream increase in intracellular PIP_2 and subsequent phosphatidylinositol phosphate-dependent kinase-1 activation. This in turn results in the translocation of glucose transporters from cytoplasmic vesicles to the cell membrane in insulin sensitive cells, facilitating intracellular glucose transport [21]. The anabolic downstream effects of insulin are far-reaching and include cellular uptake and use of glucose in adipose and muscle cells, stimulation of hepatic cells to store glucose as glycogen, promotion of hepatic FFA formation and uptake and use in other tissues, inhibition of lipolysis in adipocytes, and stimulation of protein anabolism. Furthermore, insulin is known to have direct anti-inflammatory effects and modifying effects on many counter-regulatory mechanisms [21].

Treatment of hyperglycemia in critically ill adults has become standard of care, but because of lack of outcome data, strict glycemic control in PICUs remains controversial. Indeed, even in adults it is not clear which patients should be treated with strict glycemic control. In fact, one study in adult patients with brain injury showed that intensive insulin therapy led to a reduction in glucose at the tissue level in the brain but was actually associated with increased markers of cellular stress, thus implying that normoglycemia may in fact be detrimental to certain neurologic tissues after injury [22]. Furthermore, the major adverse effect of glucose control in adults and children is hypoglycemia, which may be more deleterious in the pediatric population, as sustained low blood glucose may impact brain development. However, because of the adult literature and recent evidence that hyperglycemia is associated with increased morbidity and mortality in children [17,23–27], many PICU practitioners have begun to tentatively control blood glucose in their patients. Preliminary reports do suggest that this control may be achieved safely and effectively in this population, and currently randomized, controlled trials to assess outcome improvement in children are in progress. In an era where goal-directed therapies with clinical practice guidelines are gaining ease and popularity, safe glycemic control in PICU settings should be achievable, but until definitive evidence is available they may need to be practiced with caution.

Relative adrenal insufficiency

In 1976, a blinded, prospective study was published comparing high dose steroid therapy to placebo in clinical septic shock [28]. In 86 saline treated subjects, mortality was 38.4%, compared with 10.4% in 86 high-dose steroid treated subjects. Interestingly, the study was "confirmed" by a retrospective analysis of 328 patients from the same ICU, yielding similar results. Thus, intensive care medicine entered an era during which steroids in supraphysiologic doses (eg, infusions of methylprednisolone 30-mg/kg–75-mg/kg over 1–12 hours) were often prescribed, and ideas of adrenal insufficiency became popular. A decade later, several studies [29–31] failed to confirm this original study, and, indeed, began to identify late morbidities (infections) from such therapies, and the practice of "megadose" steroids in septic shock was largely abandoned. However, some of these studies [29] did note that reversal of shock and 5-day survival was more likely in patients who received steroids, even though these differences disappeared later in the course. This raised the question of existence of a subgroup of patients with septic shock who may benefit from steroids. A decade later in the 1990s, the practice of testing the adrenal gland in sepsis by ACTH stimulation in real time was studied [32,33], and the concept of relative adrenal insufficiency (RAI) became established based on baseline cortisol levels and adrenal response to corticotrophin stimulation [34].

In 2002, an article by Annane and colleagues [35] was published in which a placebo-controlled, randomized, double-blind, multicenter trial of "low dose" hydrocortisone and fludrocortisone in subjects with septic shock and 28-day mortality as outcome measure confirmed the hypothesis that patients with septic shock and relative adrenal insufficiency could benefit from replacement. The study was handicapped by inclusion of subjects who had received etomidate, which inhibits steroidogenesis [36] after only one dose [37] and has been associated with increased mortality [38]. However, the study established that relatively small dose glucocorticoid replacement (200-mg hydrocortisone per 24 hours in adult patients) positively affected survival and, along with meta-analysis [39], the results of this study became evidence for guidelines recommending the use of corticosteroids in septic shock [40].

Absolute and relative adrenal insufficiency were studied recently in a group of children with septic shock [41]. Using "high dose" ACTH (250 µg), RAI occurred in 26% of the subjects; 80% of these children were catecholamine resistant. No subjects with fluid responsive shock had adrenal insufficiency. There was no relation of adrenal insufficiency to mortality. The effects of therapy were not studied in this article.

Causes of RAI are unknown. Destruction of the gland is likely uncommon in pediatrics, although several infectious agents that directly infect the gland can cause adrenal insufficiency, including HIV, cytomegalovirus, fungal infections, and tuberculosis. Destruction of the gland must be extensive (greater than 90%) for adrenal insufficiency to develop. Medications, including etomidate (vide supra) and ketoconazole may affect the HPA and adrenal gland, as may pre-existing use of therapeutic steroids. Sepsis generates mediators that have been shown to affect all levels of the HPA [42]. TNFα induces the release of ACTH, yet inhibits the response of ACTH to corticotropin releasing factor. Interleukin-6 (IL-6) stimulates ACTH secretion, and deficient production of IL-6 during sepsis may occur [36]. Macrophage migration inhibitory factor [5] is a peptide released by the pituitary and activated macrophages during septic shock. It is a counter-regulator of endogenous glucocorticoids [36] and antagonizes their peripheral effects while amplifying the immune response by up-regulating toll-like receptors. By these and other mechanisms, evidence exists that all levels of the HPA are affected by mediators released during sepsis.

The concept of RAI rests on the measurement of basal cortisol levels, followed by the response to corticotrophin challenge during the acute phase of shock and critical illness. However, there are at least two methods of corticotrophin challenge, and no consensus exists on diagnostic criteria based on results of such testing. Early in stress, diurnal variation of cortisol levels disappears, and cortisol levels become tonically elevated. Based on the normal response of nonstressed patients to exogenous corticotrophin, many consider measured random levels of greater than 17 µg/dL to 25 µg/dL to represent an adequate response to stress, and thus eliminate adrenal insufficiency (versus RAI) as a cause [42]. However, a pediatric study used a basal level of less than 7 µg/dL to identify adrenal dysfunction [43]. Corticotrophin challenge testing is performed by at least two different methods. Most studies use a supraphysiologic dose of 250 µg cosyntropin (125 µg for less than 10 kg), which is greater than 100 times physiologic ACTH levels. Others [44] recommend a more physiologic 1-µg dose. Cortisol levels are measured 30 and 60 minutes after ACTH administration, and increments of greater than 7 µg/dL or peaks of greater than 17 µg/dL to 25 µg/dL are expected to demonstrate competent adrenal function. See Zimmerman [45] for an excellent discussion of the quandary surrounding adrenal testing.

Underlying the confusion of the various testing methods is concern that currently available tests all measure total cortisol concentration, including free and bound hormone [44]. Normally, 90% of cortisol is bound to cortisol binding globulin (CBG). During stress states, CBG levels decrease acutely and gradually return to normal during the prolonged phase of critical illness. The fall may be attributed to cleavage of CBG by neutrophil-derived elastase. Furthermore, approximately 20% of cortisol is bound to albumin, which commonly falls early in critical illness. A study measuring free cortisol levels in ICU patients [46] revealed normally elevated free cortisol levels in hypoalbuminemic subjects, yet in whom cosyntropin stimulation produced total cortisol levels of less than 20 µg/dL, the cutoff value suggesting adrenal insufficiency for this study. Currently, free cortisol is difficult to measure. Salivary cortisol levels reflect free serum levels and merit further study [47]. Eosinophilia is a readily available marker to suggest adrenal insufficiency [48] and may correlate with free cortisol levels. Once further studies are available using free hormone levels, interpretation and significance of the majority of existing studies in this field will need re-examination, so that the unnecessary exposure of critically ill patients to exogenous glucocorticoids may be prevented [49], and the known adverse effects of glucocorticoid therapy be avoided, including hyperglycemia and polyneuropathy of critical illness.

In January 2008, the results of a multicenter, randomized, placebo-controlled trial investigating the use of low dose corticosteroids in septic shock were published [50]. The CORTICUS (Corticosteroid Therapy of Septic Shock) trial was prompted by the 2002 Annane study [35], which demonstrated efficacy of steroids in septic shock among those patients who failed to respond to corticotrophin stimulation. In CORTICUS, 499 subjects were randomized to receive placebo or hydrocortisone 50-mg intravenously every 6 hours for 5 days, followed by a 6-day weaning period. All subjects were tested for response to 250-mcg corticotrophin; nonresponders were defined as having a cortisol response of less than or equal to 9 mcg/dL. In contrast to the Annane study, fludrocortisone was not given. Based on entry critieria, the study populations were dissimilar with

Annane's subjects, demonstrating more severe organ dysfunction upon entry. The primary endpoint was death at 28 days in nonresponders. Among those who did not respond to corticotrophin (cortisol rise less than or equal to 9 mcg/dL total, no free levels), there was no significant difference in mortality with the use of corticosteroids versus placebo; neither was there significant difference in mortality among those who did demonstrate adrenal responsiveness (cortisol greater than 9 mcg/dL). The study clearly failed to identify patients, based on corticotrophin testing, who may benefit from corticosteroids. The study did confirm earlier reversal of shock; however, this earlier reversal was not associated with improved survival. Among the steroid group there were more episodes of late onset sepsis, including new episodes of septic shock. As with Annane's 2002 study, CORTICUS was contaminated by etomidate, but similarly among groups, and the use of etomidate confirmed the observation that this drug may be associated with altered adrenal function. There is no mention of glycemic control in this study, raising the question of glycemic control preserving a possible trend toward increased survival manifest early in CORTICUS but not sustained over 28 days. Another dissimilarity between the two studies was weaning strategy, with CORTICUS subjects being exposed longer and therefore with cumulatively higher doses of corticosteroids.

The most recent guidelines for management of septic shock were released in the 2008 Surviving Sepsis Campaign [51]. The results of CORTICUS were considered, with the final recommendation for steroid use coming from a split decision among experts (see appendix [50]). "We suggest that intravenous hydrocortisone be given *only* to adult septic shock patients after it has been confirmed that their blood pressure is poorly responsive to fluid resuscitation and vasopressor therapy." Other recommendations relative to steroids in shock included: (1) ACTH stimulation test should not be used to decide who gets steroids; (2) oral fludrocortisone if hydrocortisone (and thus mineralocorticoid effect) is not available; (3) wean from steroids as soon as the vasopressors are off; and (4) do not give steroids for sepsis in absence of shock unless the patient's endocrine or corticosteroid administration history so warrants. Of course, these are guidelines for adult patients and are accompanied by attendant inherent risks of adaptation to pediatrics. The Surviving Sepsis recommendations include "pediatric considerations." Specific pediatric guidelines have not been published since 2002 but are consistent with 2008 Surviving Sepsis suggestions, and state, "Adrenal insufficiency should be suspected in catecholamine-resistant hypotensive shock in children with a history of CNS abnormality or chronic steroid use or with purpura fulminans. Use of hydrocortisone in this situation may be life-saving. Dose recommendations vary from a bolus of 1–2 mg/kg for stress coverage to 50 mg/kg for shock, followed by the same dose as a 24-hr infusion" [52].

The powerful therapeutic potential of glucocorticoid therapy tempts the clinician when dealing with life-threatening septic shock. Although testing as currently employed does not so identify, it is likely that there are clinical states and patient subsets in which such therapy is indicated. At this point in history, these indications are unclear, except for catecholamine-resistant septic shock and in septic children with clear history or evidence of adrenal insufficiency. In these scenarios, judicious use of glucocorticoids may shorten the clinical course of shock, but these agents have not yet been convincingly demonstrated to impart survival advantage in children, and have been associated with increased mortality in pediatric sepsis [53]. Specifics and complications of glucocorticoid therapy must be delineated and monitored, especially relative to critical illness hyperglycemia, and, if unattended, may negate any advantage that may result from steroid therapy. If glucocorticoids are used, they should be weaned as soon as possible. The entire pattern of hypophyseal-pituitary-adrenal response to stress needs description in terms of free cortisol levels. Guidelines themselves are subject to inherent problems and may paradoxically discourage needed research [54].

Disorders of water and solute balance: syndrome of inappropriate antidiuretic hormone and cerebral salt wasting

Brain disorders complicated by increased intracranial pressure are commonly managed with hyperosmolar therapies, either in rescue or by creating a clinical state of hyperosmolar isovolemia. Hypertonic saline may be infused for days to maintain a hypernatremic state with the design to diminish brain edema. These same neurologic and neurosurgical patients are also prone to hyponatremia. This creates clinical confusion between the disorders of the syndrome of inappropriate antidiuretic hormone (SIADH) and cerebral salt wasting (CSW) syndrome [55]. Disorders of solute and water homeostasis are common and occasionally the primary pathophysiologic mechanism leading to death or permanent disability, especially neurologic. Normal serum osmolality ranges between 280 and 295, with even more tightly maintained limits within a given individual. The primary mechanism by which this is accomplished is through sensitive relations between serum osmolality, plasma vasopressin release from the posterior pituitary gland, and the V2 receptors on the principal cells of the renal collecting ducts [56]. Small increases in serum osmolality cause immediate picomolar release of ADH from the pituitary, with serum levels of 6 pg/mL resulting in maximal renal antidiuresis. Termination of effect depends on the loss of osmotic stimulus and the brief 15-minute half-life of ADH. Serum osmolality is sensed by receptors in the anterior wall of the third ventricle, which are perfused by fenestrated capillaries; that is, these receptors are outside the blood brain barrier [57]. Increased osmolality (more accurately: hypernatremia) triggers action potentials in the magnocellular neurons, which are then propagated down the axon to the posterior pituitary. Transcription of ADH is followed by translation and posttranslational processing (glycosylation and proteolytic cleavage) of the hormone as it traverses down the axon to be stored in the neurosecretory granules of the posterior pituitary, where several days to a month or more supply of ADH exists before release is stimulated by action potentials spreading along the axons of magnocellular neurons emerging from the hypothalamus to the neurohypophysis.

ADH release is also subject to volume and pressure sensing by arterial and venous baroreceptors. High pressure and high volume states tend to diminish ADH release [58], whereas hypotension from volume depletion is a potent stimulus for ADH release in amounts far exceeding that necessary for water conservation and more associated with systemic vasoconstriction. However, hormonal protection from hypotension and hypovolemia depend primarily on renin-angiotensin-aldosterone and sympathetic nervous system mechanisms. ADH affects its action through V1, V2, and V3 receptors. V1 activation induces vascular smooth muscle vasoconstriction. V2 receptors exist on renal tubules and induce antidiuresis. V3 receptors are associated with enhanced ACTH release from the anterior pituitary, thereby linking ADH in activation of the stress response.

The renin-angiotensin-aldosterone system is primarily concerned with maintaining adequate systemic circulatory volume by manipulating sodium reabsorption and handling the potentially lethal potassium loads presented to the organism [59]. The juxtaglomerular apparatus senses low sodium, chloride, and flow in the distal loop of Henle and responds by producing renin and by regulating glomerular arteriolar resistance, thus glomerular filtration. Renin, with a usual half-life of 15 to 20 minutes, converts circulating angiotensinogen to angiotensin I. Angiotensin converting enzyme, widespread in plasma and primarily pulmonary endothelium, then converts angiotensin I to angiotensin II in picomolar quantities. With a half-life of less than 1 minute, angiotensin II then engages the AT1 receptor and proceeds to maintain normal extracellular volume and blood pressure by several mechanisms, including: (1) direct vasoconstriction, (2) enhancement of adrenergic activity both by increasing catecholamine release from the adrenal medulla and increasing central sympathetic outflow, (3) promoting ADH release, and (4) increasing aldosterone release from the adrenal cortex. Aldosterone binds a cytosolic receptor in renal connecting tubule and cortical collecting duct epithelial cells and, via genomic action, increases the population of both the apical sodium channels and basolateral sodium-potassium (Na-K) ATPase pumps, resulting in sodium reabsorption. In concert with simultaneous ADH secretion, circulatory volume is thus restored.

Natriuretic peptides are a family of molecules that are produced when states of hypervolemia and increased preload are sensed by atrial stretch receptors [60]. As a class, these molecules counter sympathetic and other stress mechanisms: central sympathetic outflow is diminished; ACTH secretion is inhibited; central venous capacitance is increased by venodilation; vascular endothelial permeability is increased, shifting fluid extravascularly; and vagal afferent input is down-regulated, blunting reflex tachycardia. A striking natriuresis is induced by increased glomerular filtration rate

(GFR) and decreased sodium reabsorption. Other sodium and volume retaining mechanisms are inhibited by reducing renin release, inhibiting aldosterone release, countering angiotensin II mediated sodium reabsorption, and diminishing both ADH secretion and collecting duct response to it. Natriuretic peptide receptors are found throughout the central nervous system, both outside, allowing engagement of circulating molecules, and within the blood-brain barrier, reflecting production of natriuretic peptides within the CNS that likely act in an autocrine and paracrine manner. In contrast to angiotensin II, these peptides have antimitogenic effects. Thus, natriuretic peptides seem to constitute a negative feedback loop, allowing modulation toward equilibrium of the adaptive responses to shock and critical illness.

The syndrome of inappropriate antidiuretic hormone

SIADH was first described in 1957 in a patient with bronchogenic carcinoma who had hyponatremia and inappropriately elevated levels of ADH [61]. Since then a myriad of disease states and drugs have been associated. Recently, the term "syndrome of inappropriate antidiuresis" [62] has been proposed, recognizing that other perturbations may produce the situation of decreased serum osmolality and concentrated urine. Robertson [63] has classified the syndromes of inappropriate antidiuresis as the following types (Fig. 2). Type A is classical SIADH in which exists dissociation between serum osmolality and ADH secretion. Type B is elevated basal ADH secretion in spite of regulation by serum osmolality. Type C is a "reset osmostat" in which ADH is totally appropriately suppressed but only when a lower set-point osmolality is reached. Type D represents concentrated urine, even in the absence of ADH, and is related to mutations of the aquaretic ADH receptor.

Clinically, concern for SIADH arises when presented with hyponatremia, a common electrolyte disorder in the ICU (Fig. 3). A first step is to compare calculated and measured serum osmolalities. Calculated plasma osmolality equals 2 (plasma Na) + (glucose mg/dl ÷ 18) + (serum urea nitrogen or BUN mg/dl ÷ 2.8), and plasma osmolality is measured by freezing-point depression. Pseudohyponatremia exists when plasma sodium is low but measured osmolality is normal, and is usually the result of hyperlipidemia or hyperproteinemia, in which these substances expand nonaqueous plasma volume, normally only 7%. Hyponatremia with high plasma osmolality may exist with hyperglycemia and relative insulin deficiency or resistance, preventing movement of glucose to the ICF, or in the presence of occult osmotically active substances such as mannitol or radiologic contrast agents.

Both measured and calculated osmolality account for glucose and urea in vitro, neither of which are normally osmotically active in vivo, as urea moves freely across cell membranes, including the osmoreceptor cells of the hypothalamus, as does glucose when in equilibrium with insulin. Thus, the osmostat "sees" only the osmolar effect of sodium, chloride, and bicarbonate, resulting in the concept of "effective osmolality," in which predominantly

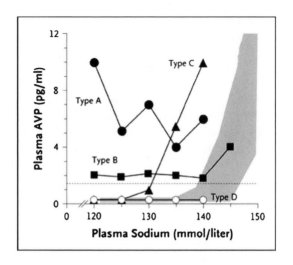

Fig. 2. Types of the syndrome of inappropriate antidiuresis. (*From* Robertson GL. Regulation of arginine vasopressin in the syndrome of inappropriate antiduresis. Am J Med 2006;19 (Suppl 1):S36–S42; with permission.)

sodium and its anions determine movement of water across cell membranes. Therefore, effective osmolality closely approximates twice the serum sodium [64].

Once pseudohyponatremia is eliminated, then serum osmolality should be compared with urine osmolality. Osmoreceptors are very sensitive, and below the effective osmolal threshold of approximately 275 mOsm/kg, ADH secretion ceases and urine osmolality should be maximally dilute and less than 100 mOsm/kg. If hyponatremia exists in the presence of urine osmolality greater than 100 mOsm/kg, then SIADH should be suspected. SIADH is a disorder of free water excretion, and therefore effective vascular volume would be expected to expand. As this occurs, the renin-angiotensin system is down-regulated, aldosterone falls, natriuresis occurs, a new equilibrium is reached, and further expansion of the extracellular fluid is prevented. In the absence of aldosterone, urinary sodium is greater than 40 mmol/L and becomes dependent upon sodium intake, a fact that may be used to clarify a diagnosis of SIADH [65]. For example, if the urine sodium is 30 mEq/L and indeterminate, then the response to a saline volume

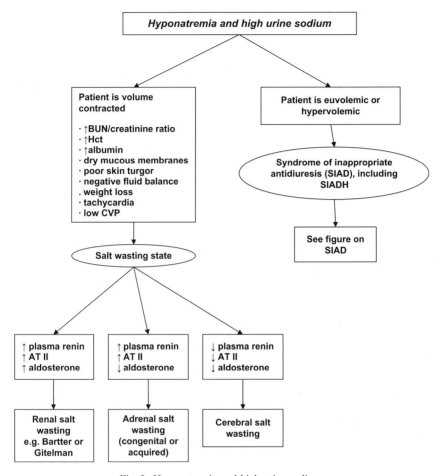

Fig. 3. Hyponatremia and high urine sodium.

challenge is illustrative. If SIADH exists, then volume expansion with intravenous saline has no effect on ADH levels, which are dissociated from serum osmolality, and the urine osmolality remains high while the administered NaCl is excreted, and the urine sodium rises above 40 mEq/L. ADH also has an effect of renal potassium clearance, thus preventing hyperkalemia during SIADH [66]. As will be discussed further with cerebral salt wasting syndrome, the clinical determination of a euvolemic state is necessary to meet criteria for SIADH.

Treatment of SIADH depends on clinical symptoms. A hypoosmolar, water intoxicated state predisposes to cerebral edema and can be catastrophic in any number of CNS conditions, which are prone to cause SIADH . Therefore, vigilance, prompt recognition, and management are mandatory, especially if brain pathology exists. At times, rapid correction of the serum sodium may be in order, and emergent administration of hypertonic saline in threatened cerebral herniation is common. Osmotic demyelination syndromes are associated with rapid osmotic corrections, which disrupt the blood brain barrier but apparently are rare in children and usually associated with chronic hyponatremic states rather than the acute pathologies of the PICU. Evidence exists that dexamethasone may protect from this potentially fatal complication [67].

Mainstays of therapy for SIADH include water restriction and NaCl administration. Water restriction can be difficult when the requirements of nutrition and medications exist, but intense restriction over brief intervals is possible by temporarily accepting hypocaloric nutrition and concentrating all medications in minimal fluid volumes. The caveat to fluid restriction is that a euvolemic state should exist and that subtle hypovolemia and complicating cerebral salt wasting does not exist. Salt administration is common therapy, but the osmolality of the saline administered must exceed that of the urine, and 0.9% saline may dangerously and paradoxically lower the serum sodium because of net water gain [68]. Therefore, correcting hyponatremia with 3% or other hypertonic saline is in order. A loop diuretic magnifies the effect of hypertonic saline by increasing free water excretion by other mechanisms. Vasopressin receptor antagonists [69] are available, but are currently quite expensive and without report of use in pediatrics.

Cerebral salt wasting

CSW was described in 1950 [70] and named as an entity in 1954 [71], before the description of SIADH in 1957 (vide supra). After SIADH was adopted as a common cause of hyponatremia in neurologic and other illnesses, CSW faded to the background as a rare or nonexistent entity. The true incidence of the disorder is unknown, and few series are published for children. Even today it continues to be confused with SIADH, with some proposing that CSW is overestimated (vide supra). Adding to the confusion is the fact that the two entities may coexist in the same patient, and each alone or together may be precipitated by the same various CNS pathologies. Teleologically, it may be speculated that a negative feedback mechanism exists by which excessive volume accumulation is modulated: thus, CSW may be overcompensation for or an inappropriate response to the consequences (intravascular volume expansion) of SIADH. Adding to the confusion is the fact that, in the absence of a definitive objective measure or diagnostic test, distinction between the two entities rests on a precise physical examination to determine if the patient is intravascular volume neutral or deplete, a clinical task which can be very difficult [72].

Pathophysiologically, CSW is proposed to occur by at least two mechanisms: disruption of sympathetic neural input into the kidney or hormonal influence of a natriuretic factor, such as brain natriuretic peptide [73]. Activation of the sympathetic nervous system decreases sodium and water excretion by decreasing GFR and by activating the renin-angiotensin-aldosterone system [74]. In CSW, renin and aldosterone do not rise, as would be expected in a hypovolemic state. Therefore, defective sympathetic activation of the kidney might lead to salt wasting. As with ADH in SIADH, natriuretic peptides (vida supra) seem logical participants in CSW. These hormones promote natriuresis by several mechanisms, including decreasing central sympathetic outflow, thereby connecting two proposed mechanisms for CSW. However, a clear relation of serum levels of natriuretic peptides to CSW is difficult to demonstrate. Other conditions may lead to renal salt wasting, including exogenous diuretics, renal tubular disorders, and pressure natriuresis [75,76], which may be associated with adrenergic overload. ADH levels in CSW are expected to be elevated, because volume depletion stimulates ADH release. CSW may exist in the absence of hyponatremia if water and sodium balances are carefully matched [77].

Diagnostically, CSW and SIADH share a similar laboratory profile: hyponatremia, normal potassium, elevated serum ADH, normal or low uric acid, and elevated urine sodium (see Fig. 3). Elevated B-type natriuretic peptide may exist, but a clear relation of serum levels of natriuretic peptides has not been established. SIADH is a volume neutral or slightly expanded state, whereas CSW is associated with hypovolemia. Therefore, an elevated BUN/creatinine ratio, hemoconcentration, or elevated serum albumin suggest salt wasting: renal, adrenal, or cerebral. However, early in the course these may not be apparent, and distinction between SIADH and salt wasting rests on the clinical determination of a contracted effective circulating blood volume. Clinical determination depends on physical signs, such as basic vital signs (tachycardia, low central venous pressure, postural hemodynamic changes), dry mucous membranes, poor skin turgor, and recent weight loss. An elevated plasma renin activity, elevated aldosterone, and elevated catecholamines would assist in the differential diagnosis of salt wasting, but none of these tests are readily available in real time. A careful investigation into recent fluid and sodium balance is most helpful, and negative balances of fluid and sodium make CSW more likely. A response to normal saline fluid challenge may be helpful: this should improve signs of hypovolemia in CSW but may actually result in further hyponatremia if SIADH exists.

Therapy of CSW requires the maintenance of intravascular volume with saline while carefully monitoring salt and water balance. Aldosterone levels are usually suppressed, and reports of successful therapy with fludrocortisone exist [78]. Caveat: if SIADH is confused with CSW, and fluid restriction is prescribed in a patient with salt wasting, then potentially disasterous hypovolemia and cerebral hypoperfusion may ensue, especially in cases of subarachnoid hemorrhage when vasospasm is more likely to occur.

Hypertensive urgencies of endocrine concern

Endocrine causes of hypertensive emergencies in pediatric intensive care are rare but important to recognize, as they can cause truly life-threatening hypertensive crises leading to encephalopathy or intracranial bleeding. While the list of endocrinologic diseases associated with hypertension is extensive, most of these disease states cause hypertension by similar mechanisms, and usually involve either catecholamine excess or adrenal dysfunction [79,80].

Catecholamine excess (dopamine, epinephrine, norepinephrine) occurs from overproduction, often by secretory tumor cells. Pheochromocytomas are the most common catecholamine-producing tumor in the pediatric critical care setting, and should be considered in the differential of any critically ill child presenting with hypertension [81,82]. They arise most commonly from chromaffin cells of the adrenal medulla, and are manifested by excess production of catecholamine metabolites in plasma and urine. They may also arise from extra-adrenal sites, such as sympathetic chains in the neck, abdomen, thorax, and the organ of Zuckerkandl at the origin of the inferior mesenteric artery [83]. Symptoms are caused by the excess of catecholamines and include intermittent or sustained hypertension, as well as tachycardia, chest pain, sweating, flushing, palpitations, and headaches. The diagnosis requires a high index of suspicion, but demonstration of increased plasma metanephrine or normetanephrine is highly sensitive (levels greater than 2,000 pg/mL are considered diagnostic) [83]. Increased levels of other catecholamine metabolites may also be seen in the plasma and urine. Glucagon stimulation testing and clonidine suppression testing can also be used for diagnosis, but are rarely needed. Direct tumor location should be pursued once biochemical evidence is available. Resection and treatment is beyond the scope of this article, but should involve a pediatric oncologist and surgeon with experience in operating on patients with catecholamine-secreting tumors [84].

Hyperthyroidism is another endocrinologic disorder that also mimics the hyperadrenergic state and, thus, can present with hypertension. In this condition catecholamines are normal, but excess thyroid hormone leads to catecholamine beta receptor up-regulation, and thus causes tachycardia and often hypertension. Hypertension is usually mild in this setting, manifests mostly as systolic elevation, and the hyperthyroid state as the cause is usually self evident. Beta-blockers are commonly used in this setting [85].

Problems with adrenal dysfunction leading to hypertension typically involve disorders of mineralocorticoid activity [79,86]. Aldosterone is the principal hormone responsible for salt retention, and increased activity from any cause leads to increased Na/K exchange in the distal tubule of the kidney, resulting in salt and fluid retention and potassium wasting.

Two adrenal enzyme deficiencies, 17-alpha-hydroxylase and 11-beta-hydroxylase, cause decreased production of cortisol and are actually forms of congenital adrenal hyperplasia, but cause hypertension because of accumulation of intermediaries in the mineralocorticoid pathway, which has intrinsic aldosterone activity. The deficency of 17-alpha-hydroxylase prevents synthesis of glucocorticoids and androgens, and presents with hypertension, undervirilization, and hypokalemia. Hypertension in this setting is treated by glucocorticoid replacement, which suppresses ACTH activity and thus suppresses the mineralocorticoid pathway [79]. Deficiency of 11-beta-hydroxylase leads to decreased glucocorticoid production but spares the androgen pathway. Although aldosterone is actually reduced in this deficiency, increased accumulation of other steroids with mineralocorticoid activity (ie, deoxycorticosterone) leads to hypertension. These patients also often present with virilization (in females) because of increased androgen production [79,80]. Both of these forms of congenital adrenal hyperplasia are associated with decreased cortisol, decreased aldosterone (but increased mineralocorticoid intermediaries), and low renin levels.

Primary hyperaldosteronism is very rare in children, but causes include aldosterone-producing tumors (typically adrenal adenomas), the autosomal dominantly inherited glucocorticoid-suppressible hyperaldosteronism, and Conn's syndrome (primarily found in adults). All three of these causes of hypertension are associated with high serum and urine aldosterone levels in the face of depressed renin activity.

One last cause of endocrine mediated hypertension that is rare but worthy of mention is a form of familial pseudohyperaldosteronism, the syndrome of apparent mineralocorticoid excess. This entity presents with normal serum aldosterone and cortisol levels, low renin levels, and elevated ratios of urinary metabolites of cortisol to metabolites of cortisone [79]. The cause of excess mineralocorticoid activity in these patients is caused by a deficiency of the enzyme 11-betahydroxysteroid dehydrogenase (11BHSD), which is responsible for converting cortisol to cortisone. Cortisol has significant affinity for and activity at the mineralocorticoid receptor, whereas cortisone does not. Cortisol is usually prevented from acting as a potent mineralocorticoid via this conversion, thus deficiency of 11BHSD leads to increased cortisol with increased mineralocorticoid activity [79,86].

The presentation of hypertension in the PICU setting can often be a diagnostic dilemma. As endocrine diseases are actually rare causes of hypertension, one must rule out other more common conditions, such as pain or anxiety, fluid overload, renovascular disease, medication administration, and increased intracranial pressure. Once these causes are ruled out, the pediatric intensivist can rely on patient and family history, clinical examination, and laboratory findings to help discern whether primary endocrine disease is the culprit. The following list of initial laboratory tests should help work through some of these endocrinologic conditions [80,83]:

Urine catecholamines
Free T4 and TSH
Renin, aldosterone, 11-DOC
Cortisol, ACTH, 17 OH progesterone
Urine NA, K
Plasma Chem 8
Urine aldosterone

Management of the patient with panhypopituitarism in the pediatric ICU

Management of the postoperative state in the patient with panhypopituitarism requires consideration of both anterior and posterior pituitary gland function. Although the patient may lack all of the hormones of the anterior pituitary, only cortisol and thyroid replacement will be essential in the immediate postoperative period. Growth hormone and gonadotrophin deficiencies may eventually need replacement, but usually not in the immediate postoperative period. Thyroid hormone has a long half-life of 7 days [87]. If preoperative thyroid levels were normal then thyroid hormone replacement can be postponed for several days until the patient can take oral medications. However, levothyroxine is available for intravenous use. Cortisol (hydrocortisone) replacement is essential and should begin before surgery and continue at stress, dosing intravenously until the patient is stable [88]. If the patient is receiving postoperative steroids (usually as dexamethasone), additional steroid replacement in the form of hydrocortisone is not needed until after the dexamethasone has been discontinued. When considering hydrocortisone therapy, several caveats should be kept in mind. Replacing thyroid hormone before replacing hydrocortisone in the patient with panhypopituitarism can precipitate adrenal insufficiency [89]. When given in stress doses, hydrocortisone can bind to aldosterone receptors and have a mineralocorticoid effect [90]. Conversely hydrocortisone deficiency can mask diabetes insipidus by impairing free water clearance by the kidney [91].

The major challenge in managing the patient with panhypopituitarism in the postoperative period is fluid and electrolyte management because of possible deficiency of ADH. The importance of meticulous management of fluid intake and output beginning before surgery, continuing during the operative period, and being addressed immediately in the postoperative period cannot be overemphasized. A common mistake is to ignore careful balancing of intake and output until after well into the postoperative period, when the patient may exhibit polyuria. During surgery, patients are often administered liberal fluids to compensate for vasodilation. In the postoperative period this excess fluid is excreted. A common error is to mistake this normal diuresis of excess fluid with the emergence of diabetes insipidus and to either give excessive fluid replacement or to initiate vasopressin therapy inappropriately. This can be avoided by careful comparison of pre-, peri-, and postoperative fluid intake and output, and by monitoring serum osmolality. If the patient has normal postoperative diuresis, the urinary output will be appropriate for the increased previous fluid intake (considering other sources of fluid loss, such as insensible water loss), and the serum osmolality will remain normal. If diabetes insipidus is developing the fluid output will exceed that expected and the serum osmolality will increase [91]. If the patient had normal posterior pituitary function before surgery but had neurosurgical intervention in the hypothalamic-pituitary area, the possible emergence of postoperative diabetes insipidus should be anticipated. This often has a triphasic evolution [91]. Initially, the patient may have blunted ADH secretion and exhibit a transient diabetes insipidus lasting only a few days. Leakage of ADH from damaged neurons can then lead to the second phase of SIADH. Eventual death of the secreting neurons then leads to a third phase of permanent diabetes insipidus.

In the immediate postoperative period, diabetes insipidus can often be managed with careful fluid replacement alone, particularly in younger children. The following protocol is described by Muglia and Mazjoub [91]. An infusion of one-fourth normal saline in D5W (5% dextrose in water) is started at 40 mL/M^2 per hour. Potassium of 40 mEq/L can be added if needed. Hourly urine output is measured. Hourly urine output less than 40 mL/M^2 per hour is not replaced. The volume of hourly urine in excess of 40 mL/M^2 hour is replaced as D5W up to a maximum fluid replacement of 120 mL/M^2 hour. Vasopressin replacement is not used at this point. With this protocol, a mild hypernatremia (to 150 mEq/L) is permitted. Falling sodium concentrations (dropping osmolality), particularly if associated with decreasing urine output, may be a signal that the patient is entering the SIADH phase. Appropriate fluid restriction is needed during this phase. Once the patient has clearly developed permanent diabetes insipidus, vasopressin therapy may be added. If the patient is not taking fluids orally, intravenous aqueous vasopressin can be used until the patient can take oral fluids and exhibits a normal thirst response. Fluid intake should be limited to 1 L/M^2 per 24 hours while on intravenous vasopressin. Intravenous desmopressin is not recommended because of its longer half-life [91]. However, once the patient can take oral fluids and exhibits normal thirst, desmopressin in either the intranasal or oral form can be used.

Standard hormone replacement of cortisol, thyroid, and other deficient hormones can be initiated once the patient is stable and taking oral fluids.

Hyperthyroidism

Hyperthyroidism is an uncommon pediatric endocrine presentation. Many cases are mild and will not require management in a critical care setting [92]. The classic clinical presentation will be a patient with weight loss, tachycardia, elevated systolic blood pressure with widened pulse pressure, tremor, and a hyperkinetic state. Usually they will also exhibit exophthalmos, lid lag, loss of convergence, tremor, and a goiter. They may also complain of weakness and diarrhea. The diagnosis can be established with an elevated free T_4 (or total T_4), elevated total T_3, and depressed TSH. Occasionally T_4 may be only mildly elevated with a disproportionate increase in the T_3 level. Patients with more severe untreated hyperthyroidism are at risk for developing "thyroid storm," which is a marked exacerbation of the hypermetabolic state and carries a risk of cardiovascular collapse with shock and heart failure [93]. Cardiac arrthymias, such as atrial fibrillation, may be precipitated. These patients will present with very elevated T_4 values, fever, flushing, sweating, marked tachycardia, marked agitation, and at times delirium. Patients with these symptoms are best managed initially in a critical care setting until stable, as symptoms can be confused with sepsis or other causes. Fortunately, cardiovascular collapse occurs only rarely in the pediatric patient.

Although the presentation of hyperthyroidism resembles a hyperadrenergic state, these patients actually have normal levels of circulating catecholamines. The elevated thyroid hormones stimulate an increase in beta adrenergic receptors, resulting in an increased sensitivity to circulating catecholamines [87].

Treatment of the hyperthyroid state involves several interventions [93]. A beta-blocker is given to relieve the cardiovascular symptoms. Propanolol has traditionally been used to treat hyperthyroidism and can be given orally or intravenously. In addition to its cardiovascular effects, it also inhibits peripheral conversion of T_4 to T_3. However, this effect takes several days and probably offers no advantage in acute management. Esmolol has a rapid onset of action and can be used intravenously to titrate rapid control of cardiovascular problems. Oral beta-blockers, such as atenolol, offer the advantages of selective beta-1 blockade and a longer duration of action that allows single daily dosing. An agent to block continued thyroid hormone production by the overactive thyroid gland is also required. Either propylthiouracil (PTU) or methimazole can be given orally. Although PTU can also inhibit the tissue conversion of T_4 to T_3, this action is not of clinical significance. Methimazole has a longer half-life, and after acute management offers the advantage of single daily dosing for maintenance therapy in most patients. Although these agents inhibit further production of thyroid hormone, neither will inhibit the release of thyroid hormone stored in the thyroid gland. An enlarged thyroid gland may continue to release excess hormone for up to 6 weeks, even after starting antithyroid therapy. Addition of a saturated solution of iodine, such as saturated solution of potassium iodide or Lugol's solution, will effectively inhibit stored T_4/T_3 release. To prevent precipitating further hyperthyroid crisis, iodine should not be started unless PTU or methimazole have also been started. In the rare patient with full thyroid storm, adding hydrocortisone should be considered, because in high doses it will impair peripheral T_4 to T_3 conversion and will suppress thyroid hormone release by the thyroid gland [87]. Similarly, the use of an iodinated radiocontrast agent, such as sodium ipodate, as a potent blocker of T_4 to T_3 conversion has been reported. However, these radiocontrast agents are not currently available in the United States.

Most patients can be managed with the combination of a beta-blocker, methimazole (or PTU), and a saturated solution of iodine. This initial therapy should be continued until the acute hyperthyroid state is controlled. At this point, the beta-blocker and iodine solution can be discontinued.

Options for long-term management include continued antithyroid medication (PTU or methimazole), radioiodine ablation, or surgery [93].

Summary

The practice of pediatric critical care involves daily encounters with patients who express manifestations of the neuroendocrine-immune stress response. This article has described the sympathoadrenergic arm of that response. Extending life beyond "natural" limits, a common occurrence in the ICU, has resulted in expressions of stress metabolism that are only now becoming evident and described and are understood in only rudimentary terms. Two of the more common such expressions are critical illness hyperglycemia and relative adrenal insufficiency. Such conditions present new challenges to the practitioner. Existing rational and empiric therapies are largely untested in pediatrics, and these therapies may conflict with and complicate one another. Beyond these currently unanswerable issues, the authors have discussed a set of common clinical issues in the daily practice of pediatric critical care.

Acknowledgments

Sincere appreciation is extended to Balint Kacsoh, MD, PhD, for his review and contributions to this article.

References

[1] Selye H. Nature 1936;32.
[2] Selye H. Diseases of adaptation. Wis Med J 1950;49(6):515.
[3] Felmet K, Carcillo J. Neuroendocrine-immune mediator coordination and disarray in critical illness. In: Fuhrman BP, Zimmerman JJ, editors. Pediatric critical care. Philadelphia: Mosby Elsevier; 2006. p. 1462–73.
[4] Van den Berghe G. Dynamic neuroendocrine responses to critical illness. Front Neuroendocrinol 2002;23:370–91.
[5] Low MJ. Neuroendocrinology. In: Kronenberg HM, Melmed S, Plolnsky KS, editors. Williams textbook of endocrinology. 11th edition. Philadelphia: Saunders; 2008. p. 85–154.
[6] Jessop DS, Harbuz MS, Lightman SL. CRH in chronic inflammatory stress. Peptides 2001; 22:803–7.
[7] Kacsoh B. The endocrine pancreas. In: Endocrine physiology. New York: McGraw-Hill; 2000. p. 360–99, 231–2.
[8] Vanhorebeek I, Van den Berghe G. The neuroendocrine response to critical illness is a dynamic process. Crit Care Clin 2006;22:1–15.
[9] Chicanza IC. Prolactin and immunomodulation. Ann N Y Acad Sci 1999;876:119–30.
[10] Devins SS, Miller A, Herndon BL, et al. Effects of dopamine on T-lymphocyte proliferative responses and serum prolactin concentrations in critically ill patients. Crit Care Med 1992; 20:1644–9.
[11] Finney SJ, Zekveld C, Elia A, et al. Glucose control and mortality in critically ill patients. JAMA 2003;290(15):2041–7.

[12] Stidham G, Bugnitz MC. The neuroendocrine response to stress. In: Rogers MC, editor. Textbook of pediatric intensive care. 3rd edition. Baltimore (MD): Williams and Wilkins; 1996. p. 1512.

[13] Van den Berghe G, Wilmer A, Hermans G, et al. Intensive insulin therapy in the medical ICU. N Engl J Med 2006;354(5):449–61.

[14] Van den Berghe G, Wilmer A, Milants I, et al. Intensive insulin therapy in mixed medical/surgical intensive care units: benefit versus harm. Diabetes 2006;55(11):3151–9.

[15] Jeremitsky E, Omert LA, Dunham CM, et al. The impact of hyperglycemia on patients with severe brain injury. J Trauma 2005;58(1):47–50.

[16] Van den Berghe G, Wouters P, Weekers F, et al. Intensive insulin therapy in the critically ill patients. N Engl J Med 2001;345(19):1359–67.

[17] Yung M, Wilkins B, Norton L, et al. Glucose control, organ failure, and mortality in pediatric intensive care. Ped Crit Care Med 2008;9(2):147–52.

[18] Institute for Healthcare Improvement. Available at: www.ihi.org/ihi/topics/criticalcare/intensivecare/changes/implementeffectiveglucose.html. Accessed October 14, 2007.

[19] Garber AJ. American Diabetes Association position statement on inpatient diabetes and metabolic control. Endocr Pract 2004;10(1):77–82.

[20] Dellinger RP. Surviving Sepsis Campaign guidelines for management of severe sepsis and shock. Campaign consortium statement. Crit Care Med 2004;32(3):858–73.

[21] Kido Y, Nakae J, Domenico A. Clinical review 125: the insulin receptor and its cellular targets. J Clin Endocrinol Metab 2001;86:972–9.

[22] Vespa P, Boonyaputthikul R, McArthur DL, et al. Intensive insulin therapy reduces microdialysis glucose values without altering glucose utilization or improving the lactate/pyruvate ratio after traumatic brain injury. Crit Care Med 2006;34(3):850–6.

[23] Faustino EV, Apkon M. Persistent hyperglycemia in critically ill children. J Pediatr 2005; 146(1):30–4.

[24] Branco R, Garcia R, Piva J, et al. Glucose level and risk of mortality in pediatric septic shock. Pediatr Crit Care Med 2005;6(No 4):470–2.

[25] Van Waardenburg DA, Jansen TC, Vos GD, et al. Hyperglycemia in children with meningococcal sepsis and septic shock: the relation between plasma levels of insulin and inflammatory mediators. J Clin Endocrinol Metab 2006;91(10):3916–21.

[26] Wintergerst KA, Buckingham B, Gandrud L, et al. Association of hypoglycemia, hyperglycemia, and glucose variability with morbidity and death in the pediatric intensive care unit. Pediatrics 2006;118(1):173–9.

[27] Srinivasan V, Spinella PC, Drott HR, et al. Association of timing, duration, and intensity of hyperglycemia with intensive care unit mortality in critically ill children. Pediatr Crit Care Med 2004;5(4):329–36.

[28] Schumer W. Steroids in the treatment of clinical septic shock. Ann Surg 1976;184(3):333–9.

[29] Sprung CL, Caralis PV, Marcial EH, et al. The effects of high-dose corticosteroids in patients with septic shock. N Engl J Med 1984;311:1137–43.

[30] Bone RC, Fisher CJ Jr, Clemmer TP, et al. A controlled clinical trial of high-dose methylprednisolone in the treatment of severe sepsis and septic shock. N Engl J Med 1987;317:653–8.

[31] Veterans Administration Systemic Sepsis Study Group. Effect of high-dose glucocorticoid therapy on mortality in patients with clinical signs of systemic sepsis. N Engl J Med 1987; 317:659–65.

[32] Rothwell PM, Udwadia ZF, Lawler PG. Cortisol response to corticotrophin and survival in septic shock. Lancet 1991;337:582–3.

[33] Soni A, Pepper GM, Wyrwinski PM, et al. Adrenal insufficiency occurring during septic shock: incidence, outcome, and relationship to peripheral cytokine levels. Am J Med 1995; 98:266–71.

[34] Annane D, Sébille V, Troché G, et al. A 3-level prognostic classification in septic shock based on cortisol levels and cortisol response to corticotrophin. JAMA 2000;283(8):1038–45.

[35] Annane D, Sébille V, Charpentier C, et al. Effect of treatment with low doses of hydrocortisone and fludrocortisone on mortality in patients with septic shock. JAMA 2002;288(7): 862–71.
[36] Wagner RL, White PF, Kan PB, et al. Inhibition of adrenal steroidogenesis by the anesthetic etomidate. N Engl J Med 1984;310:1415–21.
[37] Absolom A, Pledger D, Kong A. Adrenocortical function in critically ill patients after a single dose of etomidate. Anaesthesia 1999;54:861–7.
[38] Ledingham IM, Watt I. Influence of sedation on mortality in critically ill multiple trauma patients. Lancet 1983;1(8336):1270.
[39] Keh D, Sprung CL. Use of corticosteroid therapy in patients with sepsis and septic shock: an evidence-based review. Crit Care Med 2004;32(11):S527–33.
[40] Annane D, Bellisant E, Bollaert PE, et al. Corticosteroids for severe sepsis and septic shock. BMJ 2004;329:480–8.
[41] Pizarro CF, Troster EJ, Damaini D. Absolute and relative adrenal insufficiency in children with septic shock. Crit Care Med 2005;33(4):855–9.
[42] Zaloga GP, Marik P. Hypothalamic-pituitary-adrenal insufficiency. Crit Care Clin 2001; 17(1):25–41.
[43] Menon K, Clarson C. Adrenal function in pediatric critical illness. Pediatr Crit Care Med 2002;3(2):112–6.
[44] Beishuizen A, Lambertus GT. Relative adrenal failure in intensive care: an identifiable problem requiring treatment? Best Pract Res Clin Endocrinol Metab 2001;4:513–31.
[45] Zimmerman J. Testing the waters. Pediatr Crit Care Med 2007;8(3):305–7.
[46] Hamrahian AH, Oseni TS, Arafah BM. Measurements of serum free cortisol in critically ill patients. N Engl J Med 2004;350:1629–38.
[47] Arafah BM, Nishiyama FJ, Tlaygeh H, et al. Measurement of salivary cortisol concentration in the assessment of adrenal function in critically ill subjects: a surrogate marker of circulating free cortisol. J Clin Endocrinol Metab 2007;92(8):2965–71.
[48] Beishuizen A, Vermes I, Hylkema BS. Relative eosinophilia and functional adrenal insufficiency in critically ill patients. Lancet 1999;353:1675–6.
[49] Loriaux L. Glucocorticoid therapy in the intensive care unit. N Engl J Med 2004;350:1601–2.
[50] Sprung CL, Annane D, Keh D, et al. Hydrocortisone therapy for patients with septic shock. N Engl J Med 2008;358:111–24.
[51] Dellinger RP, Levy MM, Carlet JM, et al. Surviving Sepsis Campaign: international guidelines for management of severe sepsis and septic shock: 2008. Crit Care Med 2008; 36(1):296–327.
[52] Carcillo JA, Fields AI, Task Force Committee Members. ACCM clinical practice parameters for hemodynamic support of pediatric and neonatal septic shock. Crit Care Med 2002;30:1365–78.
[53] Markovitz BP, Goodman DM, Watson S, et al. A retrospective cohort study of prognostic factors associated with outcome in pediatric severe sepsis: what is the role of steroids? Pediatr Crit Care Med 2005;6:270–4.
[54] Finfer S. Corticosteroids in septic shock. N Engl J Med 2008;358:188–90.
[55] Singh S, Bohn D, Carlotti APCP. Cerebral salt wasting: truths, fallacies, theories, and challenges. Crit Care Med 2002;30(11):2575–9.
[56] Robinson AG, Verbalis JG. In: Kronenberg HM, Melmed S, Plolnsky KS, editors. Williams textbook of endocrinology. 11th edition. Philadelphia: Saunders; 2008. p. 263–8.
[57] Robertson GL. Physiology of ADH secretion. Kidney Int Suppl 1987;21:S20–6.
[58] Thrasher TN. Baroreceptor regulation of vasopressin and renin secretion: low-pressure versus high-pressure receptors. Front Neuroendocrinol 1994;15:157–96.
[59] Dluhy RG, Lawrence JE, Williams GH. In: Larsen PR, Kronenberg HM, Melmed S, editors. Williams textbook of endocrinology. 10th edition. Philadelphia: Saunders; 2003. p. 562–4.
[60] Levin ER, Gardnere DG, Samson WK. Natriuretic peptides. N Engl J Med 1998;339:321–8.

[61] Schwartz WB, Bennett W, Curelop S, et al. A syndrome of renal sodium loss and hyponatremia probably resulting from inappropriate secretion of antidiuretic hormone. Am J Med 1957;23:529–42.
[62] Feldman BJ, Rosenthal SM, Vargas GA, et al. Nephrogenic syndrome of inappropriate antidiuresis. N Engl J Med 2005;352:1884–90.
[63] Robertson GL. Regulation of arginine vasopressin in the syndrome of inappropriate antidiuresis. Am J Med 2006;119:S36–42.
[64] Rose BD, Post TW. Antidiuretic hormone and water balance. Available at: http://www.utd.com. Accessed August 19, 2007.
[65] Rose BD. Diagnosis of hyponatremia. Available at: http://www.utd.com. Accessed July 19, 2007.
[66] Field MJ, Stanton BA, Giebisch G. Influence of ADH on renal potassium handling. Kidney Int 1984;25:502–11.
[67] Murase T. Mechanisms and therapy of osmotic demyelination. Am J Med 2006; 119(7 Suppl 1):S69–73.
[68] Rose BD. New approach to disturbances in the plasma sodium concentration. Am J Med 1986;81(6):1033–40.
[69] Palm C, Pistrosch F, Herbrig K, et al. Vasopressin antagonists as aquaretic agents for the treatment of hyponatremia. Am J Med 2006;119(7A):S87–92.
[70] Peters JP, Welt LG, Sims EAH, et al. A salt-wasting syndrome associated with cerebral disease. Trans Assoc Am Physicians 1950;63:57–64.
[71] Cort JH. Cerebral salt wasting. Lancet 1954;1:752–4.
[72] Chung HM, Kluge R, Schrier RW. Clinical assessment of extracellular fluid volume in hyponatremia. Am J Med 1987;83:905–8.
[73] Palmer BF. Hyponatremia in a neurosurgical patient: syndrome of inappropriate antidiuretic hormone versus cerebral salt wasting. Nephrol Dial Transplant 2000;15:262–8.
[74] Guyton AC, Hall JE. Sympathetic nervous system activation increases sodium reabsorption. In: Textbook of medical physiology. Philadelphia: W.B. Saunders; 2000. p. 309.
[75] Guyton AC, Hall JE. Effect of pressure on urine output—the pressure-natriuresis and pressure-diuresis mechanisms. In: Textbook of medical physiology. Philadelphia: W.B. Saunders; 2000. p. 308.
[76] Zhang Y, Mircheff AK, Hijdra A, et al. Rapid redistribution and inhibition of renal sodium transporters during acute pressure natriuresis. Am J Physiol 1996;270:F1004–14.
[77] Gowrishankar M, Lin SH, Mallie JP, et al. Acute hyponatremia in the perioperative period: insights into its pathophysiology and recommendations for management. Clin Nephrol 1998;50:352–60.
[78] Taplin CE, Cowell CT, Silink M, et al. Fludrocortisone therapy in cerebral salt wasting. Pediatrics 2006;118(6):e1904–8.
[79] Kohane DS, Tobin JR, Kohane IS. Endocrine, mineral, and metabolic disease in pediatric intensive care. In: Rogers MC, editor. Textbook of pediatric intensive care. 3rd edition. Baltimore (MD): Williams and Wilkins; 1996. p. 1247–60.
[80] Oberfield SE, Gallagher MP, Levine LS. Endocrine hypertension. In: Finberg L, Kleinman RE, editors. Saunders manual of pediatric practice. Philadelphia: WB Saunders; 2002. p. 912–5.
[81] Chernausek SD. Pheochromocytoma and the multiple endocrine neoplasia syndrome. In: Sperling MA, editor. Pediatric endocrinology. Philadelphia: WB Saunders; 2002. p. 439–54.
[82] Styne DN. Guide to pediatric endocrine emergencies. In: Pediatric endocrinology. Philadelphia: Lippincott Williams and Wilkins; 2004. p. 305.
[83] Ross JH. Pheochomocytoma. Special considerations in children. Urol Clin North Am 2000; 27:393–402.
[84] Kwon KT, Tsai VW. Metabolic emergencies. Emerg Med Clin North Am 2007;25(4): 1041–60.
[85] Ringel MD. Management of hypothyroidism and hyperthyroidism in the intensive care unit. Crit Care Clin 2001;17:59–74.

[86] Connell JM, Fraser R. Adrenal corticosteroid synthesis and hypertension. J Hypertens 1991; 9:97–107.

[87] Kacsoh B. The thyroid gland. In: Endocrine physiology. New York: McGraw-Hill; 2000. p. 332, 340, 355.

[88] Miller WL. The adrenal cortex. In: Sperling M, editor. Pediatric endocrinology. 2nd edition. Philadelphia: WB Saunders; 2002. p. 427.

[89] Aron DC, Findling JM, Tyrell JB. Hypothalamus and pituitary gland. In: Gardner DC, Shobock J, editors. Greenspan's basic & clinical endocrinology. 8th edition. New York: McGraw-Hill; 2007. p. 138.

[90] Kacsoh B. The adrenal gland. In: Endocrine physiology. New York: McGraw-Hill; 2000. p. 447.

[91] Muglia LJ, Majzoub JA. Disorders of the posterior pituitary. In: Sperling M, editor. Pediatric endocrinology. 2nd edition. Philadelphia: WB Saunders; 2002. p. 308–10.

[92] Raine JE, Donaldson MDC, Gregory JW, et al. Thyroid disorders. In: Practical endocrinology and diabetes in children. 2nd edition. Massachusetts: Blackwell Publishing, Ltd.; 2006. p. 101.

[93] Dallas JS, Foley TP. Hyperthyroidism. In: Lifshitz F, editor. Pediatric endocrinology. 5th edition. New York: Informa Healthcare USA, Inc.; 2007. p. 419, 430–7.

PEDIATRIC CLINICS

OF NORTH AMERICA

Pediatr Clin N Am 55 (2008) 835–845

Index

Note: Page numbers of article titles are in **boldface** type.

doi:10.1016/S0031-3955(08)00127-2